# Complete Conditioning for FOOTBALL


Michael J. Arthur, CSCS
Strength and Conditioning Coach
University of Nebraska

Bryan L. Bailey, CSCS
Strength and Conditioning Coach
University of Nebraska


Human Kinetics

*To my father, Francis, who was instrumental in developing in me the passion for coaching, and to my mother, Marlyn, for her loving support and strength.—Mike Arthur*

*To my loving parents, Bill and Alta Bailey, for instilling in me the passion and determination to tackle each and every endeavor I encounter in life with a total commitment of love. And to all the University of Nebraska athletes I've had the privilege to meet and work with; you have made me the person I am today.—Bryan L. Bailey*

**Library of Congress Cataloging-in-Publication Data**

Arthur, Michael J., 1952-
Complete conditioning for football / by Michael J. Arthur and Bryan L. Bailey.
p. cm. 97-38483
ISBN 0-88011-521-1 CIP
1. Football--Training. I. Bailey, Bryan L., 1956-
II. Title.
GV953.5.A78 1998
613.7'11--dc21

ISBN: 0-88011-521-1



**Developmental Editor**: Julie Rhoda; **Assistant Editor**: Sandra Merz Bott; **Editorial Assistant**: Laura T. Seversen; **Copyeditor**: Jim Burns; **Proofreader**: Erin Cler; **Graphic Designer**: Stuart Cartwright; **Graphic Artist**: Sandra Meier; **Photo Editor**: Boyd Lafoon; **Cover Designer**: Jack Davis; **Photographer (cover)**: © AllSport/Brian Bahr; **Photographers (interior)**: Tom Slocum, Peter N. Hasselbalch, and photos on pages 7, 37, 46, 57, 86, and 237 by Joe Mixan; **Mac Illustrator**: Sara Wolfsmith; **Line Drawing Illustrator**: Tom Roberts; **Printer**: United Graphics

Human Kinetics books are available at special discounts for bulk purchase. Special editions or book excerpts can also be created to specification. For details, contact the Special Sales Manager at Human Kinetics.

Printed in the United States of America 10 9 8 7 6 5 4 3 2

**Human Kinetics**
Web site: http://www.humankinetics.com/

*United States:* Human Kinetics, P.O. Box 5076, Champaign, IL 61825-5076
1-800-747-4457
e-mail: humank@hkusa.com

*Canada:* Human Kinetics, 475 Devonshire Road, Unit 100, Windsor, ON N8Y 2L5
1-800-465-7301 (in Canada only)
e-mail: humank@hkcanada.com

*Europe:* Human Kinetics, P.O. Box IW14, Leeds LS16 6TR, United Kingdom
(44) 1132 781708
e-mail: humank@hkeurope.com

*Australia:* Human Kinetics, 57A Price Avenue, Lower Mitcham, South Australia 5062
(088) 277 1555
e-mail: humank@hkaustralia.com

*New Zealand:* Human Kinetics, P.O. Box 105-231, Auckland 1
(09) 523 3462
e-mail: humank@hknewz.com

# CONTENTS

# FOREWORD

Winning as often and consistently as we have at the University of Nebraska requires many contributing factors and individuals working together. *Complete Conditioning for Football* provides one very important piece to the puzzle.

In this book, strength and conditioning coaches Mike Arthur and Bryan Bailey present the training approach they helped develop and implement as members of our Athletic Performance Team. This program is widely recognized as one the most effective in developing athletes to their full potential.

Like most programs, strength, power, speed, agility, and flexibility are emphasized. So are proper nutrition and adequate rest. What sets this conditioning program apart from others is that it is designed to meet the specific performance needs of football players. Techniques like blocking, throwing, and cutting are improved through this tailor-made training program. More importantly, the program is based on a strong scientific foundation and was developed from sound training principles.

Many of the guiding principles of the conditioning program were established by Boyd Epley, Assistant Athletic Director and Director of Athletic Performance at Nebraska. Boyd was the first person to have the official job title of Strength Coach back in 1970 and founded the National Strength and Conditioning Association in 1978. He is universally regarded as one of the world's leading strength and conditioning experts.

*Complete Conditioning for Football* offers not only this special expertise but also very practical fitness tests, drills, workouts, and position-specific programs for each conditioning phase. If you coach or play the game, this book is as essential as a playbook or helmet.

Being in peak football shape doesn't guarantee victory, but it certainly does improve your chances. In the fourth quarter with the game on the line, you need the physical advantage. Put yourself and your team in the best possible position to win. Work hard and smart with *Complete Conditioning for Football*.

Tom Osborne
Former Head Football Coach
Assistant Athletic Director
University of Nebraska

# INTRODUCTION

The improvement of performance in football over the past few years has been phenomenal. Twenty years ago, the average lineman weighed 240 to 250 pounds and ran a 5.2-second 40-yard dash. This was considered to be nearing the genetic potential for a player. Now running backs who weigh 240 pounds are running 4.4-second 40-yard dashes. Strength training has made the single, most positive contribution to this improvement. Today sports conditioning and strength training influence every football program in the country. Players now find it necessary to lift weights and do conditioning drills to better prepare themselves for the competitive rigors of a football season.

Just a short time ago most coaches thought that strength training would cause athletes to become muscle-bound and would be counterproductive to good technique. Now it has been proven that football performance depends either directly or indirectly on qualities of muscular strength. We must remember that technique is the medium that expresses strength. If you compare two athletes who have equal technical skills and abilities, the stronger one is going to win.

The number-one purpose of complete conditioning—including the physical, technical, tactical, and psychological aspects of training—is to improve the player's ability to make the play. Strength training is an important part of complete conditioning. The primary function of the body's 600-plus muscles is to contract (shorten in length) to move body parts. Only muscle can cause movement. The stronger the muscles and the more forceful the contractions, the faster the player can run. With strength training, not only does a player get stronger, but his muscle mass also becomes larger. So the player not only runs faster but also weighs more. The combination of speed and size increases the performance potential of a football player.

A bonus of complete conditioning and strength training is injury prevention. Training strengthens the muscle attachments and increases the density of bone at the sites of muscle origins and insertions. If an injury does occur, it will probably not be as serious, and the athlete can rehabilitate faster.

In addition to physical changes, psychological changes develop from complete sports conditioning. As a player becomes bigger and faster as a result of consistent and intense workouts, he gains confidence. This increased confidence will carry over when he lines up on the football field. A player who has conditioned himself properly will be just as strong and fast in the fourth quarter as he was in the first quarter. As Vince Lombardi said, "Fatigue makes cowards of us all."

The proper application of conditioning principles is critical to maximize performance potential. This book will stimulate you to evaluate what you are doing in your program. Coaches and athletes should question why they include an exercise or drill in their program. Many will find they are doing the same drills their coach did, whether these drills are right or wrong. Make productive use of your time. Don't waste it doing things that won't improve performance. Incorporate the principles outlined in this book into your program and you'll be on the path to success.

Each player's situation is different, and you must address an athlete's past training experience, available practice time, and available equipment. The purpose of this book is to enable you to set up strength and conditioning training based on the needs of your players and situation. Sample programs will give you ideas about how to implement your own program. Multisport athletes whose primary focus is football are sometimes confused about how to implement year-round conditioning workouts and still be competitive in each sport in which they participate. Some guidelines for meeting the conditioning needs of these athletes are given in chapter 9.

Athletes are always on the lookout for new and better ways of training, but shortcuts and gimmicks are not the answer. The bottom line is hard work. This book will show you the way, but you will have to provide the work.

CHAPTER 1

# PERFORMANCE NEEDS FOR FOOTBALL

Many factors make up a good football player. Some players are born with the natural talent to play football, while others have to work harder to make up for a lack of ability. But regardless of your level of talent, you can become a better player. There are no shortcuts to becoming the best player you can be, however; it takes lots of hard work and dedication. This book provides you with a conditioning program that has been proven to work for thousands of football players, including the 1994 and 1995 National Championship team at the University of Nebraska. The hard work will come as you condition, using this program: the dedicated effort must come from you.

The performance pyramid shown in figure 1.1 was inspired by John Wooden's "Pyramid of Success." John Wooden believed success is not how much money, power, or prestige you can attain, but knowing within yourself that you have done everything possible to be the best person you're capable of becoming. The performance pyramid represents

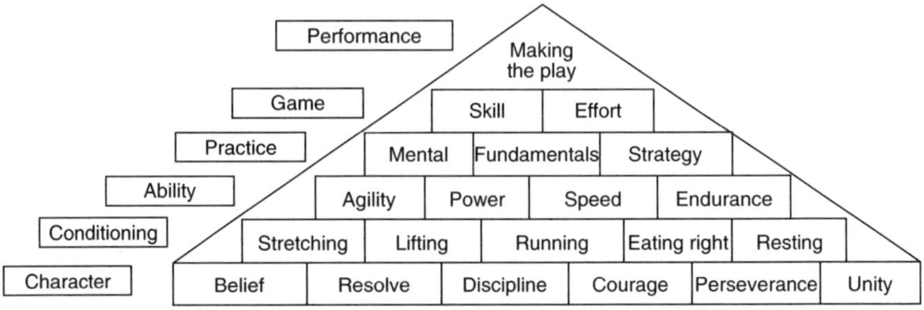


**Figure 1.1** Performance pyramid.

the entire training process followed by the University of Nebraska football program or any other successful team. The purpose of this training process is to develop players' athletic performance potential to the maximum. Each block signifies a different component of training, arranged by level according to the desired training effect. The training process starts at the bottom, with each succeeding level building on the one below it.

Character is at the foundation because it creates the greatest changes, which in turn affect everything above it. For example, as you develop character you become more consistent in your workout habits at the conditioning level. Better conditioning leads to greater athletic ability by improving power and endurance. Then as gains in power and endurance increase, practices become more effective. More effective practices lead to improved football skills. Ultimately these skills improve your potential to make more plays in performance.

# CHARACTER

A sound character is the basis for being the best player you can be; it assures a solid foundation. Character is a person's attitudes and behaviors, based on the individual's values. A person's values reflect his view of reality.

At the extremes, two opposing views of reality are evident in today's world, and each of us falls some place between the two. These views govern the values, attitudes, and behaviors that in turn determine our character. One view holds that each person is to do his own thing. That is, there is no absolute truth; rather, whatever a person does can be rationalized to meet the needs of the situation. This view holds that life is short, so get the most pleasure as possible out of it right now; the end result is more important than the means. The other view holds that there are infinite and unchanging absolute truths and natural laws that govern all people, and that you must live in harmony with these fundamental principles to achieve your maximum human potential. To know yourself, you must have a philosophy of life that does not change according to the situation, a philosophy that gives you a true personal identity. Through knowing yourself you acquire self-mastery, and through self-mastery you can delay gratification and make sacrifices.

The first of these fundamental views fosters someone who isolates himself from the world, whose attitude is "What is in it for me?" and whose emphasis is on getting ahead. The second view leads to the kind of character needed to play good football. A person with this view believes in an ultimate truth, is at peace with himself, and lives in unity with others. As John Wooden said, "[Know] within yourself you have done everything possible to be the best person you're capable of becoming."

Coach Tom Osborne of the University of Nebraska stresses six character qualities and values during team meetings, which we will discuss next. The most significant aspects of his messages are the cornerstones: belief and unity. There are many different character qualities and values that vary with the individual. John Wooden's pyramid consisted entirely of character traits and values: industriousness, enthusiasm, sympathy, judgment, self-control, initiative, cooperation. The list can go on. What is important is that you select a few basic character traits that provide a code of conduct based on your own personal values and an ultimate meaning of life for you.

## Belief

In order for any football program to work, you must first believe in it. For example, the Nebraska football team believes that if they are the most physical football team they will win games. Based on this belief, the offensive and defensive philosophies are to play a physical style of football called *power football* in which the offense is based on a very strong running game and the defense forces the action by attacking the opponent's offense. The players believe in this approach and feel it will win any game before they even take the field. We are convinced that when an opponent gets physically beat, they start making mental mistakes. Their execution then breaks down, and they turn the ball over.

Many programs fail because the athletes do not believe in them. They question what the coach is trying to accomplish or feel something else will work better. The same is true with a conditioning program; if an athlete does not believe in the program he will not be motivated to put full intensity into his workout. Belief is best instilled in the players by coaches whose actions reflect what they communicate to the team. A coach with a strong belief has the ability to demonstrate his knowledge and understanding of the program to the team. There is a consistency in the program that doesn't change and is successful from year to year. It is not based on how many games are won, but on the success of each player in becoming the best he is capable of becoming.

## Unity

"Unity"—a cornerstone of the performance pyramid—is the University of Nebraska football team's motto. Some teams use intimidation, talk trash, or use revenge or hate as motivation. In the heat of the battle when the game is on the line, the outcome is not going to be based on these tactics; it's going to be based on the team's unity. A team that has strong unity unleashes the greatest effort possible from each player and coordinates it so the team works together as a unit. A team without unity may get great effort from each player, but the efforts are not in harmony with the rest of the team.

Unity means putting your teammates first and yourself second. The success of the team depends on you doing your part. Determine what your strengths are and how you can contribute to the team. This doesn't allow every player to be in the limelight. You cannot worry about your teammate getting more ink than you. Respect your teammates, coaches, teachers, and those against whom you compete.

Success does not always challenge the unity of a team; often adversity does. For example, if a team loses or a player is involved in an unfortunate incident, it reflects on the whole team. The team can respond by falling apart or by pulling together in spite of the adversity. Playing well under adversity is the true test of team unity.

## Resolve

After losing a heartbreaker to Florida State for the National Championship in the 1994 Orange Bowl, the University of Nebraska coaches and team resolved to win the National Championship the following year. The rallying cry of resolve was, "Unfinished Business." Resolve is a fixed purpose of mind to focus all actions on the accomplishment of a specific goal. The basic question asked was, what actions are we doing now that are counterproductive to winning the National Championship? What actions are we currently not doing that would be productive to winning the National Championship? A decision was made to stop the actions that were counterproductive and replace them with productive actions. This resolve did not focus on winning the National Championship, but focused on what it takes each day to get the job done. This involved sacrificing certain comforts and making a commitment each day to prepare thoroughly and work hard. If everyone concentrated on doing his part each and every day, the National Championship would take care of itself. To achieve this resolution required a systematic approach. Everybody was on the same page in setting training objectives, procedures, and timetables. If anybody screwed up, there was a price to pay; everybody knew they were in it together.

The team was reminded daily of their resolve during the long, hot summer months. A reminder was put on the scoreboard during each running session: 36 seconds on the clock and the slogan "Unfinished Business." Thirty-six seconds was the amount of time left when Florida State took the lead during the Orange Bowl. We had been that close to winning the championship; now each player was responsible for reaching down deep within, giving it all he had, and making sure it wouldn't happen again.

## Discipline

Discipline means following through on your resolve. Today there are many young people who encounter little tangible and consistent discipline in their lives; athletics provide a beneficial disciplined structure for many young people. The simple disciplines of coming to practice at a certain time every day, doing certain workouts in the weight room in the off-season, and making a consistent effort on the playing field enable players to begin to gain some control over their lives and to become disciplined in other endeavors.

Discipline is doing the right thing at the right time. Are you willing to give up activities that are counterproductive—watching too much television, staying out late, using alcohol and / or drugs—to become the best you can be? Are you willing to consistently push yourself through painful workouts, eat properly, and get plenty of rest to become the best you can be? Discipline is a matter of replacing bad habits with good habits. A sign over the doorway to our weight room says, "Your workout habits determine your future." This sign reminds players that reaching their goals isn't going to be accomplished in one workout. It takes discipline to come into the weight room day after day to work out until it becomes a habit.

## Courage

Everyone has to deal with the problems of everyday life. These problems can have a negative effect on performance if you do not deal with them correctly. Because of fear some try to deal with a problem by avoiding it and hoping it will go away. The best way to deal with fear is to face it head-on with courage, doing what you believe is right and not giving in to the popular view of others. The first time a problem is met face-to-face you're not sure how you are going to measure up. For example, it takes courage to not use steroids if all of your friends are taking them. Courage enables you to conquer your fear. You can begin to understand more about yourself based on how you react to fear. Do you run from it? Do you go with the flow? Do you meet it head-on? If you meet it head-on, soon the fear is conquered, the problem solved, and you discover that you do have courage. Each time a problem is met head-on and defeated, courage is strengthened. Eventually, encountering problems is seen as an opportunity to exercise and strengthen your courage.

## Perseverance

Perseverance is the ability to continue to believe in yourself when facing adversity. There are a variety of adverse situations that can discourage you and cause you to give up on yourself. Often in major college football the race doesn't go to the swiftest, but to the one who is the most persistent and most determined in his pursuit of a spot on the team. We consistently see players who come in as freshmen with less ability than other players, but who eventually earn more playing time than their more talented teammates. Some players get a serious injury that sets them back for long periods of time. But through diligent rehabilitation, they struggle step-by-step each day to make it back on the field and compete again.

Jared Tomich is an example of a player who worked hard and persevered. Jared's situation was unique in that he was a great player, but poor grades kept him from getting an athletic scholarship. He could have let this discouragement defeat him and given up on football. Instead, he enrolled in classes at the University of Nebraska and paid his own way. During the first year he was diagnosed with a learning disability. He worked hard on his schoolwork, overcame the learning disability, and became scholastically eligible to play football. The following school year he walked on and became a redshirt—meaning he spent his time practicing as a scout team player running the opponents' plays against the top units. His third year out of high school he received a scholarship and played in every game as an alternate. The next two years he was selected as a first team all-American, and during his senior year nominated as an Outland and Lombardi Trophy candidate. He was voted by his teammates as the 1996 Lifter of the Year and Team Captain. He was drafted by the New Orleans Saints in the second round of the 1997 NFL draft. But his greatest achievement was persevering in the classroom and graduating from college with a degree in communication studies.

You need perseverance in all aspects of your life, including conditioning for football. Every player has reached a plateau in his training in which no further progress seems possible regardless of unrelenting endeavor. Don't become discouraged when you reach a training plateau; they are normal and necessary for your progress. Most of your time is going to be spent on a plateau. Though the goal is seemingly impossible you must continue to persevere, because a burst of progress is just beyond the horizon. There are no shortcuts or secrets to achieving your maximum performance potential. You must take one step at a time, one step building to the next step. Sometimes you must take a step or several steps back and go around in order to reach your goal.

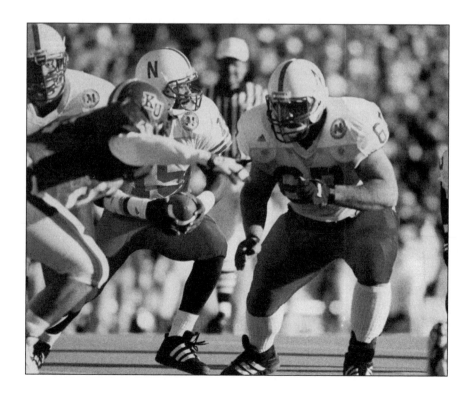

# CONDITIONING

The performance pyramid uses the basics of conditioning to build on the character foundation. This book deals with this conditioning level of the pyramid. We give a brief description of conditioning here and go into greater detail in subsequent chapters. Conditioning is often confused with training. However, training is the entire process of improving performance, and it has many components. Conditioning, on the other hand, is concerned with improving the body's force capability, energy utilization, and energy recovery. In order to optimally condition your body to play good football, you must include stretching, lifting, running, proper nutrition, and ample rest in your training program. Performing specific exercises and drills with the correct volume, intensity, and variation is crucial to maximizing the effectiveness of your conditioning program.

Regardless of your natural speed and strength, you can become better through a good conditioning program. Adam Treu is an example of a player who made such tremendous physical progress that he was drafted in the fourth round of the 1997 NFL draft. He came to Nebraska as a walk-on offensive lineman in 1992. He weighed 248 pounds, ran a 5.49-second 40-yard dash and had a 22.5-inch vertical jump. With consistent effort using the program outlined in this book he made tremendous improvement. During his last year he weighed 305 pounds, ran a 5.10 40-yard dash, and had a 26.5-inch vertical jump. This type of progress is possible for anyone with the desire to become the best he can be.

## Stretching

In the past we frequently heard coaches complain about certain players "playing tight" and needing more stretching, so we focused on stretching these players until they developed good flexibility. But the coaches later came back to us to say that the player was still playing tight. This caused us to take a closer look at what we were doing with our stretching program. We learned that what these players were lacking was mobility. We were using primarily static stretches, but these were not functional for football players' dynamic activities on the field. So we started doing "mobility drills," or functional stretching that takes the joints of the body through full ranges of motion while doing functional, football-specific movements. These drills have proven successful in our program, and best of all, we don't hear much complaining from the coaches about players being tight anymore.

## Lifting

The basis of any football conditioning program is lifting weights, which includes using barbells, dumbbells, and exercise machines in the weight room. The purpose of lifting for football is not to look like a bodybuilder or to become brute strong like a power lifter, but to train your muscles to become more powerful and improve your speed to become a better football player. We call this type of lifting *strength training.*

Analyzing test data taken at the University of Nebraska supports the hypothesis that increasing muscle hypertrophy or size is highly correlated with improving speed and power. Improving muscle strength also has a significant correlation with improved speed and power. The key word here is *improvement;* strength and muscular size are relative to the individual. You probably have observed large players who display tremendous strength, but out on the field have two left feet. Other players have little muscular hypertrophy and strength in the weight room, but are tremendous football players. Grant Winstrom is a current all-American on our team who, because of his lanky build, does not have the ability to display great strength lifting weights. But his long levers (arms and legs) give him a tremendous strength advantage on the playing field. Just remember that improving muscular size and strength is what counts, not how strong you are relative to other players on your team.

Players who strength train also tend to have fewer injuries. Strength training strengthens the muscle attachments and increases density of bones at the sites of muscle origins and insertions. If an injury does occur to a player who has been conditioning with proper strength training, it will probably not be as serious and will tend to heal faster.

## Running

A football running program should be developed in accordance with the demands of a football game. The running program should develop football-specific endurance using football-related skills. Endurance as related to football is the ability to sustain maximum speed, agility, and power on each play for an entire game. You want to be as fresh on the last play as you were on the first. While endurance can be limited due to either a neuromuscular or cardiovascular factor, the limiting factor of endurance for football is neuromuscular fatigue rather than cardiovascular failure. Therefore, building an aerobic base is not necessary for football endurance. Furthermore, scientific research shows that long, slow distance running causes an athlete's muscles to take on aerobic characteristics. This effect may be desirable for a long-distance runner, but it is counterproductive to developing the explosive, powerful muscle contractions needed for football.

The running program in this book uses interval training, as opposed to continuous long-distance runs, to develop endurance. Interval training incorporates work intervals followed by a specific rest interval. The work-to-rest ratio should be specific to the game of football. A game consists of plays lasting an average of 5 seconds with an average rest period of 50 seconds. That is, football has a work-to-rest ratio of 10:1. To be specific to football, therefore, the work intervals should last approximately 5 seconds with a rest interval of roughly 50 seconds.

The work intervals consist of football-specific speed and agility drills. Getting into position to block or tackle your opponent demands the basic motor skills of changing directions, starting, stopping, and jumping. Therefore, it is important to incorporate into your running program agility and speed drills that utilize these basic motor skills. Throughout this book, interval training—utilizing speed and agility drills—makes up the running program to develop endurance, just as strength training—utilizing barbells, dumbbells, exercise machines, and plyometrics—makes up the lifting program to develop power.

## Eating Right

Having enough energy to work out and practice is a primary concern of any athlete who wants to become a better player. Usually a decrease in performance can be traced to improper nutrition; what you eat determines how you supply energy to the body before workouts and practices. Likewise, to speed up recovery after your workout or practice you need to replenish the nutrients you have utilized.

While nutrition plays a crucial part in achieving maximum performance potential, it is one area where most athletes are confused. You are bombarded every day with new nutrition products that claim to be the answer to maximum performance. You are often willing to try anything new that promises the slightest chance to improve your performance, and often waste money on products that do nothing. It is important to educate yourself on how to make proper healthy food selections and what products can actually improve performance. We provide a three-step guide and shopping list in chapter 8 to help you eat right.

## Resting

Any athlete who does not get enough rest is only fooling himself. Rest is on a par with working out and diet in developing your maximum performance potential. The body cannot recover between workouts without enough rest. Eventually, not getting enough rest leads to overtraining and injuries. Getting enough rest should be high on your priority list, especially during periods of physical and mental stress.

The primary context of rest as it relates to conditioning is regular sleep. There are two primary principles of sleep: to sleep eight hours a day during times of hard conditioning and to wake up and go to bed the same time each day. Other aspects of rest to consider in conditioning are the lengths of time between workouts to prevent overtraining, the rest periods between exercise sets, and active rest. These aspects are covered in greater detail in chapter 2.

## ATHLETIC ABILITY

This book's primary mission is to demonstrate how to improve athletic ability through conditioning. To clearly understand a football player's conditioning needs we must look in depth at what athletic abilities are important in the game of football. Athletic abilities are a set of attributes that an athlete has or achieves that relate to the ability to perform during a game. There are over 100 types of athletic abilities, but each sport has certain ones specific to it. Some of these athletic abilities include maximum speed, acceleration, agility, balance, muscular strength, power, muscular endurance, aerobic endurance, anaerobic endurance, speed endurance, and flexibility.

Athletic abilities can be objectively measured using field tests. Several years ago we administered a battery of field tests that measured several of the athletic abilities mentioned above. By statistically analyzing the test data we determined which athletic abilities were most specific to football performance. We first had the players complete several field tests, then we divided players according to their actual ability to play football during a game. The players who played the most were ranked number one. Players who played occasionally were ranked number two. Players who played only when the outcome of the game was already decided or not at all were ranked three. The field tests were then correlated with each player's assigned ranking.

Players ranked number one (those who played the most in game situations) correlated highest with the athletic abilities of speed (10- and 40-yard dashes), agility (pro agility run), and power (vertical jump). Surprisingly, muscular strength (squat and bench press), muscular endurance (sit-ups, dips, pull-ups), aerobic endurance (1.5-mile run), anaerobic endurance (300-yard shuttle run), flexibility (sit and reach, shoulder elevation), and upper body power (seated shot put) didn't correlate as well with the number-one ranked players.

One test that we have been unable to develop is an endurance test that correlates well to the actual ability to play football. The only test we have for endurance is the outcome of the football games. And we seem to be doing pretty well; we don't get beat because of a lack of endurance conditioning.

The 10-yard dash, 40-yard dash, pro agility run, and vertical jump are used to determine the athletic abilities of each football player at the University of Nebraska. Therefore, our conditioning program is geared to improving these parameters. Other tests do not seem as strongly to determine a football player's performance potential; it would be counterproductive to develop a conditioning program based on parameters, such as long-distance running, that do not indicate football performance potential. A player's goal is to improve these performance indicators each and every time he tests. Now let's investigate speed, agility, power, and endurance more closely.

**Speed.** Speed is the ability to cover a certain distance from point A to point B in the shortest time possible.

**Agility.** Agility is the ability to stop, start, and change directions quickly while maintaining good body control.

**Power.** Power refers to an athlete's ability to generate the greatest combination of strength and speed while executing a skill.

**Endurance.** Endurance as related to football is the ability to sustain maximum speed, agility, and power on each play for an entire game.

## Speed

Speed, expressed in how many yards are covered per second, can be determined by dividing the distance run by time. For example, if a player runs a 40-yard dash in 4.6 seconds, he is running at an average speed of 8.7 yards per second.

$$\frac{\mathbf{40\ yd}}{\mathbf{4.6\ s}} = \frac{\mathbf{8.7\ yd}}{\mathbf{s}}$$

That is, 8.7 yards per second is the average speed over a distance of 40 yards. This number doesn't indicate top speed or acceleration. A player who averages 8.7 yards per second runs at different speeds during the 40 yards. Let's take a closer look at the 40-yard dash and time it in 5-yard splits. The first three columns of table 1.1 show that as a player runs 40 yards his speed is initially slower and gradually gets faster during the course of the run.

A graphic view of this 40-yard dash gives a different perspective (figure 1.2). Even though the player is getting faster and faster, the

**Table 1.1 Time, Speed, and Acceleration Over 40 Yards**

| Interval (yd) | Split time (s) | Speed (yd/s) | Acceleration (yd/s/s) |
|---|---|---|---|
| 0 | 0.00 | 0.00 | 0.00 |
| 5 | 0.96 | 5.21 | 5.21 |
| 10 | 0.70 | 7.14 | 2.76 |
| 15 | 0.59 | 8.47 | 2.26 |
| 20 | 0.53 | 9.43 | 1.81 |
| 25 | 0.49 | 10.20 | 1.57 |
| 30 | 0.46 | 10.87 | 1.45 |
| 35 | 0.44 | 11.36 | 1.12 |
| 40 | 0.43 | 11.63 | 0.61 |

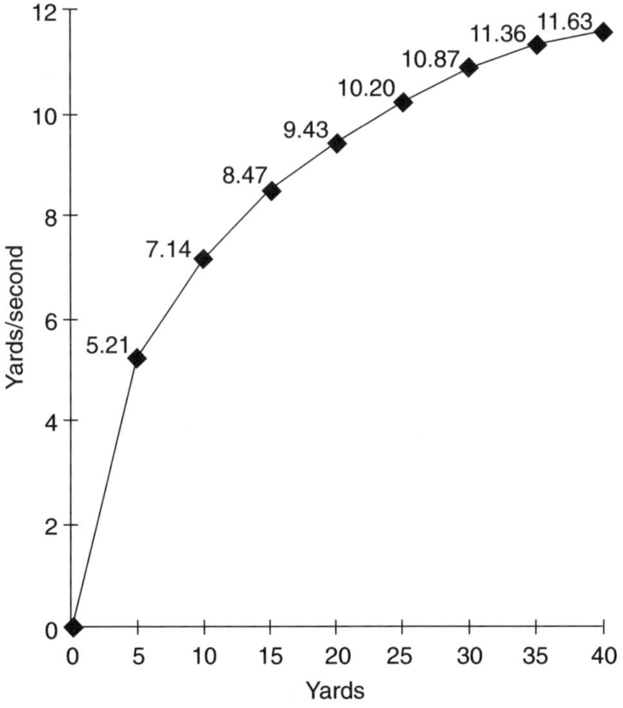


**Figure 1.2** Acceleration over 40 yards.

greatest gain in speed (greatest acceleration) is made at the beginning. Acceleration is the rate of change of speed. It is figured by subtracting the initial speed from the final speed and dividing by time.

$$\frac{8.7 \text{ yd/s} - 0 \text{ yd/s}}{4.6 \text{ s}} = \frac{8.7 \text{ yd/s}}{4.6 \text{ s}} = 1.89 \text{ yd/s/s}$$

The final column of table 1.1 shows acceleration in 5-yard segments. You can see that acceleration is greatest at the initial portion of the run, and as the speed increases the acceleration decreases. So the greatest rate of change of speed happens during the initial stages of the 40-yard dash. As shown in figure 1.2, the steeper the curve, the greater the acceleration.

How important is acceleration when compared to top speed? Let's look at figure 1.3, showing two athletes running the 40-yard dash. One athlete runs it in 4.6 seconds (dotted line), and the second athlete runs it in 4.5 seconds (solid line). You can see that the athlete who ran 4.6 actually has greater top speed, but didn't run the faster 40-yard dash, because the athlete who ran the 4.5 accelerated to his top speed faster—

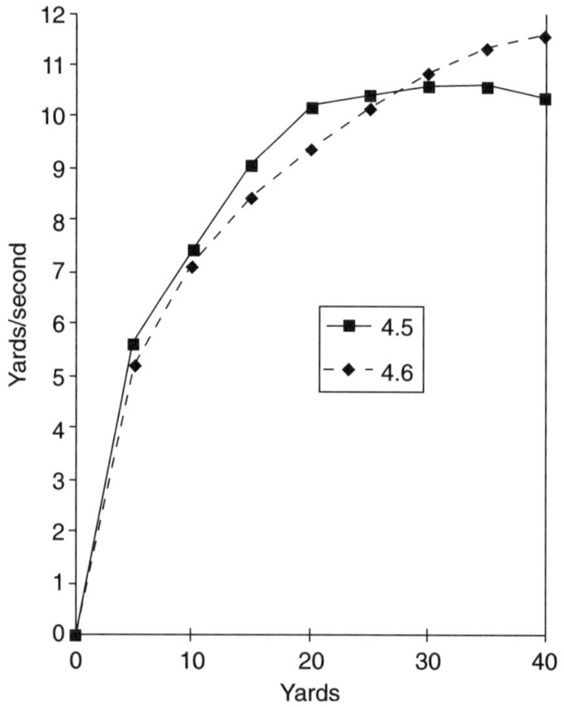


**Figure 1.3** Acceleration versus speed in two athletes running 40 yards.

shown by how steep the curve is the first 20 yards. So it isn't always the athlete with the greatest top speed who wins the race. Therefore, speed is relative to the distance run. If the distance is short, such as 10 to 40 yards, the person with the greatest acceleration is going to have the greatest speed. As the distance gets longer, 100 to 400 yards, the athlete with the greatest top speed is going to have the greatest speed. Players with the greatest acceleration have speed that is relevant for most distances run during a football game.

Now let's compare what actually happens in a game situation to a player's 40-yard dash time. Figure 1.4 compares our quarterback's 40-yard time and a touchdown play covering 40 yards. You can see that the player does not reach his top 40-yard speed (10.87) during the game play. Rather, the top speed he attains as he outruns the pursuit into the end zone is 8.82 yards per second. Furthermore, the data points of the play show many periods of acceleration and deceleration. An average play for most players covers a total distance of 15 to 20 yards, though this distance might be shorter for a lineman and longer for a receiver or defensive back. Figure 1.4 makes it clear that being able to accelerate

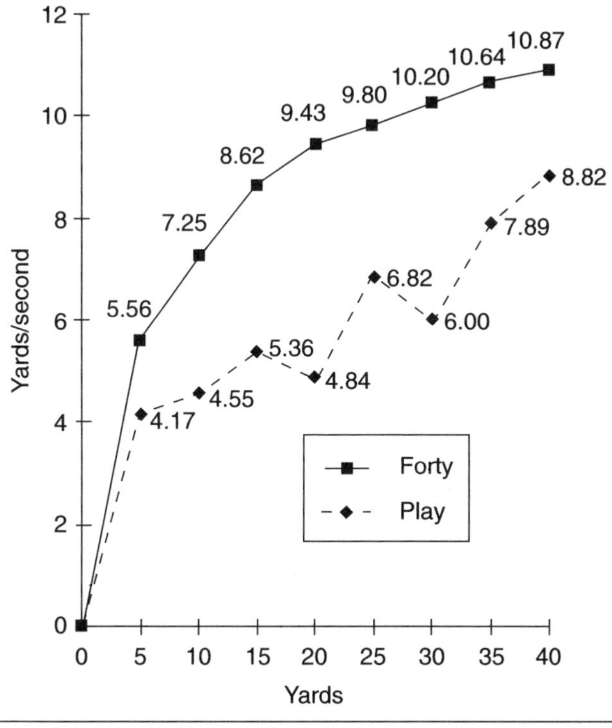


**Figure 1.4** Comparison of quarterback's 40-yard time and a 40-yard touchdown play.

quickly is more important than attaining top speed during a football game.

## Agility

The reasons for the changes in speed during the play illustrated in figure 1.4 may be divided into the movements shown in table 1.2.

In the visual view of the play in figure 1.5, the distance from the line of scrimmage to the end zone is 22 yards, but the play covered an actual distance of at least 40 yards. Six changes of direction, one about every 7 yards, occurred during the play.

**Table 1.2 Changes in Speed During a Play**

| Yards | Split | Speed | Description of play |
|---|---|---|---|
| 0 | 0.00 | 0.00 | Ball snapped |
| 5 | 1.20 | 4.17 | Reverse pivot, runs down the line of scrimmage |
| 10 | 1.10 | 4.55 | Sees hole, cuts up the field; breaks arm tackle |
| 15 | 0.93 | 5.36 | Cuts back across the grain |
| 20 | 1.03 | 4.84 | Breaks arm tackle |
| 25 | 0.73 | 6.82 | Cuts back up the field and turns on the jets |
| 30 | 0.83 | 6.00 | Cuts to the outside, cuts back up the field |
| 35 | 0.63 | 7.89 | Outruns pursuit |
| 40 | 0.57 | 8.82 | Outruns pursuit |

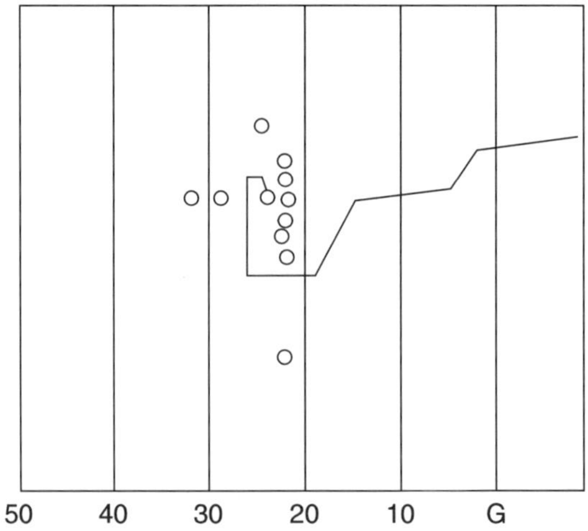


**Figure 1.5** Forty-yard touchdown play.

From the runner's point of view, the ability to read a defensive player's movements determines what direction to run. When he sees an opening, the ability to react, change direction, and accelerate to the open field is crucial. Other times he must fake to get the defensive player to move one direction so that he can cut in the opposite direction. Regardless of what position you play, being able to change directions and accelerate is fundamental to football. The acceleration and agility drills (see chapters 6 and 7) will help you improve these skills.

## Power

To understand power you must first know what force is. Force (external or internal) is defined as the cause or the agent that produces or tends to produce motion. External forces are those forces acting externally on the body, such as friction caused by the resistance of motion between two bodies, air resistance, and the pull of gravity. In strength training the external force is the weight that is attempted or actually lifted. Internal forces are efforts or movements caused by muscular contractions. In strength training the internal force of muscle contraction must overcome the external force of the weight being lifted.

Net force is the sum of all forces involved. The net force is what determines the strength of the lifter. For example, if bench pressing 100 pounds, you need to generate at least 101 pounds of force through muscle contraction; thus, the net force of 1 pound enables you to lift the barbell. If you generate 100 pounds of force, the net force is zero and there is no movement. If your muscles can only generate 90 pounds of force, the net force is –10 and you are not able to lift the barbell. Strength is, therefore, the internal force of muscle contraction.

Often strength is confused with power. Power is the rate at which work is done. Work is the application of strength (force) through a distance. Therefore power is strength times speed. Power is often referred to as explosive strength (strength that can be expressed in a short time frame).

$$\textbf{Work} = \textbf{Strength} \times \textbf{Distance}$$

$$\textbf{Speed} = \textbf{Distance/Time}$$

$$\textbf{Power} = \textbf{Strength} \times \textbf{Speed}$$

Therefore:

$$\textbf{Power} = \textbf{Strength} \times \textbf{Distance/Time} = \textbf{Work/Time}$$

Power can be expressed in foot-pounds per second. That is, if a muscle can lift one pound one foot in one second, it is said to have a power of one foot-pound per second.

You may hear a sportscaster say, for example, that a certain player can bench press 400 pounds. But, does this player have more power than one who only bench presses 300 pounds? Let's compare the two athletes. The first athlete bench presses 300 pounds for a distance of two feet in two seconds. The second athlete bench presses 400 pounds for a distance of two feet in four seconds. Which athlete develops the most power?

**Athlete #1** $$P = \frac{300 \text{ lb} \times 2 \text{ ft}}{2 \text{ s}} = \frac{600}{2} = 300 \text{ ft/lb/s}$$

**Athlete #2** $$P = \frac{400 \text{ lb} \times 2 \text{ ft}}{4 \text{ s}} = \frac{800}{4} = 200 \text{ ft/lb/s}$$

From these examples you can see that strength is different than power. Even though the second athlete lifted more weight or displayed more strength, he did not display more power than the first athlete.

So the next time a television announcer says a particular player can bench press 400 pounds in two seconds, you can be impressed. Therefore, strength is related to power, but strength is not concerned with the amount of time it takes to be expressed. Power is concerned with how much strength can be expressed within a specified period of time.

Let's take a closer look at strength and speed. There is an inverse relationship between the speed and the amount of strength needed to do a movement. As the need for strength decreases the speed of movement increases. For example, an athlete can throw a marble faster and farther than a 16-pound shot. Because the weight of the shot is greater, it requires greater strength to throw. It is impossible to use a great amount of strength to throw a marble, but it can be thrown with great speed. Figure 1.6 shows this strength-speed relationship.

In football, the team or player who can block and tackle the best is usually the victor. These skills are most effective when executed with as much power (speed and strength) as possible. To develop maximum isometric strength (internal force = external force) takes approximately .6 to .8 second. At maximum isometric strength, no movement takes place, and the speed of movement is zero. Therefore no power is produced (zero multiplied by anything is zero) even though maximum strength is being expressed. With movements at top speed, the ability to use strength is minimal and the amount of power produced is insignificant. Looking at a power curve, the greatest power is at 30 to 50 percent of maximum strength (figure 1.7). Since it takes approximately .6 seconds to develop maximum strength, maximum power is developed in .2 second. The amount of time to apply force (to extend the legs) during a block or tackle is .2 to .3 second. Therefore, the amount of time it takes

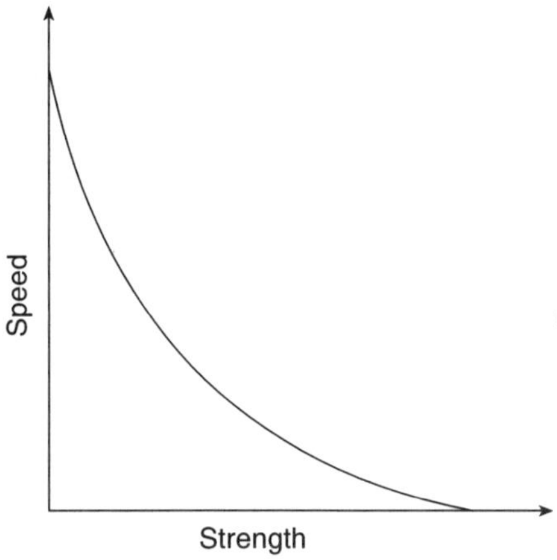


**Figure 1.6** The strength-speed relationship.

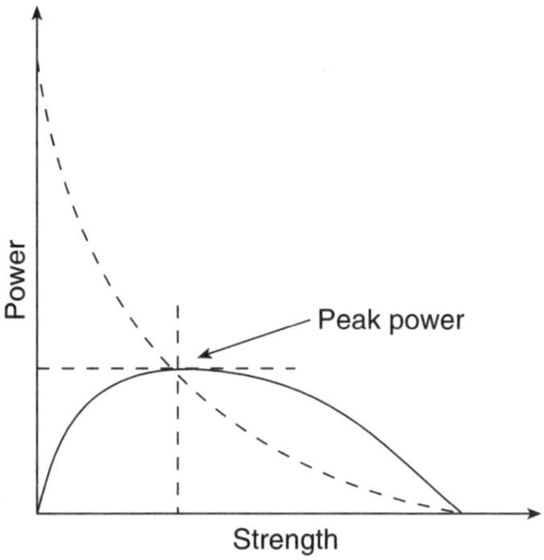


**Figure 1.7** The strength-power relationship.

to apply strength during a tackle or block corresponds to the time it takes to produce maximum power.

In timing athletes with varying 10-yard dash times, we have found that the time it takes to extend the legs and the amount of time the foot is in contact with the ground is virtually the same. A fast runner does not extend his legs any faster or have a quicker footstrike than a slower runner. The average time to extend the legs during the 10-yard dash is .3 second for the first step and .2 second for steps two and three. Again, maximum power is developed during the acceleration phase of sprinting. The same is true with the vertical jump, which is a simple test of power. Every player extends the legs at the same rate, .2 second, but there is a difference in the height jumped. The limiting factor in these movements is not the speed of leg extension, but the amount of force that can be applied within .2 to .3 second. Therefore, the focus of the strength and conditioning program is to develop strength within this time frame to develop maximum power for football skills; exercises must be incorporated that require the expression of strength in .2 to .3 second. Chapter 5 describes these "explosive exercises."

Though in football we are more concerned with power than strength, the form of training used to develop power is still classified under strength training. When the term "strength training" is used in this book it signifies training for maximum strength and power (explosive strength).

## Endurance

Whether a player is a running back accelerating through a hole, a guard pulling around end to block, or a linebacker blitzing the quarterback, his success largely depends on speed, agility, and power. Still, it is not sufficient to be able to run fast and change direction quickly for only a few plays. That is, a player must be able to sustain maximum speed, agility, and power on each play for an entire game. Training the body to maintain maximum performance throughout the game is where endurance comes in.

To develop a better understanding of endurance and how it relates to football players, let's take a closer look at energy and how it is supplied to the muscles. Energy is defined as the ability to perform work. As we have mentioned previously, work is the application of strength through distance. Muscular contraction is determined by the power needs (energy per unit time) or the work capacity (amount of energy available). As you can see, power and energy are closely related.

The following is a simple look at a complex process that requires many enzymes and chemical reactions. Energy is initially supplied through the food we eat. This food cannot be used immediately; rather it must be broken down into adenosine triphosphate (ATP). ATP is the immediate energy source for all muscle contraction. ATP consists of an adenosine component and three phosphate bonds.

$$\textbf{Adenosine—}P_1 - P_1 - P_1$$

When acted on by the enzyme adenosine triphosphatase (ATPase), ATP is broken down into adenosine diphosphate (ADP), inorganic phosphate ($P_1$), and energy is released to do work (muscle contraction).

$$\textbf{ATP + ATPase = ADP + } P_1 \textbf{ + Energy}$$

There is a limited amount of ATP in the muscle cell at any one moment, and it is constantly being utilized and resynthesized. Energy is required to regenerate ATP for muscle contraction and is supplied by the interaction of three energy-yielding systems. These energy systems are represented in figure 1.8 as a hydraulic model of three interconnected storage tanks. These "tanks" are found close to the contractile mechanisms in each muscle fiber. The tank that directly provides energy to the contractile mechanism represents the phosphagen energy system. The other two tanks (lactic acid and oxygen) are connected to the phosphagen tank. Therefore, the ATP supplied from the lactic acid and oxygen tanks is first dumped into the phosphagen tank, which ultimately supplies the energy from the breakdown of ATP to the contractile mechanism. Which energy source the muscle uses to replenish ATP depends upon the intensity (rate of ATP utilization) and duration (amount of ATP needed) of the work bout.

There is enough ATP stored in the phosphagen tank to supply about one second worth of energy during high-intensity, short-duration

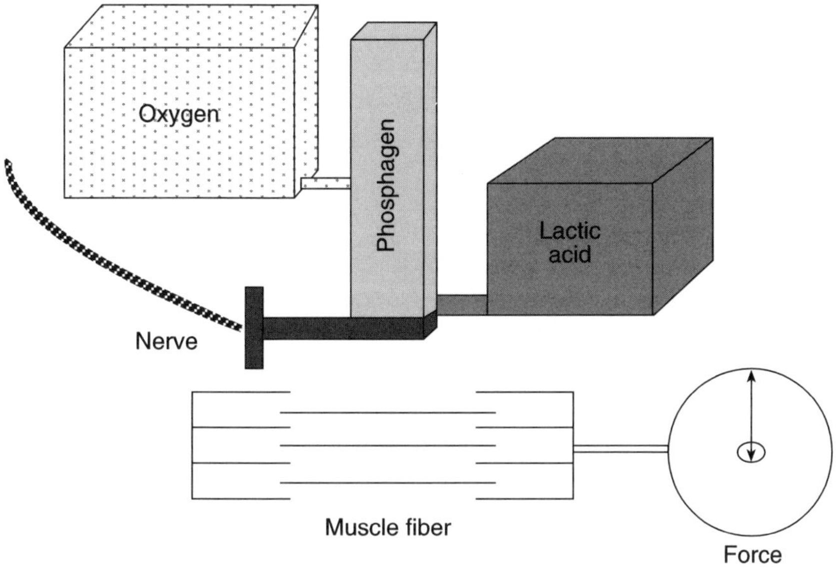


**Figure 1.8** A model of the three energy-yielding systems: oxygen, phosphagen, and lactic acid.

activities such as the 40-yard dash or lifting heavy weights. As ATP is broken down during muscle contraction it is replenished immediately from energy supplied from the breakdown of the compound phosphocreatine (PC). When acted upon by the enzyme creatine kinase (CK), PC is broken down into creatine, $P_{1.}$

$$\mathbf{PC + CK = C + P_1 + Energy}$$

The energy released is then used to combine the $P_1$ to an ADP molecule to regenerate an ATP molecule.

$$\mathbf{Energy + ADP + P_1 = ATP}$$

Football demands a rapidly available supply, rather than a large amount, of ATP. The process of transferring energy from PC to form ATP occurs in less than a second. It is a simple one-step process and does not require any special cellular functions. Without the phosphagen system, football players would not be able to perform explosive movements.

The amount of PC stored in the muscle exceeds that of ATP, but is also limited. During high-intensity exercise PC is depleted within six seconds. Thus, energy from the phosphagen system is utilized for only short maximum bursts of power (figure 1.9).

If intense exercise is continued for more than six seconds, the energy is supplied from the lactic acid energy system (figure 1.10). The release

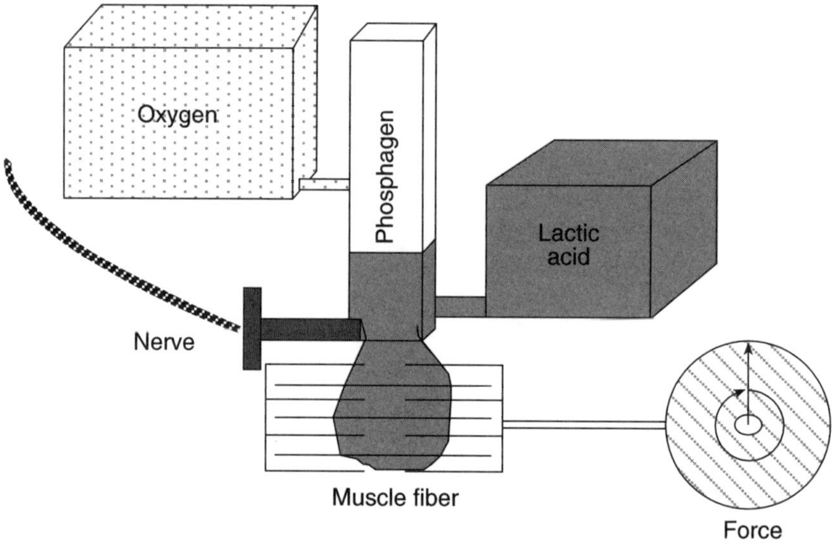


**Figure 1.9** Energy from the phosphagen system is utilized for short maximum bursts of power, such as those used in football.

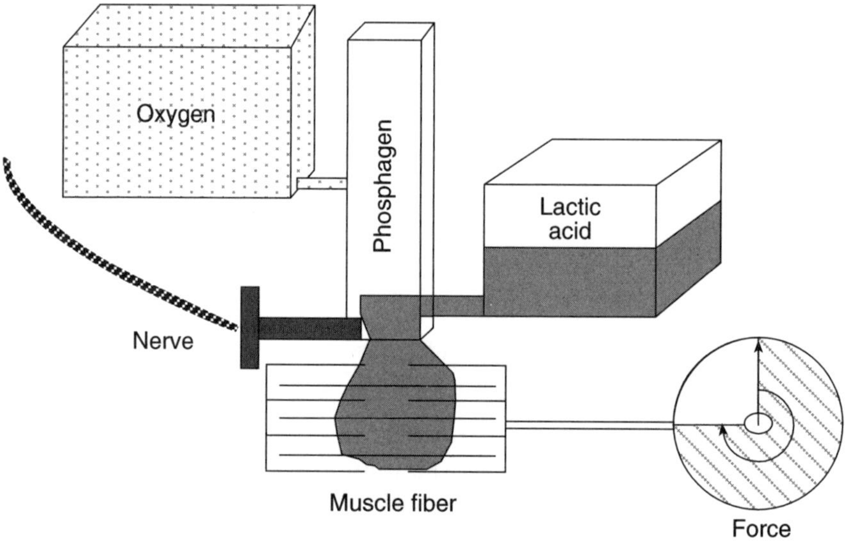


**Figure 1.10** The lactic acid system helps supply energy after the phosphagen system's energy is depleted (after about 6 seconds of maximal work).

of energy to the contractile mechanism is now slower because the opening in this system's outlet is smaller than the phosphagen tank outlet. Therefore, the amount of force generated is reduced. ATP from this tank is released from the breakdown of glycogen and glucose in the absence of oxygen through a process called anaerobic glycolysis. Through this process a metabolic by-product called lactic acid accumulates in the muscle. The highest accumulation of lactic acid is reached during high-intensity activities that last from one to three minutes. If this tank is emptied, too much lactic acid accumulates in the muscle causing pain and resulting in a loss of coordination and force production; this often happens at the end of 400- or 800-meter races. Because football plays last no more than eight seconds and there is adequate recovery between them, lactic acid does not accumulate to a great degree. Thus, the lactic acid system plays a very small role in football.

Another tank represents the oxygen system. This system is more specific to activities requiring endurance over a long duration at low intensity. After about three minutes of low-intensity exercise, ATP is supplied almost completely from this tank (figure 1.11). The ATP in the other two tanks levels off. The diameter of the outlet from this third tank is very small, reducing the flow of ATP even more and generating less force.

Each play in a football game involves an effort of 100 percent intensity for roughly 5 seconds. Between each play there is an average of 50 seconds rest, including time-outs and penalties. The demand for ATP is high during a play, and as the play ends, the phosphagen tank is almost

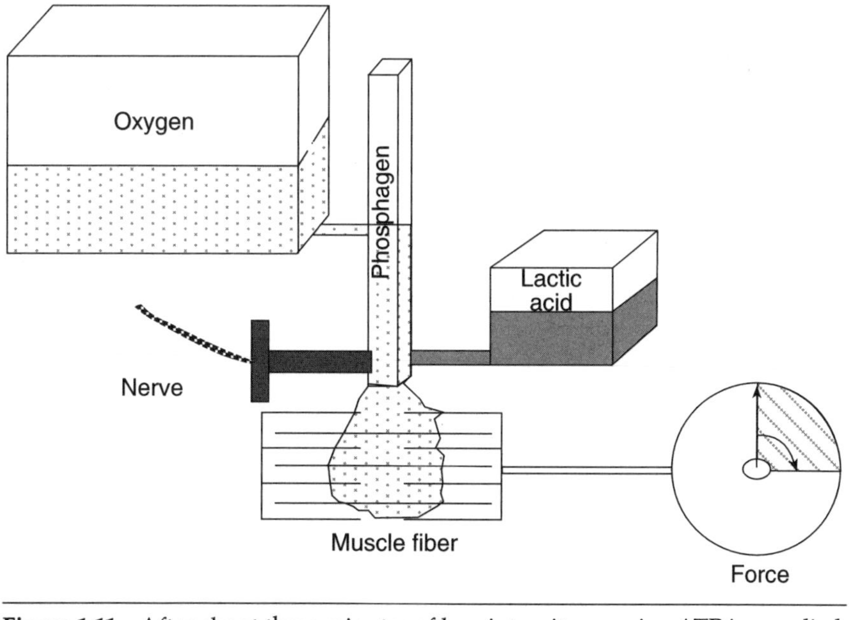


**Figure 1.11** After about three minutes of low-intensity exercise, ATP is supplied from the oxygen (aerobic energy system) "tank."

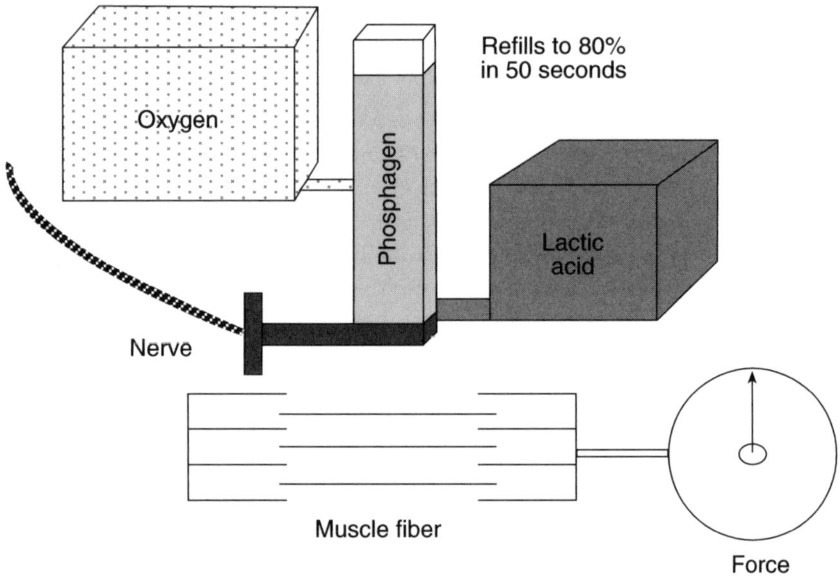


**Figure 1.12** The phosphagen energy system is utilized by the short bursts in football play, but has a chance to refill between plays.

drained (refer to figure 1.9). The tank refills to almost maximum capacity between plays, allowing maximum intensity for the next play (figure 1.12). Therefore, the energy supplied during a football game is predominantly from the phosphagen energy system. The limiting factor of a player being able to give 100 percent effort for each play for an entire football game depends on how efficiently he is able to replenish the phosphagen tank. The interval training described earlier in this chapter gives a brief overview on how to train the phosphagen energy system. The principal concept of interval training is to develop the ability to recover completely within the specified rest interval so that maximum intensity is possible with each work interval. A specific program to develop football endurance is covered in chapter 9.

## PRACTICE

How well you play in a game depends on how well you practice. The game is won or lost by the end of Thursday's practice, because the game is simply executing what you have practiced during the week. The three elements covered in practice are fundamentals, strategies, and mental aspects. Practice also builds on your foundation of character, conditioning, and athletic ability.

## Fundamentals

Every great coach is a firm believer in the fundamentals of blocking and tackling. Technique is the medium through which the power of these skills is expressed; the better a player's technique, the more power he can generate when executing a skill. Conversely, if a player doesn't have the ability to effectively generate power his technique is limited. A great football player has the ability to generate high power *and* express it effectively through good technique.

## Strategies

Strategy is a general game plan based on your team's offensive, defensive, and kicking philosophies; both these philosophies and strategy are determined by the head coach and the type of players available on the team. Plays are then devised to take advantage of the team's strengths. Then you determine your opponents' weaknesses and attack them with your strengths.

The majority of the time the team that implements its strategy with the fewest mistakes wins. To eliminate mistakes each player must know his assignments until they become second nature. The team must also be prepared to adjust to different situations such as weather and field conditions. Repetition in practicing the plays is the key to a well-disciplined and well-prepared team.

## Mental Training

Each time a team takes the field the team members must have no doubt that they are going to win the game. This confidence comes from knowing you have prepared your body well, that you have mentally conditioned yourself to give 100 percent on each and every play, that you know your assignments, and that your team is better conditioned than your opponent's.

Most great athletes admit a great percentage of their success is due to mental factors. Recent research has shown that a mental training technique called visualization can improve physical performance, as our subconscious is unable to distinguish between what is vividly imagined and what is real. For example, a former Nebraska player told me of an experience he had in a game in which a long pass was thrown to him and everything seemed to move in slow motion. It felt like it took five minutes for the ball to get to him. He had plenty of time to get himself into the best possible position to make the catch. As he watched the ball go into his hands he could read the lettering on it. He attributed this experience to visualizing himself over and over again in a game situation catching a long pass. The key to this technique is to get into a relaxed state of mind and visualize the game situation in detail. While specific visualization and mental training techniques are not covered in this book, mental training sources include Charles Garfield's *Peak Performance* (1985), Dorothy Harris' *The Athlete's Guide to Sports Psychology* (1984), George Leonard's *Mastery* (1991), Dan Millman's *The Warrior Athlete, Body, Mind & Spirit* (1979), and Kay Porter's *Visual Athletics* (1990).

## GAME

How an individual plays in a game situation depends on factors that can't be objectively measured with a stopwatch or tape measure. The intangibles separate who plays in the game and who doesn't. The two basic criteria that Coach Tom Osborne and his staff at the University of Nebraska look for when recruiting a player are skill and effort.

### Skill

A player may have the basic athletic abilities of speed, power, agility, and endurance, but this doesn't guarantee success in football. Athletic abilities are only the underlying parameters of being a skillful football player. Learning football techniques through practice combined with athletic ability enhances a player's skill level. A coach is not concerned with how fast or powerful a player is, but how fast and powerfully he plays. Practice doesn't always make perfect; some players may lack the genetic abilities to execute football skills properly. Body control, hand-eye coordination, concentration, timing, and reactions are some of the intangibles that can't always be coached. For example, no matter how much you throw and catch the football, chances are you're not going to be able to throw with the accuracy of Steve Young or make catches like Jerry Rice.

### Effort

Effort comes from giving 100 percent on each and every play. Never save yourself for later in the game. Take one play at a time. When things don't go your way, never give up. Play the next play with all you have, from the time the ball is snapped until the whistle is blown. Play from sideline to sideline. Once your block is made, look downfield for someone else to block. Effort is a common thread throughout all the levels of the pyramid. It takes effort to improve character, to condition yourself, and to practice effectively. Give 100 percent effort during practice in order for it to be carried over into a game situation.

Combine effort with ability to execute your assignment. A 100 percent effort doesn't do much good if you blow your assignment. Mental mistakes in a crucial situation can hurt the team's momentum. Effort doesn't mean fighting; show composure and keep your head in the game. If an opposing player starts swinging, are you able to walk away without fighting back? It is usually the one who retaliates who gets the flag, and a penalty against your team in a crucial situation could lose the game.

## PERFORMANCE

The apex of football performance (and the pyramid) is the ability to *make the play*. Making the play means making more tackles, rushing for more yards, intercepting more passes, making more pancake blocks, causing more fumbles, and scoring more touchdowns. If you are able to make more of these kinds of plays you help your team win more games. Making the play is the culmination of a player's character, conditioning, athletic ability, practice habits, skill level, and effort. If you can make the play, your future in football is promising.

Our primary mission in this book is to show you how to improve athletic ability through strength and conditioning. If you can become more agile, faster, more powerful, and develop endurance you will become a better football player. The next chapter deals with strength and conditioning guidelines and principles to enhance your athletic ability. The rest of the book describes drills and exercises and organizes them into daily programs that are most effective in developing athletic ability. Character development is described briefly in chapter 8. There are many books that cover character development in greater detail at your local library and bookstore. This book will not cover the details of practice, games, and performance shown on the rest of the pyramid. This is the responsibility of the football coach and not the strength and conditioning coach. Again, there are plenty of books that cover these levels of the pyramid. This book concentrates on conditioning to improve athletic ability.

CHAPTER 2

# CONDITIONING PRINCIPLES

In chapter 1 we established what you need to become the best football player you possibly can be. This chapter guides you in developing and implementing a program to allow you to peak the four athletic indicators of speed, agility, power, and endurance.

Thousands of conditioning programs have been developed over the years. Scientific facts formulate the basis of some of these programs, and some elicit initial gains that may be—in the end—detrimental to sports performance. Many coaches and athletes adopt a system because a champion sprinter or weightlifter was successful with it. While these programs develop speed and strength, they often do not have in mind the goals of a football player. The best alternative takes the basic concepts developed by sprinters and weightlifters and applies them specifically to improving football performance.

## ADAPTATION

The primary principle in any conditioning program is the principle of *adaptation*—the body's ability to change according to the demands of the physical environment. The primary focus of strength training and interval training is to cause adaptations to the nervous, muscular, and energy systems. The body adapts to strength training by increasing muscle size and strength, and ultimately power, speed, and agility. The adaptations brought on by interval training are increases in power, speed, agility, and endurance capacity. However, it is important to temper the demands of training with moderation (and rest) so that maximum adaptation takes place with the least expenditure of time and energy. Unnecessary demands on the body can lead to overtraining and possible injury. You can read more about overtraining in chapter 8.

As scientific breakthroughs bring more insight as to how the body adapts to different programs, they also raise more questions. The program we recommend today will most likely be different in the future. We provide you with guidelines here, but you must modify them to fit your situation and each athlete's potential. We hope our guidelines stimulate you to evaluate what you are currently doing in your program and to open your minds and ask yourselves why you are doing what you're doing. We feel that applying the following principles together unlocks a player's potential to achieve peak performance.

This chapter introduces three basic principles of adaptation:

**Specificity.** How much of the training adaptation is transferred to a gain in competitive performance? What is the correct selection of exercises and drills to get a high transfer of training? The primary focus is the adaptation of the nervous system.

**Overload.** Adaptation takes place when the magnitude of training is greater than normal, and is achieved by prescribing the correct number of sets, repetitions, and intensity of effort. The primary focus is the muscular and energy systems' adaptation to the overload.

**Periodization.** Training phases must be planned so that speed, agility, power, and endurance will peak during the most important competitions.

## SPECIFICITY

We determined in chapter 1 that speed, agility, power, and endurance are the athletic abilities important for football. A training program must not only allow the body to adapt to the loads placed upon it in order to become better conditioned, it must also adapt the body specifically for playing football. Swimming or bicycling long distances do not duplicate the requirements needed to play football. Of course, the most specific way to become a better football player is by playing football, but most coaches and athletes understand that other modes of training can improve the abilities of athletes to become better football players.

The key to determining what training is best for football is to ask: Does an exercise or drill improve the athlete's ability to perform better in his sport? Coaches often confuse the difference between physiological (strength and endurance) and performance improvement. Exercises and drills must specifically match the biomechanical needs of football. The sequential activation of muscle groups must be timed in the proper motor unit recruitment patterns, with the proper force production, so that movements can be done powerfully with coordination and balance. For example, a player who does a lot of leg extensions or leg curls may improve his strength in these movements, but there is little transfer of training specific to the proper motor unit recruitment patterns of sprinting and jumping performance.

Many athletes are more concerned with how they look on the beach than how they perform on the field. Exercises done in front of a mirror that isolate and pump the arms, chest, and shoulders become the focus of these athletes' strength programs. However, there is no single best exercise or drill; rather, a variety of exercises and drills complement each other in order to make the best training progress. The goal of any program is to get the greatest return (performance improvement) on your investment (proper selection of exercises and drills). The following biomechanical guidelines determine the core exercises and drills of the strength and interval training programs used in this book.

## Ground-Based Activities

The most important principle to remember when selecting lifting exercises and running drills is that they should allow you to apply force against the ground with your feet. This principle carries through to the other principles described in this chapter. The first step in analyzing a movement is to determine the position of the feet and hands. Do this by determining whether the movement is an open or closed chain movement. In an open chain movement the hands or feet can move freely, such as the feet moving forward when punting a football or the movement of the hand when throwing a football. In a closed chain movement the feet or hands are fixed, such as the hands when doing a push-up or the feet pushing against the ground during sprinting or jumping.

No athletic movement is a totally closed or open chain movement, but a combination of the two. Most movements start with a closed chain movement and finish with an open chain movement. Movement of the body is impossible without first applying force against the ground (closed chain movement). Exerting force against the ground with the feet causes an equal and opposite reaction in the direction of movement (figure 2.1). Any exercise or drill initiated by a closed chain movement is called a ground-based exercise.

Football skills such as sprinting, blocking, tackling, and throwing are ground-based exercises. Depending on the skill, the hands act in an open chain or combination open/closed chain movement. With sprinting the feet are closed chain when applying force against the ground, but the movement is open chain during the swing phase when the feet move forward. The hands are open chain because they swing freely during the entire sprinting action. During tackling and blocking the hands are at times moving freely, and at other times their movement is closed chain because they become somewhat fixed when contact is made with the opponent.

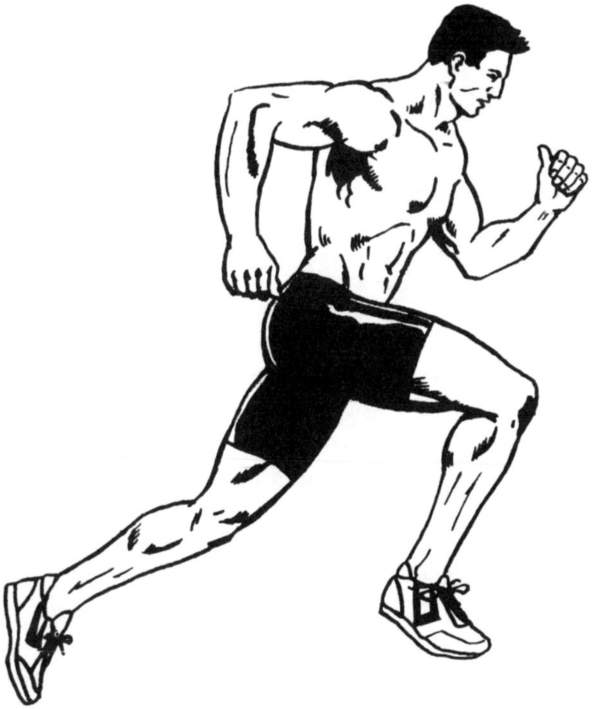

**Figure 2.1** Exerting force against the ground allows the body to move.

Try this experiment. First throw the football as you normally would with your feet on the ground. Next, jump straight up in the air, as high as you can, and throw the football. Which method allows you to throw the greatest distance?

Did you find that you could throw much farther with your feet on the ground? You must have your feet on the ground to express maximum force. The more force you apply against the ground, the faster you run and the more effectively you block and tackle.

The body's ability to stabilize joint actions contributes to proper neuromuscular coordination of the multiple joint actions needed for football. For example, the initial action of throwing a football originates from the muscular contractions of the hips and legs exerting a force against the ground in a backward direction. The earth, being more stable because of its large mass, does not move, and the reaction to this force is exerted through the athlete in a forward direction. As the athlete extends his legs against the ground his ankle, knee, and hip joints stabilize as the reaction force transfers to the torso (stomach and lower back). The torso rotates and then stabilizes as the muscular force is relayed to the chest and shoulders, and then to the arms and wrist, which display the greatest motion. The force applied to the football is possible because the muscles effectively stabilize the joints as they sequentially contract. Thus, jumping in the air and throwing the ball, as illustrated in the experiment, does not allow the leg and hip joints to effectively stabilize.

Let's now look at ground-based activities in relation to joint actions, muscle actions, and contractions.

## Multiple Joint Actions

If a tug-of-war contest pitted three strong men against one man, who would you pick to win the contest? The summation of forces produced by three men pulling in the same direction exceeds the force generated by one man pulling in the opposite direction. The same is true with joint actions. The greater the number of joint actions working together, the greater the force development. Football skills involve multiple joint actions of the hips, knees, and ankles, with the muscular forces added together. This multiple joint action of the hips, knees, and ankles working in concert is known as the *triple extension,* the most powerful movement of the body. Two conditions must be met for the summation of force to be effective. First, as mentioned earlier, each joint action must be firmly stabilized for the force to be conducted through the body. Second, the forces from each joint action must be timed in the correct neuromuscular recruitment patterns. Not as much force can be developed when doing single joint actions such as the leg extension or leg curls, and the timing of muscle recruitment patterns cannot be developed. Therefore, there is little transfer of training in performance improvement.

Figure 2.2 shows the acceleration phase of the 40-yard dash. When executed correctly, the body is positioned in a straight line at the ankle, knee, and hip joints, resulting in the triple extension. Compare this body position with that of an athlete doing a power clean (figure 2.3). During the extension phase the body is also positioned in a straight line at the ankles, knees, and hips. Both of these movements are powerful because of the amount of force produced by the triple extension. Notice the similarities between the two skills if you change the angle of the lifting figure (figure 2.4).

## Multiple Plane Movements

Football skills involve movements in several planes simultaneously. For example, the hip and shoulder joints allow forward, backward, rotational, and side-to-side movements, while a sprint action is primarily done in one plane—forward. But as we discussed in chapter 1, football is not

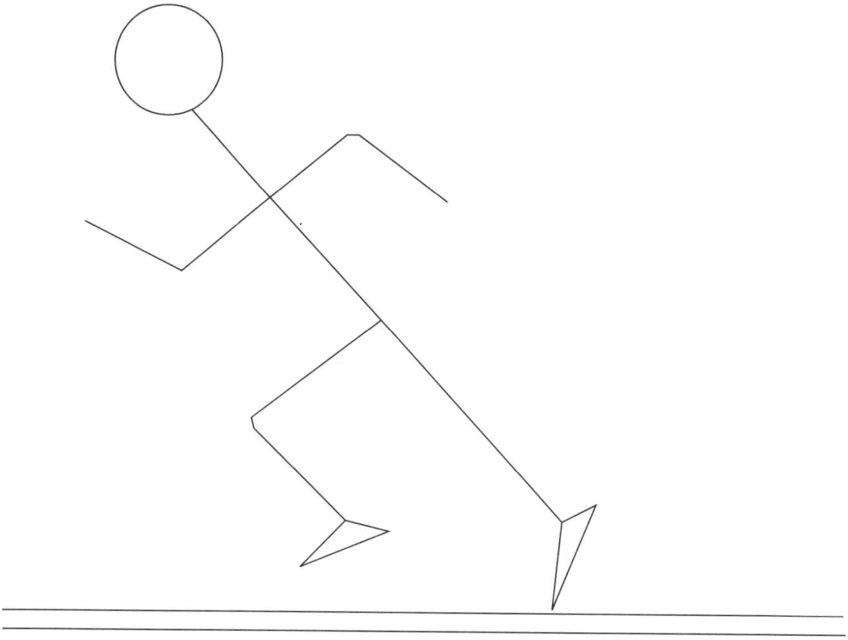

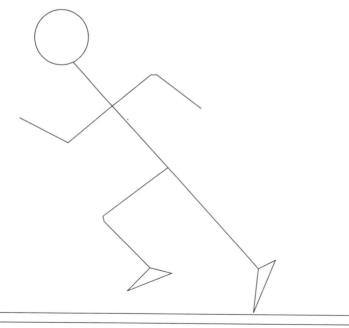

**Figure 2.2** The acceleration phase of the 40-yard dash.

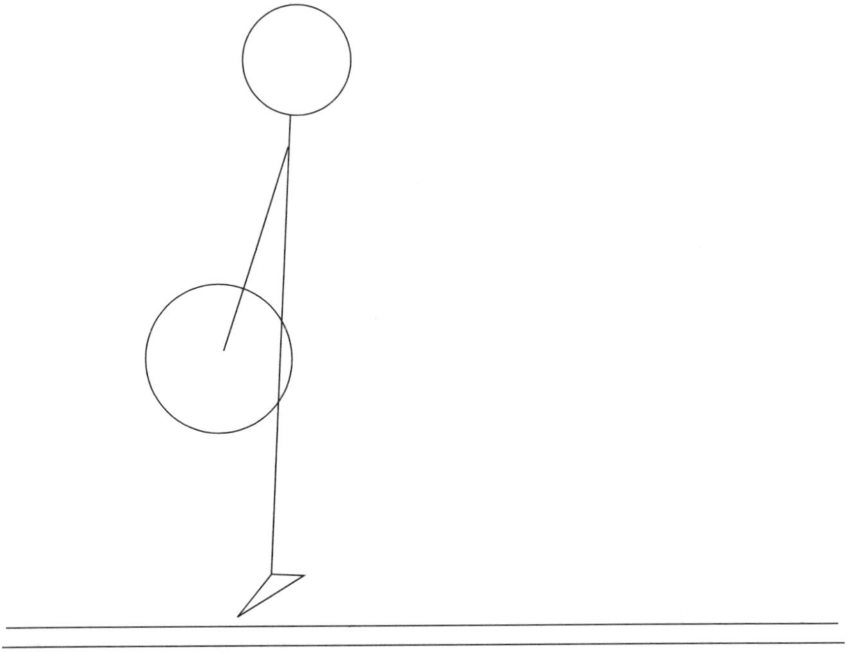

**Figure 2.3** The correct body position while performing the power clean.

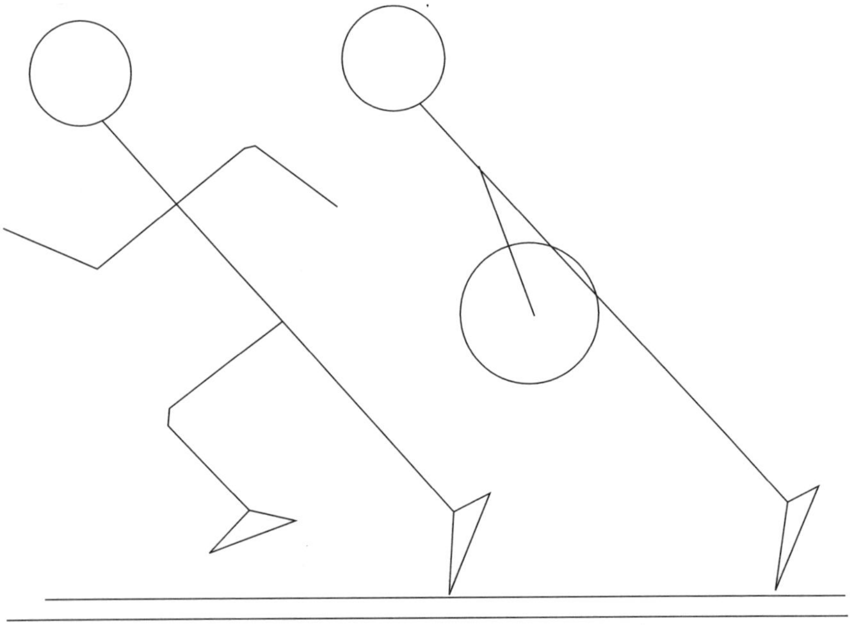

**Figure 2.4** Notice the similarities in body position between the acceleration phase of running the 40-yard dash and the power clean.

played simply by moving forward, but requires changes of direction in which cutting maneuvers (side steps or crossover steps) are used. Making a cut requires movements in three planes at the hip joint (forward, rotational, and sideways), two planes at the knee joint (forward and rotational), and two planes at the ankle joint (forward and rotational). Therefore, it is important to include exercises in your strength program that incorporate multiple plane movements. Chapter 5 includes several exercises that meet the needs of multiple plane movements. Your running program should also incorporate a combination of movements including changes of direction. Chapter 7 describes agility drills that utilize multiple plane movements. Multiple plane movements are only possible with ground-based exercises. Open chain, single joint actions restrict movement in one plane only.

## Synergism

Synergism occurs when several muscles act together to produce a coordinated joint action by neutralizing each other's individual secondary activity. Only exercises using free weights allow synergism. For example, when doing power presses (see chapter 5) the shoulder joint muscles must control and balance the barbell. Many smaller synergistic muscle groups of the shoulder girdle assist in coordinating joint actions and preventing unwanted movements. Muscle synergism is required as the body constantly changes position relative to an opponent during tackling and blocking. The synergistic muscles allow for split-second adjustments during movements so that maximum force can be applied to the opponent. Only free weight exercises allow muscle synergism to regulate and coordinate the movement of the resistance. Weight machines, on the other hand, use lever arms, guide rods, and pulleys to dictate the path of movement and balance the resistance, requiring the muscle only to provide the force. Therefore, machines limit the development of muscle synergism.

All speed and agility drills allow for synergism by the nature of their movements. No outside forces are required to change the movement patterns of the body during speed and agility drills. Only the internal adjustment of synergetic muscles assists movement changes and keeps the body in balanced positions to allow maximum force development. The multiple plane movements of free weights also help prevent major joint injuries. The balancing action of synergistic muscles develops joint integrity better than machines. For example, exercises using benches or seats as support restrict the body from stabilizing properly; when doing leg presses the adjustable board substitutes as the stabilizer. The back and stomach muscles are not required to stabilize the action, as when blocking and tackling. However, squatting using free weights requires the back and stomach muscles to stabilize the torso isometrically. This need to stabilize the body allows the legs and hips to work with the back and stomach muscles as a unit to perform the lift.

## Stretch-Shortening Cycle

Both eccentric contractions (stretching a muscle) and concentric contractions (shortening a muscle) occur when executing many sport skills that require a maximum rate of force development. An eccentric contraction followed by a concentric contraction is known as the stretch-shortening cycle. When the muscle is stretched, it builds elastic energy. The muscle then fights to return to its normal resting length (similar to the stretching of a rubber band). If the muscle shortens immediately after the stretch, greater force and power can be generated. For example, as your foot strikes the ground when sprinting, the muscles of the hips and legs eccentrically contract and then concentrically contract, accelerating your body in the direction of the applied force.

## Acceleration

According to Newton's second law, if a given period is available to apply force to an object, the acceleration of the object is directly proportional to the amount of force applied. In other words the greater the force applied, the greater the acceleration. Acceleration of a joint action is a key factor in the proper execution of blocking, tackling, sprinting, and throwing. The body's ability to exert force depends upon its position. For example, you can exert more force at the finish of a full squat than at the bottom (see chapter 5 for description of squat). The body position when executing the triple extension during football movements is the same position as the finish of a squat action. As the muscles contract during a triple extension, the body has better leverage to apply force, allowing greater acceleration of the joint actions.

As discussed in chapter 1 the amount of time to apply force (to extend the legs) during a block or tackle is .2 to .3 second. Therefore, a football program must include exercises that extend the legs .2 second. Traditional lifts like heavy squats and the bench press don't allow acceleration to take place at the end of the exercise. The bar must be decelerated or slowed as it comes to a complete stop at the finish of the lift. You can't accelerate at the end of these lifts, even though you are stronger and have the greatest capability to develop acceleration.

You can overcome the problem of deceleration by using light weights and jumping into the air as high as possible at the end of a squat. This allows acceleration to take place throughout the range of motion. Similarly with the bench press, if you use a light weight and the bar is thrust as high as possible, acceleration takes place throughout the range of motion. The practice of jumping with weights on your back or throwing weight upward and catching it on the way down is dangerous and not recommended. The speed and agility drills avoid this problem by allowing the athlete to explode or apply maximum force through the full range of motion. But an effective force cannot be applied when doing speed and agility drills. Explosive or Olympic-style lifts such as hang cleans and power presses (see chapter 5) allow acceleration to take place at the finish of the movement. The greatest benefit of the Olympic lifts is that the triple extension matches the time frame of .2 second.

Many machines designed with cams, lever arms, and pulley systems don't allow acceleration during the full range of motion. These machines accommodate by increasing the resistance as the body goes through favorable leverage positions. The body adapts to these machines only by increases in muscular size and strength. Isokinetic machines allow only constant velocity movements. If the velocity does not increase during

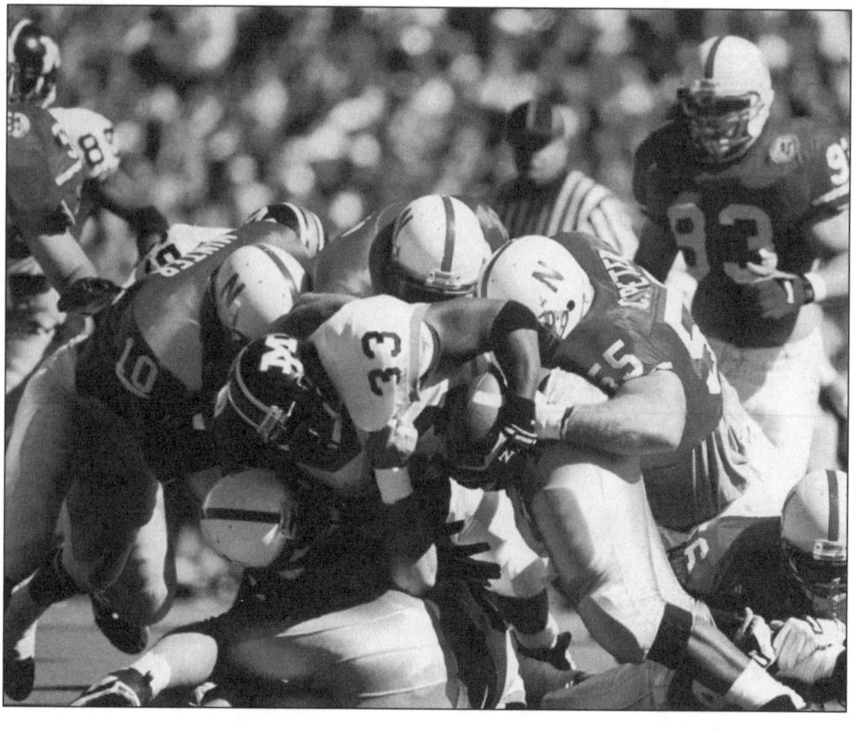

the movement, acceleration is not possible. While these machines may have some application in exercise testing, there is little transfer of training to football skills. Only explosive exercises such as the Olympic lifts and speed and agility drills allow acceleration through a full range of movement.

## Specialty Exercises

Single-jointed exercises, such as biceps curls, leg curls, or leg extensions contribute little to improving athletic performance, but they do meet the specific needs of the program. They are primarily used as specialty exercises because of their ability to isolate muscle groups. They are used by bodybuilders to build muscle mass and are included in this program to help build muscle size. Single-jointed exercises may be used to correct specific muscle weaknesses or to rehabilitate an injured muscle.

Single-jointed exercises can play a major role in maintaining muscle balance. Your body is arranged so there are muscles on both sides of a joint—where two bones join together and work like hinges so movement can occur. All muscles work in pairs, one flexing or pulling toward the body, the other extending or pulling away from the body. Therefore, it is important that your conditioning program includes exercises that work both sides of a joint or both muscles working as a pair and not just one of them. Some common muscle groups that work in pairs are the quadriceps (front of thigh) and hamstrings (back of thigh), as well as the chest and back muscles. A balanced conditioning program such as the one provided in this book includes at least one exercise for each major muscle group in your body.

# OVERLOAD

In order to facilitate optimal training adaptation, imposed overloads must be of a magnitude to force the body to adapt and must be consistently applied and gradually intensified over an extended period of time. How the load is applied determines the type of adaptation. In this program we apply overload through strength training and interval training. Strength training increases muscular size and strength (and therefore power capability) through a resistance overload. Interval training overloads the energy system (and therefore increases endurance capacity) by controlling the work-to-rest interval.

## Load Variables

The variables of strength and interval training loads include intensity, volume, duration, rest periods, and frequency. Different combinations of the load variables translate into different adaptations by the body. As discussed in chapter 1, the primary conditioning objectives for football are to develop muscular size, strength, power, and endurance. Following are examples that show how load variables can be manipulated to bring about these desired adaptations for both strength training and interval training.

### Strength Training

The load variables for strength training are intensity, volume (sets and reps), and the amount of rest between sets.

**Intensity.** Intensity is expressed as the percentage of the maximum muscular performance. The units to measure the load intensity vary depending on the type of training. When lifting, intensity is the amount of weight lifted relative to the maximum weight one is able to lift. In plyometrics intensity is expressed as the height or distance achieved relative to maximum height or distance jumped.

The percentage of a one-repetition maximum (1RM) is the most common method to figure intensity for strength training. One hundred percent intensity is the maximum load that a person can lift for one repetition (rep). The percentage of the 1RM determines the weight prescribed for a workout. So if 300 pounds is the maximum load that a person can lift, 75 percent intensity is 225 pounds, 50 percent intensity is 150 pounds, and so on.

An XRM is a maximum load that can be executed for X number of repetitions. A 10-repetition maximum (10RM) is a load that can be lifted no more than 10 times. The first nine reps of a 10-repetition set are not of sufficient force to cause a maximal muscular effort. It is only the last repetition, even though it may not generate as much force as when a muscle is fresh, that causes a maximum muscular effort. So as the load becomes heavier, fewer repetitions are possible.

Increase the intensity of speed, agility, and jumps by adding resistance to the athlete using harnesses, weight jackets and pants, parachutes, etc. Running hills and stadium steps is another way to increase the intensity.

**Volume.** Volume is a quantitative gauge of training load. Measure volume depending on the type of training. In strength training the most common way to determine volume is by counting the total number of repetitions and multiplying it by the poundage of each exercise.

The volume of the training load plays an important role in the long-term planning of a strength program. Excessive load volume can cause drops in strength gains and eventually lead to potential injury. Remember that volume has limitations; stay within a proper range to get the maximum benefits. The correct volume is related to the intensity of the workout.

The number of repetitions per set varies depending on the skill level of an exercise. For example, the snatch exercise requires a high skill level, so the number of repetitions should not exceed three. Doing more than three repetitions causes a breakdown in technique. The hang clean does not involve as much skill as the snatch, so as many as five repetitions can be done. Biceps curls require a low level of skill, and 10 repetitions can be safely achieved.

## Relative Volume and Total Repetitions

Relative volume is figured by multiplying the number of repetitions by the number of sets.

Repetitions (Reps) = The number of times you repeat an exercise movement

Sets = Exercise bouts specified by a given number of reps

Example: 3 sets of 10 repetitions

Volume = $(3 \times 10) = 30$ repetitions

## Absolute Volume or Total Poundage

Absolute volume is figured by multiplying the number of repetitions by the number of sets by the poundage.

Poundage = Resistance used for each set

Volume = Sets $\times$ Reps $\times$ Load

Example: 3 sets of 10 repetitions at 300 pounds on the squat

Volume = $(3 \times 10) \times 300 = 9{,}000$ pounds

**Rest Periods.** For strength and power development at least three minutes of rest between sets is required at intensities over 70 percent of the 1RM. To maximize the release of growth hormone, the primary stimulus for muscle size, a one-minute rest period at intensities of 50 to 60 percent is more effective than longer rest periods.

## Strength Training Adaptations

Strength training uses barbells, dumbbells, exercise machines, and plyometrics to do lifting exercises specific to football. The number of sets and reps, the intensity, and the length of rest periods have a profound effect on the desired adaptations.

Muscle size increases through the process of tearing down and rebuilding muscle tissue. Strength training stresses individual muscle fibers and causes a breakdown of the contractile proteins. The body then adapts through the addition of a greater number of new contractile proteins, and the muscle increases its cross-sectional size to meet the demands of the future workouts. As your muscles increase in size, you are able to train the next time with greater loads. Your muscles respond again by growing larger yet. This process continues in small increments until you reach your peak.

There is a positive correlation between the cross-sectional size of a muscle and the amount of force it can apply. Therefore, the larger the muscle fibers become through strength training, the greater their capability to apply force. Muscle size can be accomplished only by increasing the size, not the number, of muscle fibers. However, certain individuals are born with more muscle fibers than others, and the more fibers a person has, the greater the potential to increase the cross-sectional size of the muscle.

Bodybuilders have developed very large muscles, and maybe we can learn something from them. They do high-volume workouts with short rest periods—workouts that scientific studies support as the best method for building muscle mass. However, high-volume workouts won't stimulate muscle growth unless the intensity is adequate. Three sets of 10 repetitions is the standard protocol for attaining muscle size. Programs that utilize 5-repetition sets are not as effective as doing sets of 10. Remember that the last few repetitions of the set must cause maximum muscular effort. As you become stronger, increase the weight and not the number of repetitions. A rest period of one minute is the optimal time between sets and exercises to elicit a muscle size adaptation.

## Strength

Strength is not only improved by increasing the size of the fibers, but also by the ability of the nervous system to recruit more motor units. A motor unit is the basic functional unit of skeletal muscle. A single motor nerve and all the muscle fibers it innervates constitute a motor unit. The human body has approximately 500,000 motor units, and the demand of everyday activities requires only a small number of these motor units. The number of motor units required for any given activity depends on the amount of force required to get the job done. When the load placed on muscles is greater than normal, the body adapts by recruiting more motor units, making the body capable of producing more force.

An individual's initial strength gains are due to the nervous system activating new motor units. Further strength gains are induced through muscle size. Thus, it is important to develop initial conditioning levels by learning proper lifting and running techniques for each exercise and drill. The motor units recruited are specific to the movement. The motor units recruited while performing incorrect movement patterns become ingrained in the nervous system. Unsound movement patterns are difficult to correct and can lead to potential injuries. Begin a program by keeping the overload light, and gradually increase it as proper technique patterns become instilled in the nervous system.

Two types of motor units—fast- and slow-twitch—vary in how force is generated, and thus regulate force required for a given activity. Constant low-level force production for endurance activities (sitting, standing, walking, jogging, etc.) is the main characteristic of slow-twitch fibers, while speed of force development for power activities (sprinting, lifting heavy weights, etc.) is mainly supplied by fast-twitch muscle fibers.

The manipulation of volume and intensity is different for basic strength development than it is for stimulating size. Power lifters are the strongest athletes when it comes to lifting maximum loads. Most power lifters agree that three to five sets of four to six repetitions work best to develop maximum strength. Most of the repetitions should be in the range of 80 to 85 percent intensity. To develop maximum strength, rest periods of three to five minutes or until you feel you are completely rested are best before doing a new set.

## Power

As discussed in chapter 1, power is the combination of speed and strength. Recall how movement speed and load relate to each other: As the load increases, the speed of movement decreases. For example, if executing a jumping squat, use different loads, starting with the weight of the bar and finishing with the maximum possible weight. Place the barbell on your shoulders, lower your body to a quarter-squat position, and jump into the air as high as possible. Jumping with the bar is the fastest movement because the load is the lowest (45 pounds). As the load becomes heavier the movement becomes slower (figure 2.5). Eventually the load becomes so heavy you cannot move the bar.

The power developed at the different loads can be figured by multiplying the amount of the load by the speed of movement. Figure 2.6 shows the various loads plotted on a graph comparing power (foot-pounds per second) to intensity of the load. The highest power outputs are at the top of the curve at about 30 percent of the load maximum (1RM). At lighter loads under 15 percent of 1RM, the velocity of the movement is very fast, but the power generated is low. This is because the load is too light to generate effective power. As the intensity goes over 65 percent, power decreases rapidly. The load becomes so heavy that the speed of movement is too slow to generate power. Therefore the highest power outputs are in the range of 15 to 65 percent of a person's 1RM, and intensity is related to the velocity at which the load can be lifted to develop maximum power. Thus, to develop power the intensity of training must be adjusted to the speed of movement.

To develop power using the explosive lifts (see chapter 5) such as the power clean and snatch, 75 to 85 percent intensity for three to five repetitions is best. Do slower multiple joint movements such as the squat

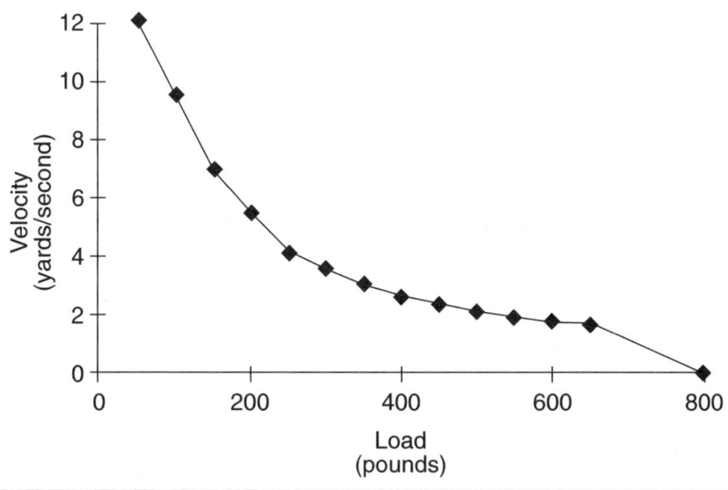


**Figure 2.5** The relationship between load and velocity.

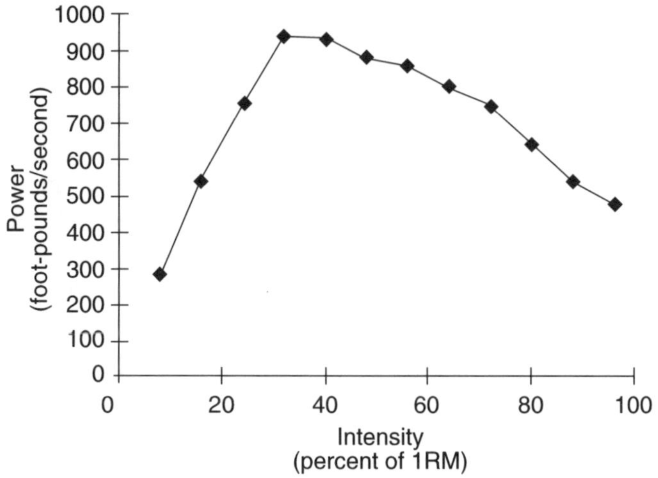


**Figure 2.6** The relationship between intensity and power.

and bench press at 50 to 60 percent for three to five sets of three to five repetitions. Do jump squats at 30 percent intensity for three to five sets of three to five repetitions. Use body weight for the resistance in plyometric exercises for three to five sets of three to five repetitions. To develop maximum power, rest periods of three to five minutes or until you feel you are completely rested are best before doing a new set.

## Interval Training

The load variables for interval training are the intensity and volume of work intervals and the rest intervals.

### Intensity

Interval training is concerned with the intensity of the work interval. Intensity is a percentage of an individual's maximum muscular performance determined by the rate of energy utilization (refer to chapter 1). Most interval training programs are interested in doing the drills within a percentage of your best time by controlling the distance and duration of the run. With this program the agility and speed drills dictate the distance of the work interval; each drill has a recommended distance to run (see chapters 6 and 7). Do not be concerned with your duration of the work interval, but do each speed and agility drill at maximum speed in the shortest period of time possible. Every drill can be completed in less than six seconds. Work bouts longer than six seconds are only possible at a submaximal intensity.

### Volume

In interval training, repetitions are the number of work intervals (i.e., speed or agility drills) to be completed. The number of repetitions determines the length of a running workout. Chapter 9 discusses the required number of repetitions to do for each drill, based on your position and the time of the year.

### Rest Intervals

Maximum muscular performance is only possible when you are completely rested. You aren't capable of running as fast when fatigued as when you are fresh. During interval training an adequate rest interval must follow each work bout to allow maximum intensity during the next work interval. A common training error coaches make in running programs is making rest intervals too short, which allows players to become fatigued and incapable of running as fast as when completely recovered. If the rest period is too short, the amount of ATP-PC replenished is not sufficient to meet the demands of the next maximum-intensity effort, and force output will be reduced. Coaches who make the rest interval too short are reducing the force and training slow-twitch muscle fibers rather than fast-twitch fibers. Yet, to develop football-specific endurance you want to train the fast-twitch fibers to be able to perform throughout the game. With too little rest, players start to pace themselves so they can survive the workout. This workout might develop mental toughness but does little to improve performance.

At the University of Nebraska, the principle concept is to develop the ability to recover as completely as possible within the specified rest interval to allow maximum intensity for each work interval. The players then have the ability to recover completely between plays in a game.

The amount of rest between sets plays a role in how the load is applied and how the body adapts. The purpose of rest between sets is to restore energy stores that have been depleted during the previous exercise bout. The length of the rest period following an exercise bout determines the intensity of the following bout. High-intensity bouts can deplete the ATP-PC stores of a muscle in less than 10 seconds, and it takes approximately 10 to 12 seconds of rest per each second of work to replenish those stores. Each drill in chapters 6 and 7 includes a recommended rest interval.

## Interval Training Adaptations

Interval training uses speed and agility drills specific to the movement patterns and skills used for football. The volume, intensity, duration,

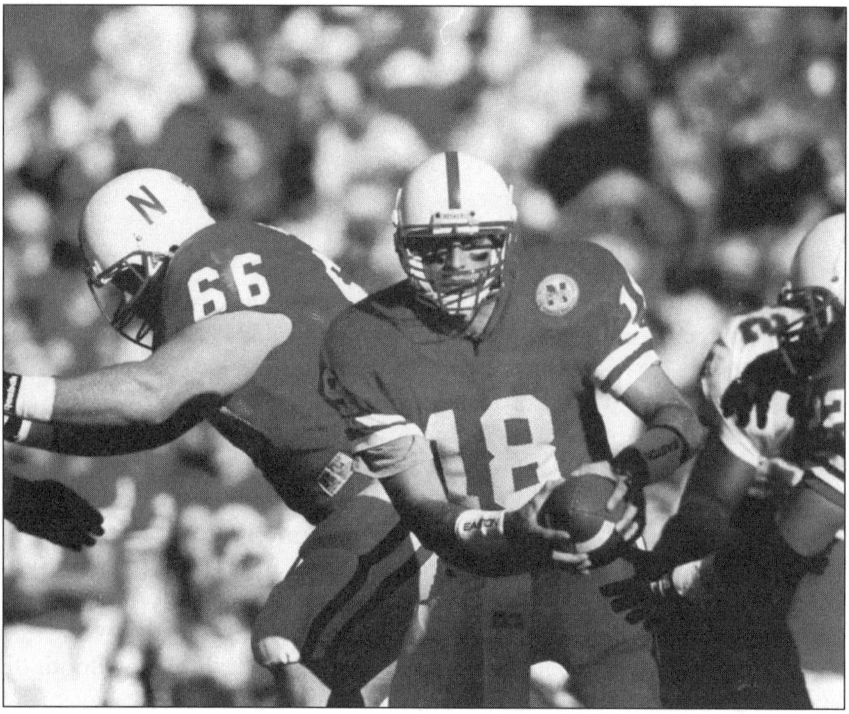

and length of rest periods are not only critical to developing speed and agility, but are also endurance-specific to a football game.

So far we have discussed the muscle and neural adaptations that occur in response to the demands placed on the body. Whether the demands are met also depends upon the supply of energy necessary for muscle contraction so that movement takes place. If the energy demands of the body exceed the energy supply, fatigue results. This energy supply can make a real difference in the fourth quarter. A football player's endurance capacity to supply energy without fatigue depends directly on how overload is applied. Many studies show that a continuous maximum overload (work interval) can only be tolerated a few minutes before fatigue sets in. If the same overload is applied for short periods of time with rest intervals, it can be tolerated much longer, and the body adapts to this overload by improving its endurance specific to football.

## PERIODIZATION

If there is no variation in the training stimulus, performance gradually levels off and leads to overtraining. An approach to offset this problem is a system of training called periodization. Periodization adds variety to the program by using different combinations of intensity, volume, exercises, and drills throughout the training season. This variation helps avoid overtraining and stimulates peak performance.

The general adaptation syndrome (GAS), which depicts how the body adapts to stress, supports periodization. There are three distinct stages of adaptation during the long-term application of the training load.

1. **Alarm stage:** This stage occurs during the first couple of weeks of a strength training program. The most noticeable consequence is muscle soreness which may cause a temporary decrease in performance.

2. **Resistance stage:** During this stage the body begins to adapt to the stress of the strength and conditioning program by increasing muscular size, becoming stronger and more powerful, and achieving greater endurance. Performance begins to improve.

3. **Exhaustion stage:** Performance eventually plateaus and diminishes when the same strength and conditioning regimen is used over an extended period (figure 2.7). The neuromuscular system simply becomes accustomed to the same stimulus and becomes stale. Confusion of what to do often causes the athlete to never reach his performance potential.

## Annual Plan

Training for football is a year-round process. Lifting and running programs must be combined systematically to improve the power, speed, agility, and endurance necessary to play championship football.

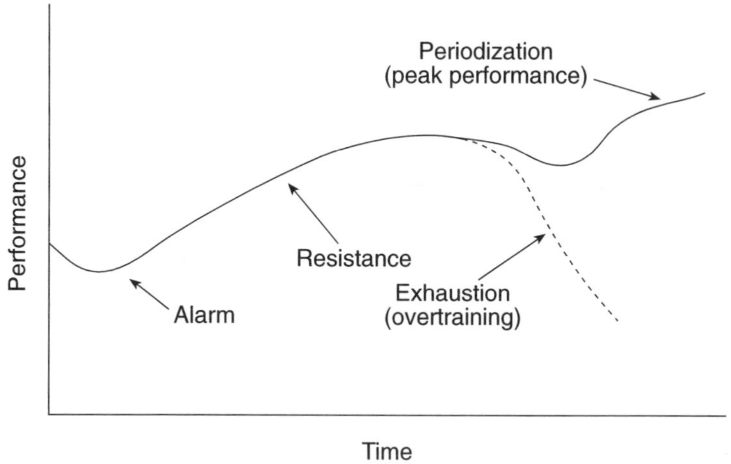


**Figure 2.7** The three stages of adaptation.

The training plan for an entire year is known as the annual plan. At the University of Nebraska the annual plan is broken into two segments: off-season and in-season (table 2.1). The first segment consists of a three- to four-week transition period during January right after the regular season. Winter conditioning occurs during February and March, and the segment finishes with spring ball during the month of April. The second segment starts in May with another two-week transition period. Summer conditioning starts in the middle of May and continues into the first few weeks of August until fall camp or two-a-days, which lasts for two weeks. The regular-season period starts late in August. The second segment ends at the bowl game, normally on January 1.

If your program does not have spring ball, as in most high school situations, the annual plan is not divided into segments, but consists of off-season, in-season, and transition periods (table 2.2). A transition period starts during December after the in-season period. The off-season starts the first part of January and continues until the season starts in August. Fall camp starts in August and lasts for two weeks. The in-season starts in early September with the play-offs in late November.

**Table 2.1 Annual Plan With Two Segments**

| First segment | | Period | Phase |
|---|---|---|---|
| January | Active rest | Transition | Active rest |
| February | Winter conditioning | Off-season | Base |
| March | Winter conditioning | Off-season | Base |
| April | Spring ball | In-season | Maintenance |
| **Second segment** | | **Period** | **Phase** |
| May | Active rest | Transition | Active rest |
| June | Summer conditioning | Off-season | Base, development, and peak |
| July | Summer conditioning | Off-season | Base, development, and peak |
| August | Fall camp | Transition | Contact |
| September | Regular-season | In-season | Maintenance |
| October | Regular-season | In-season | Maintenance |
| November | Regular-season | In-season | Maintenance |
| December | Bowl preparation | In-season | Peak |

Table 2.2 Annual Plan With Three Periods

| Month | Period | Phase |
|---|---|---|
| December | Transition | Active rest |
| January | Off-season | Base |
| February | Off-season | Development |
| March | Off-season | Base |
| April | Off-season | Development |
| May | Off-season | Base |
| June | Off-season | Development |
| July | Off-season | Peak |
| August | Transition | Contact |
| September | In-season | Maintenance |
| October | In-season | Maintenance |
| November | Play-offs | Maintenance |

## Off-Season Periods

The primary objective of the off-season period is to bring athletes to a strength and conditioning peak. The off-season usually cycles through three phases of different variations of training loads and exercises. Each phase has conditioning objectives and procedures that lay the foundation for the next phase. Usually a cycle starts with a base phase, progresses to a development phase, and finishes with a peak phase (figure 2.8). Each phase will be discussed in greater detail.

The area of each building block of the pyramid in figure 2.8 represents the volume of the strength training load. The base phase represents the greatest capacity of volume but the lowest intensity. The top of the pyramid, or peak phase, represents the least amount of volume but the highest intensity. During the base phase, when the focus is on strength training, back off the interval training program. The amount of running is increased during the development phase, with the greatest amount of running done during the peak phase.

**Base Phase (3-6 Weeks).** The primary objective of this phase is to build lean muscle mass and improve work capacity. The base consists of high-volume, low-intensity workouts that develop muscle size.

- Increase muscle mass.
- Increase work capacity.
- Improve technique of explosive lifts.

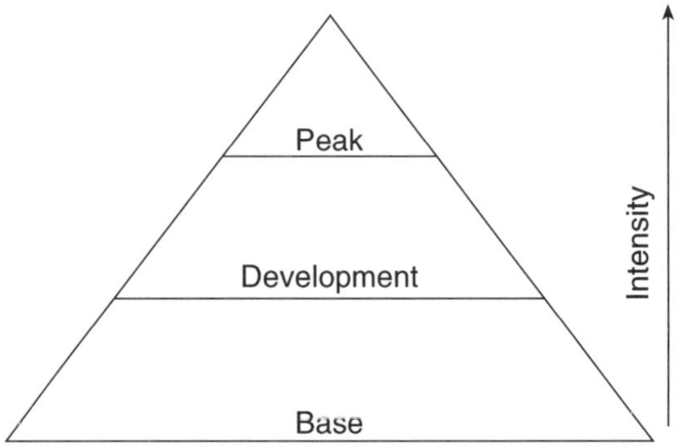


**Figure 2.8** The three phases of the off-season conditioning cycle.

- Maintain sport skills.
- Maintain agility.

You must first build muscle mass in order to build strength in the next phase. By doing high-volume workouts you increase the work capacity of your body in preparation for the higher intensity workouts of the later phases. Single-jointed exercises help stimulate muscular growth. Explosive lifts are done during this phase by concentrating on technique and keeping weight light. Speed and agility drills are optional and should be kept to a minimum, as too much speed and agility work during this phase is counterproductive to increasing both muscle size and speed.

Winter conditioning lasts only six weeks, so the base phase is all we accomplish during the first cycle before starting spring ball. The development and peak phases are accomplished during summer conditioning when there is more time before the regular season starts.

**Development Phase (4-8 Weeks).** The primary objective of this phase is to build on the base phase by decreasing the volume and increasing the intensity of conditioning.

- Develop maximum strength.
- Develop acceleration and speed.
- Develop agility.
- Maintain sport skills.

A greater volume of speed and agility drills is introduced at this time. Cleans, snatches, heavy squats, and pressing exercises form the core of the strength program. Do no more than three explosive exercises during a workout. Keep single-jointed exercises to a minimum. A few single-jointed exercises help maintain muscle size, but doing too many compromises strength gains of the multiple-jointed exercises. Do no more than one single-jointed exercise per body part during a workout, working no more than three body parts per workout. Three sets of 10 repetitions per body part are plenty to maintain muscle size.

**Peak Phase (3-6 Weeks).** The primary objective of this phase is to peak for the football season by doing more football-specific speed and agility drills.

- Develop explosive power.
- Peak acceleration and speed.
- Peak agility.
- Maintain sport skills.

Keep heavy squats and pressing movements to a minimum so that speed and agility are developed to the maximum. Keep doing the explosive lifts to improve power. Drop single-jointed exercises completely to conserve energy and to prevent overtraining.

## In-Season Periods (12-16 Weeks)

During the in-season the emphasis shifts from the strength and conditioning program to football practice. Since most time and effort in this phase is spent on improving sport skills and knowledge, the primary objective of the strength and conditioning program during the in-season is to maintain the strength and conditioning levels achieved during the off-season.

- Improve sport skills.
- Increase knowledge of football strategies and tactics.
- Increase sport-specific endurance.
- Maintain muscle size, strength, and power.

A common mistake many athletes make is to stop strength training after they enter the football season, thinking they will retain their strength. Strength is lost at the same rate as it is gained. If strength is built over a long period of time it becomes secured and tends to be lost very slowly. That is, once muscle size, strength, and power is gained, it can be easily maintained with minimal effort. However, a common mistake is to stop strength training after the football season starts. Stopping strength training will cause you to lose strength gradually over the course of the season. At the end of the season your size and power gains will be lost and this loss will adversely affect performance.

## Transition Periods (2-4 Weeks)

There are two types of transition periods: one that occurs after and one that occurs before the in-season period.

**After In-Season.** If an athlete goes right into an off-season program after an in-season period he loses all enthusiasm to work out at an intensity level necessary to bring about a conditioning response. Thus, a period of active rest is best during this time. "Active rest" means resting your mind and body from your usual workout routine but staying active.

- Recuperate physically and psychologically.
- Maintain conditioning through "active rest."

Do activities other than football, such as basketball, racquetball, tennis, swimming, or cycling on a noncompetitive basis. Active rest allows the body to recuperate physically and psychologically after a stressful season. It also allows you to maintain a certain level of conditioning.

**Before In-Season.** Most coaches feel that fall camp is the time to get in as many football repetitions—practicing twice a day with lots of hitting and contact—as possible. The focus of the training phase before in-season should be to:

- improve sport skills,
- increase knowledge of football strategies and tactics,
- increase sport-specific endurance, and
- prevent overtraining and possible injury.

Players have had no contact for a long period of time. The bruises and contusions associated with contact put a new demand on the body that you can't specifically condition for during the off-season. The body needs time to recover from and get reaccustomed to this stress. Besides the contact from practice, athletes are required to do wind sprints and then go into the weight room and lift. This can place too great a demand on the body. It is during this time of the year, second only to actual game situations, that many injuries occur. If an injury occurs it may not be serious, but it may keep the player from being able to give full effort, and these injuries often linger on for most of the season. For this reason, we recommend not lifting during two-a-days. Allow your body to recover from practices. Keep extra wind sprint running to a minimum. This approach helps prevent injuries and allows for better efforts during practice.

## Weekly Schedule

Most strength training programs usually include three workouts per week, every other day—Monday-Wednesday-Friday, or Tuesday-Thursday-Saturday. This approach is designed to give your muscles a rest day between sessions to recover and rebuild.

For football we use a strength training program called a split routine. This approach is very efficient and widely used to stimulate gains. It simply involves splitting your program and doing different exercises on alternate days. Working different exercises on separate days creates shorter workouts, as opposed to drawn-out workouts that work all the exercises in one day. The split routine allows your body to recover and rebuild from one type of exercise movement while you work a different type of exercise movement. With the split routine you get at least two full days of recovery between different types of exercise movements. You may opt for a four-day program utilizing two workouts or a six-day program utilizing three workouts (see table 2.3).

The split routine can be divided by body parts, explosive and strength exercises, or speed and agility drills. The split routine also allows different combinations of exercises and drills without overtraining. For example, combine the speed drills with the explosive exercises one day, and agility drills with the strength exercises on the next day (table 2.4).

You can make more progress over longer periods of time if you do not work at maximum loads during each workout. With the "hard-easy system" there is only one hard workout per week for each set of exercises used with the split routine. The other days are light workouts. With only one heavy workout load a week per body part, you will be ready both physically and mentally as the loads become greater. Table 2.4 shows

**Table 2.3 Split Routine Strength Training Program**

| Day | 4-day split | 6-day split |
|---|---|---|
| Monday | Workout 1 | Workout 1 |
| Tuesday | Workout 2 | Workout 2 |
| Wednesday | Rest | Workout 3 |
| Thursday | Workout 1 | Workout 1 |
| Friday | Workout 2 | Workout 2 |
| Saturday | Rest | Workout 3 |
| Sunday | Rest | Rest |

**Table 2.4 Split Routine With Various Exercises and Drills**

| | | | |
|---|---|---|---|
| Monday | Explosive lifts | Speed drills | Hard |
| Tuesday | Strength lifts | Agility drills | Hard |
| Wednesday | Rest | Rest | Rest |
| Thursday | Explosive lifts | Speed drills | Easy |
| Friday | Strength lifts | Agility drills | Easy |

**Table 2.5 Adjusting Workout Load by Reducing Intensity**

| | Sets | Reps | Intensity (percent) | 1RM (pounds) | Volume (pounds) |
|---|---|---|---|---|---|
| Hard | 1 | 10 | 65 | 300 | 1950 |
| | 2 | 10 | 70 | 300 | 2100 |
| | 3 | 10 | 75 | 300 | 2250 |
| | | | Average 70 | | Total 6300 |
| Easy | 1 | 10 | 55 | 300 | 1650 |
| | 2 | 10 | 60 | 300 | 1800 |
| | 3 | 10 | 65 | 300 | 1950 |
| | | | Average 60 | | Total 5400 |

hard workouts on Monday and Tuesday and easy workouts on Thursday and Friday.

You can easily reduce the workout loads by volume, intensity, or both. Table 2.5 shows a hard workout load made easy by adjusting only the intensity. By reducing the intensity 10 percent, the absolute volume is reduced by 14 percent.

Now that you understand the principles of strength and interval training, we can start setting up a program. Follow these steps to set up your year-round conditioning program:

1. Test yourself (chapter 3).
2. Evaluate your test results (chapter 3).
3. Set some goals (chapter 3).
4. Follow the conditioning programs (chapters 4 through 9) to help you reach your goals.

# CHAPTER 3

# TESTING, EVALUATING, AND GOAL SETTING

Every conditioning program should begin with the coach's testing and evaluating the strengths and weaknesses of each player. By learning their strengths and weaknesses it is much easier to achieve maximum results. This chapter outlines step-by-step procedures on how to safely test and evaluate athletes' fitness and athletic abilities so you can develop the objectives and specifics of your conditioning program. Once you have tested and evaluated each player, you can set goals to give the conditioning program direction.

Coaches and athletes often misconstrue the purpose of sports conditioning performance tests, believing that the results measure or predict future athletic success. While tests *can't* predict the future, conducting the right tests at the proper time *can* give the coach and athlete the following important data:

- Is the current program effectively achieving the goals desired?

- Does the athlete have obvious physical weaknesses that could lead to injury?
- If injured, has the athlete reconditioned himself to safely participate in games again?
- And most importantly, how is the athlete progressing?

By testing throughout the season and recording the results each time, you'll have concrete proof that following a strength and conditioning program results in bigger and faster football players.

## ENSURING CONTROL

Unless testing is done properly, the results are meaningless to the coach and athlete. In order to ensure control, the strength coach must do an accurate job of taking measurements. Accurate measurements are not a problem if you are conscious of validity, reliability, and objectivity.

### Validity

Validity concerns whether the test used to measure performance potential is specific to the sport in which the athlete participates. Some research (see chapter 1) found the following tests to have a high direct correlation with a player's ability to perform well in football. The tests are ranked according to which test correlates highest with performance levels in football.

1. 10-yard dash—to test acceleration
2. 40-yard dash—to test speed and acceleration
3. Pro agility run—to test agility
4. Vertical jump—to test anaerobic power

We do not have a field test to measure football endurance that is valid and easy to administer; therefore we use the 300-yard shuttle run test to give some idea of the player's endurance level. However, this test does not correlate well with the player's ability to play football.

### Reliability

Reliability means making sure the testing conditions and results are consistent each time you test. There are several factors to take into consideration here.

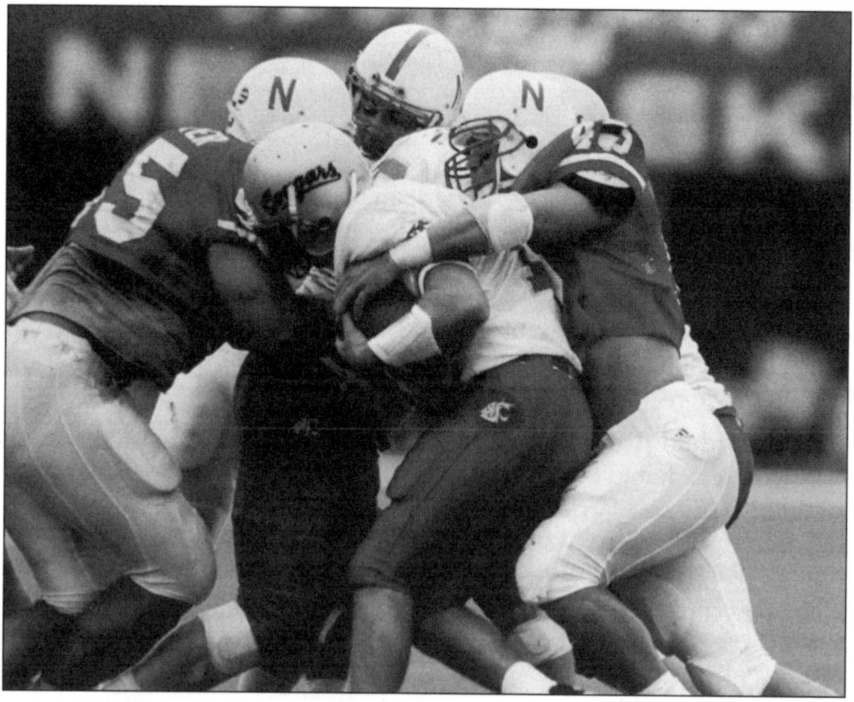

• **Environment.** The testing results will be different if you test outside in the grass one time and test inside on the basketball court another time. The condition of the field, the time of day, wind, rain, temperature, etc., all can affect test results. Thus, it is best to stick with the same testing environment each time you test. If available, a football field is the best environment in which to test the agility run and 10- and 40-yard dashes, since these are the tests most applicable to game situations. The vertical jump can be tested in a weight room or on a basketball court, as long as there is a firm surface from which to jump.

• **Testing order.** The order in which the tests are given is something you can control that will affect the results. For example, if athletes run a 40-yard dash followed by a 300-yard shuttle run during one testing period, but run the 300-yard shuttle run before the 40-yard dash during another period, the results of the 40-yard dash are guaranteed to be different. Be sure the testing order is the same each and every time. Here is a suggested testing order:

Height

Body weight

Body composition

Vertical jump

Pro agility run

10-yard dash

40-yard dash

300-yard shuttle run

• **Testing equipment.** Some tests can be administered with different equipment, which can give you different results. For example, the 40-yard dash can be done with electronic timers or with stopwatches. An electronically-timed 40-yard dash is usually about .2 second slower than a hand-held time with a stopwatch (e.g., 5.0 electronic is comparable to 4.8 hand-held). Always use the same testing equipment for each test; we recommend an electronic timing system if possible.

• **Individual differences.** There may be a lack of consistency each time you test due to the athlete's frame of mind, lack of sleep, personal problems, minor injuries, anxiety, or a lack of motivation during each test. These factors may be difficult to detect or prevent. Players should treat the night before the test like the night before a game, getting plenty of rest, giving themselves some time to get mentally motivated, and eating an easy-to-digest meal.

### Objectivity

A good rule of thumb is to have the same person administer the same test each time if possible. If this is not possible, different people should be able to administer the same test and end up with the same results. To do this, each must follow the instructions given for each test as closely as possible.

## ANNUAL TEST CYCLE

The combination of your testing periods forms an "annual test cycle." We recommend that you hold tests the week before the conditioning period starts. Testing establishes initial performance levels and determines the level of progress attained during the previous conditioning period.

In order to get the best effort each time you test, do not test too often. Athletes testing every couple of weeks won't be able to give their best effort. The chance of making progress over just a few weeks or one month is not that great. If you make a big deal out of testing and do it only three or four times a year, the chance of having best efforts is magnified. For football your annual test cycle may be scheduled as follows:

**Test 1—early January.** The football season usually ends in November or December. Allow your players some time, until early in January, so that they can let their bodies recover from the rigors of the season. Encourage them to remain active by participating in other activities that are relaxing and fun and at the same time keep them in reasonable shape. This first testing period is the start of the postseason conditioning period.

**Test 2—mid-March.** Conduct this test after an eight-week off-season cycle to give you some important information on how your players are doing and to give you some data before they start the next off-season cycle.

**Test 3—late May.** Conduct this test after the second eight-week off-season cycle to again evaluate how your players are doing.

**Test 4—mid-August.** This testing period allows you to evaluate how your players did over the summer and gives you some important information on their conditioning levels before the season starts.

## TESTING PROTOCOLS

Descriptions of the field tests used in measuring athletic abilities (as discussed in chapter 1) are given below. The description of a few simple measurements to determine body composition are also included. All these tests are valid and reliable measures of athletic ability, providing valuable feedback on the athletes' levels of athletic ability when compared to the norms shown later in this chapter. Be sure to keep accurate records so their progress in improving their athletic abilities can be determined.

An example test score card (table 3.1) that athletes can carry with them as they move from test to test is shown on page 60. Before being tested, the athlete hands the card to you, and you then test the athlete and write the score in the appropriate space. After the athlete receives the card back from you, he moves to the next test area. The data from all these cards can be entered on a master test sheet that is filed in the player's folder for future reference.

### HEIGHT TEST

**Equipment and Materials Needed:**

1. Flat wall against which the athlete stands
2. Measuring tape or marked area on wall
3. Device to place on the head to form a right angle with the wall

**Table 3.1 Test Score Card Example**

**Test Score Card**

Date 3/19/97

Name Bill Jones

Position RB Waist 32
(nearest 1/2 in.)

Height 5'11" Weight 195
(nearest 1/2 in.) (nearest 1/2 lb.)

| Tests | Score | | |
|---|---|---|---|
| Vertical jump | Reach | 94 | 30 |
| | Jump | 124 | |
| Pro agility run | 4.53 | | 4.50 |
| 10-yard dash | 1.75 | | 1.77 |
| 40-yard dash | 4.89 | | 4.95 |
| 300-yard shuttle run | 58.5 | | 59.7 |

**Procedure:**

1. Take shoes off.
2. Stand with heels, buttocks, back, and head against the wall.
3. Place device on head so that a right angle is formed with the wall.
4. Measure to the nearest half inch and record height.

## BODY WEIGHT TEST

**Equipment and Materials Needed:**

1. Scale

**Procedure:**

1. Weigh in with only T-shirt, shorts, and socks (no shoes, sweats, or equipment).

2. Weigh prior to any activity to avoid fluctuations due to dehydration.
3. Round body weight to the nearest half pound.

## WAIST MEASUREMENT TEST

**Equipment and Materials Needed:**

1. Flexible tape measure (cloth, vinyl, etc.)

**Procedure:**

1. Stand relaxed with arms at side.
2. Place tape around waist at level of navel.
3. Pull tape measure until taut, but not stretched or twisted.
4. Record to the nearest quarter inch.

## VERTICAL JUMP TEST—VERTEC

**Equipment and Materials Needed:**

1. Vertec (make sure it's calibrated)
2. Adjustment rod

**Procedure:**

*Reach*

1. Stand with side to wall, making sure feet and hips are next to wall.
2. Athlete then reaches as high as possible, keeping the feet flat on the floor.
3. Record the height reached to the nearest half inch.

*Jump*

1. The athlete goes to the Vertec and positions himself for jump.
2. The athlete jumps, hitting the highest possible vane. No steps are allowed before the jump.
3. Allow athlete three jumps; if third jump is higher than second let him continue until he cannot improve any more.

## Body Composition

By using your waist measurement as a guide, you can determine if changes in body weight are increases in lean muscle or fat. Use the following body composition profile. To get a more accurate reading of your body composition, consult a health professional in your area.

Follow this procedure to evaluate your body composition.

1. Take your score from the waist measurement test.
2. Find your height in the left-hand column of table 3.2 and your weight at the top of the chart.
3. Locate where your height and weight measures intersect. This location on the table indicates the average waist measurement for a player who is 10 percent body fat.

If the waist measurement of where your height and weight intersect equals the same that is seen on table 3.2, you are approximately 10 percent body fat. Therefore, a player who is six feet tall and weighs 190 pounds with a 34-inch waist is approximately 10 percent body fat (19 pounds of fat and 171 pounds of lean body mass). If your waist measurement is lower, then you are below 10 percent body fat. A higher waist measurement means you are above 10 percent body fat. Running backs, receivers, and defensive backs should have a waist measurement slightly lower than that depicted for their height and weight on table 3.2 (and therefore lower body fat). For linemen a slightly higher waist measurement is all right, but not more than two inches greater is desirable. Ten percent body fat is acceptable for linebackers and tight ends.

4. Record the height jumped to the nearest half inch using vertical jump conversion chart. We developed this conversion chart to help you figure the vertical jump height quickly.
5. Using the vertical jump chart (supplied with the Vertec), subtract the height reached from the height jumped to obtain the vertical jump height. For example:

   Height jumped—124″

   Height reached—94″

   Vertical jump—30″

Table 3.2 Average Waist Measurements

| | Weight | | | | | | | | | | | | | | | | | | | | | |
|---|---|---|---|---|---|---|---|---|---|---|---|---|---|---|---|---|---|---|---|---|---|---|
| **Height** | **110** | **120** | **130** | **140** | **150** | **160** | **170** | **180** | **190** | **200** | **210** | **220** | **230** | **240** | **250** | **260** | **270** | **280** | **290** | **300** | **310** | **320** |
| 5′2″-5′4″ | 29.5 | 30 | 30.5 | 31 | 32 | 32.5 | 33.5 | 34 | 34.5 | 35 | 36 | 36.5 | 37 | 37.5 | 38.5 | | | | | | | |
| 5′5″-5′7″ | | 30 | 30.5 | 31.5 | 32 | 32.5 | 33 | 34 | 34.5 | 35 | 36 | 36.5 | 37 | 37.5 | 38.5 | 39 | | | | | | |
| 5′8″-5′9″ | | | 30.5 | 31 | 32 | 32.5 | 33 | 34 | 34.5 | 35 | 35.5 | 36 | 37 | 37.5 | 38.5 | 39 | 39.5 | | | | | |
| 5′10″-5′11″ | | | | 31 | 31.5 | 32 | 33 | 33.5 | 34 | 34.5 | 35.5 | 36 | 36.5 | 37.5 | 38 | 38.5 | 39.5 | 40 | | | | |
| 6′0″-6′1″ | | | | | 31.5 | 32 | 32.5 | 33 | 34 | 34.5 | 35 | 36 | 36.5 | 37 | 37.5 | 38.5 | 39 | 39.5 | 40.5 | | | |
| 6′2″-6′3″ | | | | | | 32 | 32.5 | 33 | 33.5 | 34.5 | 35 | 35.5 | 36 | 37 | 37.5 | 38 | 39 | 39.5 | 40 | 40.5 | | |
| 6′4″-6′6″ | | | | | | | 32.5 | 33 | 33.5 | 34 | 34.5 | 35.5 | 36 | 36.5 | 37 | 38 | 38.5 | 39 | 40 | 40.5 | 41 | |
| 6′7″-6′9″ | | | | | | | | 33 | 33.5 | 34 | 34.5 | 35.5 | 36 | 36.5 | 37 | 38 | 38.5 | 39 | 40 | 40.5 | 41 | 41.5 |

6. Record the best jump.

**Causes for Disqualification:**

1. Feet and hips not next to wall when reaching
2. Standing on tiptoes when reaching
3. Taking a step or shuffle step before jumping

## PRO AGILITY RUN TEST

**Equipment and Materials Needed:**

1. An electronic timer or stopwatch
2. A course of three lines each five yards apart (figure 3.1)
3. One coach to take times and record them, two managers to watch lines

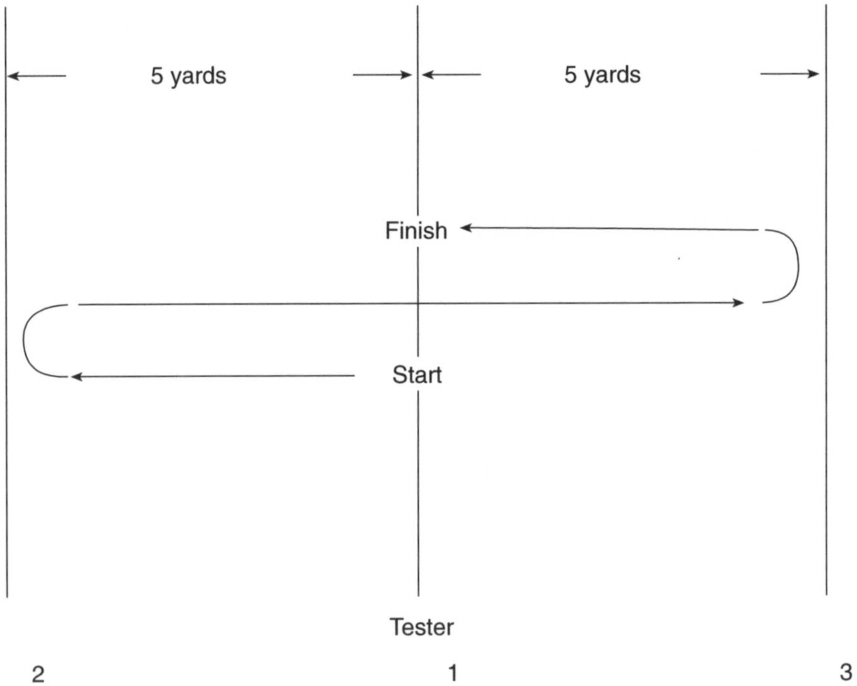


**Figure 3.1** The pro agility run test.

**Procedure:**

1. From a two-point stance straddle line 1 facing timer.
2. Start by running to the right to line 2.
3. Touch line 2 with right hand.
4. Sprint back across line 1 to line 3 to the left.
5. Touch line 3 with the left hand.
6. Stop time when player crosses line 1.
7. Record two times, circle the best time.

**Causes for Disqualification:**

1. Not touching line 2 with right hand
2. Not touching line 3 with left hand

## 10- AND 40-YARD DASH TESTS

**Equipment and Materials Needed:**

1. Electronic timing system
2. Sixty yards of flat running surface
3. Two coaches, one to time and record and one to watch for incorrect starts

**Procedure:**

1. Athlete stretches and warms up (see chapter 4).
2. Athlete places one hand on start switch.
3. Athlete starts when ready. The timer starts the watch when the athlete's hand releases the start switch.
4. Record two trials and circle the best time.

**Causes for Disqualification:**

1. Not having opposite hand and foot on starting line
2. Rocking
3. Stepping through with back foot before releasing start switch
4. Placing hand or foot in front of starting line

# 300-YARD SHUTTLE RUN TEST

**Equipment and materials needed:**

1. Three stopwatches (split timers)
2. One measured course (25 yards with two lanes; figure 3.2)
3. Two coaches to time shuttle runs: one to time rest intervals, one to watch lines
4. Recording charts for rest times

**Procedure:**

1. Record the names of the athletes on the recording sheet for the rest times.
2. Two athletes line up for the first shuttle run in lane 1 and start on starter's command.
3. The athletes sprint to the 25-yard line, turn, and come back to the starting line for six round trips (12 × 25 yards = 300 yards). Athletes must make foot contact with the 25-yard line and the starting line each time they change directions.
4. Coaches call out times and how many laps have been completed each time an athlete comes back to the starting line.
5. Timers stop the split button when the first runner crosses the line after 300 yards have been completed and the stop button when the second runner finishes. Record times for both runners.
6. Upon completion of the first shuttle run, the rest timer starts his watch to measure five minutes rest between the first and second runs. The athletes may walk, stretch, etc., as long as they are ready to start their second run after five minutes.
7. The rest timer verbally counts down the time left of the five minutes before they start.
8. The timer in the first lane starts another pair of athletes approximately one and a half minutes after the completion of the run just before them. It is the timer's responsibility in the first lane to tell the rest timer when a group has completed a run so the rest time can be recorded.
9. After both runs are completed, there should be two times recorded. Record times to the nearest tenth of a second.

**Cause for Disqualification:** Not touching the 25-yard line or starting line with foot

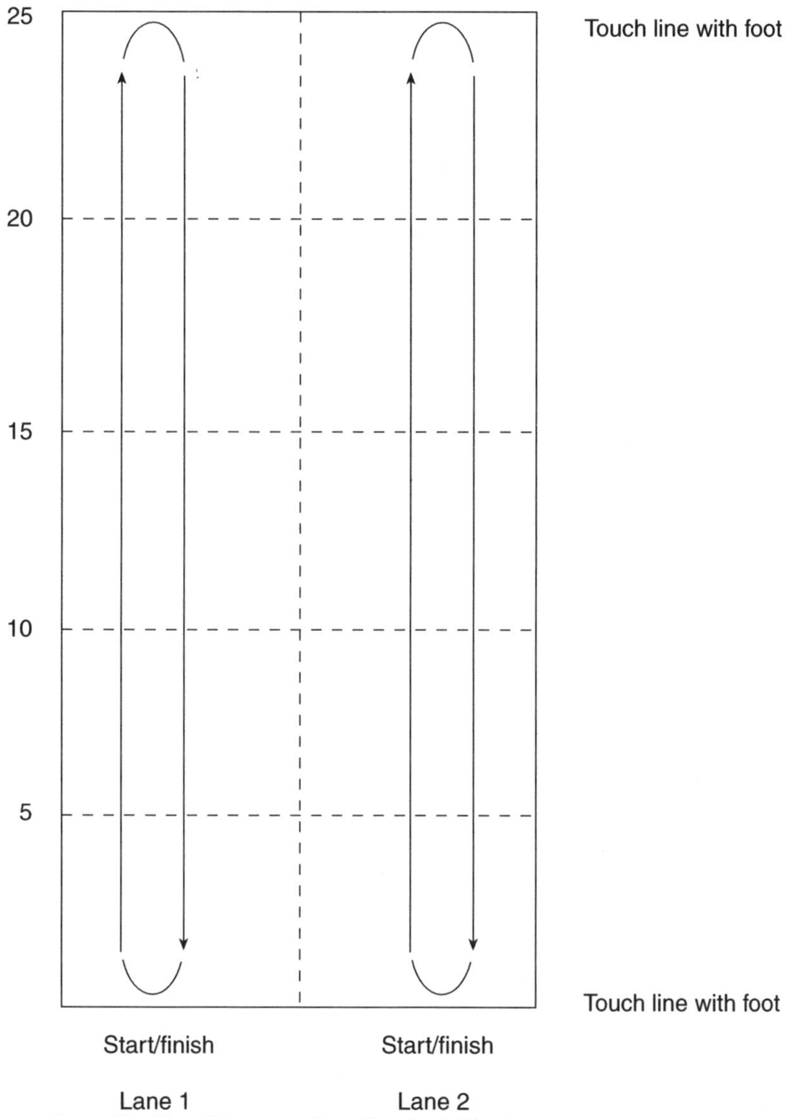


**Figure 3.2** Set-up for the 300-yard shuttle run test.

## EVALUATING TEST SCORES WITH PERFORMANCE PROFILES

After you have collected the test score cards (on table 3.1), evaluate the players using the performance profiles in tables 3.3 through 3.11 (high school players) or 3.12 through 3.27 (college players). These tables allow you to compare scores for the 10-yard dash, the 40-yard dash, the pro agility run, and vertical jump with other athletes according to their position and level of play. A range of performance scores is included, with the high scores at the top and low scores at the bottom.

The 300-yard shuttle run test is not a good predictor of a football player's ability to play football, so we evaluate this test with minimum times according to a player's position. These minimum times are used to determine their endurance levels. If they cannot make the minimum times, they are required to run the 300-yard shuttle run test again until they can make them. Following is a list of positions and the minimum times (average of two runs):

Running backs, receivers, and defensive backs—less than 59 seconds

Tight ends, rush ends, and linebackers—less than 61 seconds

Defensive and offensive linemen—less than 65 seconds

As we mentioned in chapter 1, improvement in lean body mass (usually a weight gain with waist measurements staying the same or getting lower), correlates well with increases in the performance test. If an athlete is not making improvements in his performance test, the first thing to look at is his change in body weight and waist measurement. If his waist measurement is getting too high in relation to height and weight, he may have a body composition problem. This problem can be corrected through appropriate nutrition habits (see chapter 8). Other areas to evaluate are a player's sleep patterns and amount of sleep per night (see chapter 8).

Performance scores alone don't tell you on which tests athletes performed better and worse than on other tests. The performance profiles, however, take the performance scores and compare them to norms. The performance scores are converted into norms using percentile rankings shown to the left of the conditioning profile in tables 3.3 through 3.27. A percentile indicates the point at which a certain percentage of scores falls either above or below the player's performance score. For example, a player receiving a percentile score of 80 knows that 20 percent of his teammates scored higher and 80 percent scored lower. This gives instant feedback to determine at which level each player presently stands physically.

The performance profiles also allow an athlete to compare the quality of his performance among the different components. Using the performance profiles, he can compare his speed, agility, and power rankings with those of other players. In the example given in table 3.28, Bill Jones, a running back, has pretty good speed, an excellent vertical jump, and is average in the pro agility run. His weakness seems to be his agility, so he should construct a program concentrating on developing his

Table 3.3 Defensive Backs—High School

| Percentile rank | 10-yard dash | 40-yard dash | Pro agility run | Vertical jump |
|---|---|---|---|---|
| 100 | 1.56 | 4.65 | 4.07 | 35.5 |
| 95 | 1.61 | 4.69 | 4.11 | 35.0 |
| 90 | 1.67 | 4.82 | 4.24 | 33.0 |
| 85 | 1.71 | 4.92 | 4.30 | 30.0 |
| 80 | 1.75 | 4.96 | 4.39 | 28.0 |
| 75 | 1.78 | 5.00 | 4.43 | 26.0 |
| 70 | 1.80 | 5.04 | 4.46 | 25.5 |
| 65 | 1.81 | 5.07 | 4.48 | 25.0 |
| 60 | 1.84 | 5.11 | 4.51 | 24.5 |
| 55 | 1.84 | 5.17 | 4.54 | 24.0 |
| 50 | 1.88 | 5.23 | 4.60 | 23.5 |
| 45 | 1.89 | 5.28 | 4.64 | 23.0 |
| 40 | 1.89 | 5.34 | 4.70 | 22.5 |
| 35 | 1.92 | 5.39 | 4.72 | 22.5 |
| 30 | 1.93 | 5.45 | 4.77 | 22.0 |
| 25 | 1.94 | 5.50 | 4.83 | 21.5 |
| 20 | 1.97 | 5.57 | 4.86 | 20.5 |
| 15 | 1.99 | 5.62 | 5.01 | 20.0 |
| 10 | 2.01 | 5.70 | 5.10 | 18.0 |
| 5 | 2.14 | 5.85 | 5.15 | 14.0 |

Table 3.4 Running Backs—High School

| Percentile rank | 10-yard dash | 40-yard dash | Pro agility run | Vertical jump |
|---|---|---|---|---|
| 100 | 1.52 | 4.36 | 3.99 | 36.0 |
| 95 | 1.62 | 4.53 | 4.22 | 33.5 |
| 90 | 1.70 | 4.62 | 4.29 | 32.0 |
| 85 | 1.72 | 4.71 | 4.35 | 29.5 |
| 80 | 1.75 | 4.89 | 4.38 | 27.0 |
| 75 | 1.77 | 4.95 | 4.41 | 26.5 |
| 70 | 1.78 | 5.00 | 4.45 | 26.0 |
| 65 | 1.80 | 5.04 | 4.48 | 25.5 |
| 60 | 1.82 | 5.08 | 4.50 | 25.0 |
| 55 | 1.85 | 5.11 | 4.53 | 24.5 |
| 50 | 1.86 | 5.14 | 4.56 | 24.0 |
| 45 | 1.87 | 5.18 | 4.58 | 23.5 |
| 40 | 1.88 | 5.20 | 4.62 | 23.0 |
| 35 | 1.90 | 5.23 | 4.65 | 22.5 |
| 30 | 1.91 | 5.26 | 4.68 | 22.0 |
| 25 | 1.92 | 5.35 | 4.72 | 21.5 |
| 20 | 1.93 | 5.42 | 4.76 | 21.0 |
| 15 | 1.94 | 5.49 | 4.81 | 20.5 |
| 10 | 1.97 | 5.57 | 4.89 | 20.0 |
| 5 | 2.15 | 5.75 | 5.00 | 12.5 |

Table 3.5 Quarterbacks—High School

| Percentile rank | 10-yard dash | 40-yard dash | Pro agility run | Vertical jump |
|---|---|---|---|---|
| 100 | 1.56 | 4.69 | 4.15 | 34.0 |
| 95 | 1.68 | 4.80 | 4.30 | 33.5 |
| 90 | 1.73 | 4.94 | 4.39 | 32.0 |
| 85 | 1.75 | 5.05 | 4.41 | 30.0 |
| 80 | 1.77 | 5.12 | 4.43 | 27.0 |
| 75 | 1.79 | 5.14 | 4.46 | 26.0 |
| 70 | 1.81 | 5.18 | 4.49 | 25.5 |
| 65 | 1.82 | 5.21 | 4.52 | 25.0 |
| 60 | 1.84 | 5.22 | 4.54 | 24.5 |
| 55 | 1.86 | 5.26 | 4.57 | 24.0 |
| 50 | 1.89 | 5.30 | 4.60 | 23.5 |
| 45 | 1.90 | 5.33 | 4.62 | 23.0 |
| 40 | 1.91 | 5.36 | 4.64 | 22.5 |
| 35 | 1.92 | 5.39 | 4.68 | 22.0 |
| 30 | 1.94 | 5.44 | 4.75 | 21.5 |
| 25 | 1.95 | 5.50 | 4.78 | 21.0 |
| 20 | 1.96 | 5.57 | 4.80 | 20.5 |
| 15 | 1.98 | 5.65 | 4.85 | 20.0 |
| 10 | 2.05 | 5.72 | 4.96 | 19.5 |
| 5 | 2.12 | 5.80 | 5.03 | 14.5 |

Table 3.6 Wide Receivers—High School

| Percentile rank | 10-yard dash | 40-yard dash | Pro agility run | Vertical jump |
|---|---|---|---|---|
| 100 | 1.59 | 4.64 | 4.06 | 34.5 |
| 95 | 1.64 | 4.74 | 4.17 | 33.5 |
| 90 | 1.67 | 4.91 | 4.28 | 31.5 |
| 85 | 1.69 | 4.95 | 4.35 | 29.0 |
| 80 | 1.71 | 4.96 | 4.40 | 28.0 |
| 75 | 1.72 | 5.01 | 4.43 | 26.5 |
| 70 | 1.74 | 5.05 | 4.47 | 25.5 |
| 65 | 1.76 | 5.09 | 4.48 | 25.0 |
| 60 | 1.78 | 5.11 | 4.50 | 24.5 |
| 55 | 1.80 | 5.14 | 4.53 | 24.0 |
| 50 | 1.82 | 5.18 | 4.55 | 23.5 |
| 45 | 1.84 | 5.20 | 4.59 | 23.0 |
| 40 | 1.86 | 5.22 | 4.63 | 22.5 |
| 35 | 1.86 | 5.25 | 4.65 | 22.0 |
| 30 | 1.88 | 5.29 | 4.68 | 21.5 |
| 25 | 1.90 | 5.31 | 4.70 | 21.0 |
| 20 | 1.93 | 5.37 | 4.73 | 20.0 |
| 15 | 1.96 | 5.47 | 4.80 | 19.5 |
| 10 | 2.00 | 5.63 | 5.42 | 18.0 |
| 5 | 2.20 | 6.43 | 6.15 | 15.5 |

Table 3.7 Outside Linebackers—High School

| Percentile rank | 10-yard dash | 40-yard dash | Pro agility run | Vertical jump |
|---|---|---|---|---|
| 100 | 1.60 | 4.68 | 4.18 | 33.0 |
| 95 | 1.68 | 4.76 | 4.20 | 32.5 |
| 90 | 1.73 | 4.90 | 4.35 | 31.5 |
| 85 | 1.78 | 5.01 | 4.47 | 29.5 |
| 80 | 1.80 | 5.11 | 4.50 | 27.5 |
| 75 | 1.81 | 5.21 | 4.51 | 26.0 |
| 70 | 1.83 | 5.24 | 4.55 | 24.5 |
| 65 | 1.85 | 5.28 | 4.58 | 23.5 |
| 60 | 1.86 | 5.30 | 4.61 | 23.0 |
| 55 | 1.87 | 5.36 | 4.65 | 22.5 |
| 50 | 1.88 | 5.38 | 4.67 | 22.0 |
| 45 | 1.91 | 5.42 | 4.73 | 21.5 |
| 40 | 1.93 | 5.45 | 4.77 | 21.0 |
| 35 | 1.96 | 5.50 | 4.83 | 20.5 |
| 30 | 1.97 | 5.55 | 4.86 | 20.0 |
| 25 | 1.98 | 5.60 | 4.90 | 19.5 |
| 20 | 2.00 | 5.66 | 4.92 | 19.0 |
| 15 | 2.02 | 5.71 | 4.96 | 18.5 |
| 10 | 2.07 | 5.79 | 5.20 | 18.0 |
| 5 | 2.09 | 5.91 | 5.50 | 17.0 |

Table 3.8 Linebackers—High School

| Percentile rank | 10-yard dash | 40-yard dash | Pro agility run | Vertical jump |
|---|---|---|---|---|
| 100 | 1.56 | 4.79 | 4.16 | 34.5 |
| 95 | 1.65 | 4.88 | 4.22 | 34.0 |
| 90 | 1.70 | 4.99 | 4.34 | 32.0 |
| 85 | 1.77 | 5.08 | 4.45 | 30.0 |
| 80 | 1.80 | 5.16 | 4.47 | 29.5 |
| 75 | 1.81 | 5.21 | 4.50 | 28.0 |
| 70 | 1.83 | 5.24 | 4.53 | 25.5 |
| 65 | 1.86 | 5.28 | 4.57 | 24.0 |
| 60 | 1.87 | 5.31 | 4.60 | 23.5 |
| 55 | 1.88 | 5.33 | 4.61 | 23.0 |
| 50 | 1.89 | 5.36 | 4.65 | 22.5 |
| 45 | 1.90 | 5.40 | 4.69 | 22.0 |
| 40 | 1.91 | 5.44 | 4.72 | 21.5 |
| 35 | 1.92 | 5.47 | 4.77 | 21.0 |
| 30 | 1.94 | 5.51 | 4.78 | 20.5 |
| 25 | 1.96 | 5.54 | 4.82 | 20.0 |
| 20 | 1.98 | 5.59 | 4.86 | 19.5 |
| 15 | 2.00 | 5.67 | 4.91 | 19.0 |
| 10 | 2.06 | 5.78 | 5.21 | 18.5 |
| 5 | 2.15 | 5.95 | 5.45 | 17.0 |

Table 3.9 Tight Ends—High School

| Percentile rank | 10-yard dash | 40-yard dash | Pro agility run | Vertical jump |
|---|---|---|---|---|
| 100 | 1.65 | 4.87 | 4.25 | 33.0 |
| 95 | 1.72 | 4.95 | 4.33 | 31.0 |
| 90 | 1.76 | 5.09 | 4.45 | 30.0 |
| 85 | 1.80 | 5.17 | 4.50 | 28.5 |
| 80 | 1.81 | 5.24 | 4.53 | 27.0 |
| 75 | 1.84 | 5.28 | 4.57 | 25.0 |
| 70 | 1.85 | 5.30 | 4.59 | 24.5 |
| 65 | 1.86 | 5.32 | 4.63 | 24.0 |
| 60 | 1.88 | 5.37 | 4.65 | 23.5 |
| 55 | 1.90 | 5.41 | 4.72 | 22.5 |
| 50 | 1.91 | 5.43 | 4.74 | 22.0 |
| 45 | 1.92 | 5.46 | 4.76 | 21.5 |
| 40 | 1.93 | 5.50 | 4.80 | 21.0 |
| 35 | 1.95 | 5.54 | 4.82 | 20.5 |
| 30 | 1.96 | 5.63 | 4.87 | 20.0 |
| 25 | 1.97 | 5.65 | 4.91 | 19.5 |
| 20 | 1.98 | 5.69 | 4.96 | 19.0 |
| 15 | 2.02 | 5.74 | 4.99 | 18.5 |
| 10 | 2.09 | 5.88 | 5.18 | 16.5 |
| 5 | 2.19 | 5.98 | 5.40 | 16.0 |

Table 3.10 Defensive Linemen—High School

| Percentile rank | 10-yard dash | 40-yard dash | Pro agility run | Vertical jump |
|---|---|---|---|---|
| 100 | 1.62 | 4.71 | 4.31 | 31.5 |
| 95 | 1.63 | 4.72 | 4.36 | 31.0 |
| 90 | 1.77 | 4.99 | 4.46 | 28.0 |
| 85 | 1.87 | 5.27 | 4.64 | 24.0 |
| 80 | 1.90 | 5.37 | 4.68 | 23.0 |
| 75 | 1.92 | 5.43 | 4.73 | 22.5 |
| 70 | 1.93 | 5.49 | 4.76 | 22.0 |
| 65 | 1.94 | 5.52 | 4.81 | 21.5 |
| 60 | 1.96 | 5.55 | 4.83 | 21.0 |
| 55 | 1.97 | 5.60 | 4.86 | 20.5 |
| 50 | 1.99 | 5.64 | 4.90 | 20.0 |
| 45 | 2.00 | 5.67 | 4.96 | 19.5 |
| 40 | 2.02 | 5.72 | 5.01 | 19.0 |
| 35 | 2.03 | 5.79 | 5.03 | 18.5 |
| 30 | 2.05 | 5.86 | 5.09 | 18.0 |
| 25 | 2.07 | 5.91 | 5.13 | 17.5 |
| 20 | 2.09 | 5.99 | 6.16 | 17.0 |
| 15 | 2.13 | 6.06 | 5.23 | 16.5 |
| 10 | 2.30 | 6.20 | 5.30 | 16.0 |
| 5 | 2.77 | 6.40 | 5.60 | 14.5 |

Table 3.11 Offensive Linemen—High School

| Percentile rank | 10-yard dash | 40-yard dash | Pro agility run | Vertical jump |
|---|---|---|---|---|
| 100 | 1.65 | 4.85 | 4.20 | 31.0 |
| 95 | 1.79 | 5.11 | 4.43 | 30.5 |
| 90 | 1.86 | 5.34 | 4.58 | 30.0 |
| 85 | 1.89 | 5.40 | 4.69 | 29.0 |
| 80 | 1.91 | 5.45 | 4.73 | 28.0 |
| 75 | 1.92 | 5.50 | 4.77 | 25.0 |
| 70 | 1.94 | 5.54 | 4.79 | 23.0 |
| 65 | 1.96 | 5.58 | 4.83 | 22.0 |
| 60 | 1.98 | 5.64 | 4.86 | 21.5 |
| 55 | 1.99 | 5.67 | 4.90 | 21.0 |
| 50 | 2.01 | 5.72 | 4.93 | 20.0 |
| 45 | 2.02 | 5.76 | 4.96 | 19.5 |
| 40 | 2.04 | 5.81 | 5.00 | 19.0 |
| 35 | 2.05 | 5.84 | 5.04 | 18.5 |
| 30 | 2.07 | 5.87 | 5.08 | 18.0 |
| 25 | 2.10 | 5.92 | 5.13 | 17.5 |
| 20 | 2.12 | 6.00 | 5.18 | 17.0 |
| 15 | 2.14 | 6.06 | 5.34 | 16.5 |
| 10 | 2.25 | 6.53 | 5.68 | 15.5 |
| 5 | 2.53 | 6.65 | 5.85 | 15.0 |

Table 3.12 Wingbacks—College

| Percentile rank | 10-yard dash | 40-yard dash | Pro agility run | Vertical jump |
|---|---|---|---|---|
| 100 | 1.47 | 4.37 | 3.98 | 40.0 |
| 95 | 1.48 | 4.39 | 3.99 | 38.5 |
| 90 | 1.51 | 4.40 | 4.01 | 37.0 |
| 85 | 1.53 | 4.42 | 4.03 | 34.5 |
| 80 | 1.54 | 4.50 | 4.04 | 34.0 |
| 75 | 1.56 | 4.57 | 4.05 | 33.5 |
| 70 | 1.58 | 4.59 | 4.06 | 33.0 |
| 65 | 1.59 | 4.64 | 4.07 | 32.5 |
| 60 | 1.60 | 4.65 | 4.09 | 32.0 |
| 55 | 1.61 | 4.68 | 4.13 | 31.5 |
| 50 | 1.62 | 4.69 | 4.16 | 31.0 |
| 45 | 1.63 | 4.71 | 4.20 | 30.5 |
| 40 | 1.64 | 4.73 | 4.24 | 30.5 |
| 35 | 1.65 | 4.77 | 4.26 | 30.0 |
| 30 | 1.66 | 4.84 | 4.29 | 29.5 |
| 25 | 1.71 | 4.91 | 4.30 | 29.0 |
| 20 | 1.73 | 4.92 | 4.31 | 28.5 |
| 15 | 1.76 | 4.96 | 4.32 | 28.0 |
| 10 | 1.77 | 5.05 | 4.34 | 27.0 |
| 5 | 1.79 | 5.06 | 4.39 | 26.0 |

Table 3.13 Split Ends—College

| Percentile rank | 10-yard dash | 40-yard dash | Pro agility run | Vertical jump |
|---|---|---|---|---|
| 100 | 1.42 | 4.42 | 3.87 | 36.0 |
| 95 | 1.47 | 4.50 | 3.89 | 35.5 |
| 90 | 1.53 | 4.55 | 3.96 | 35.0 |
| 85 | 1.59 | 4.60 | 3.97 | 34.5 |
| 80 | 1.60 | 4.67 | 4.03 | 34.0 |
| 75 | 1.62 | 4.69 | 4.05 | 33.5 |
| 70 | 1.63 | 4.71 | 4.07 | 33.0 |
| 65 | 1.64 | 4.72 | 4.12 | 33.0 |
| 60 | 1.65 | 4.73 | 4.14 | 32.5 |
| 55 | 1.66 | 4.75 | 4.18 | 32.0 |
| 50 | 1.67 | 4.76 | 4.21 | 32.0 |
| 45 | 1.68 | 4.79 | 4.22 | 31.5 |
| 40 | 1.69 | 4.82 | 4.25 | 31.0 |
| 35 | 1.70 | 4.84 | 4.27 | 30.5 |
| 30 | 1.71 | 4.85 | 4.29 | 30.5 |
| 25 | 1.72 | 4.86 | 4.31 | 30.0 |
| 20 | 1.73 | 4.87 | 4.33 | 29.5 |
| 15 | 1.74 | 4.90 | 4.35 | 29.0 |
| 10 | 1.75 | 5.10 | 4.45 | 28.0 |
| 5 | 1.77 | 5.20 | 4.55 | 26.5 |

Table 3.14 Fullbacks—College

| Percentile rank | 10-yard dash | 40-yard dash | Pro agility run | Vertical jump |
|---|---|---|---|---|
| 100 | 1.52 | 4.50 | 3.99 | 37.0 |
| 95 | 1.54 | 4.56 | 4.02 | 36.5 |
| 90 | 1.56 | 4.60 | 4.06 | 36.0 |
| 85 | 1.58 | 4.64 | 4.12 | 35.5 |
| 80 | 1.60 | 4.70 | 4.15 | 35.0 |
| 75 | 1.62 | 4.73 | 4.17 | 34.0 |
| 70 | 1.64 | 4.81 | 4.18 | 33.5 |
| 65 | 1.66 | 4.82 | 4.20 | 32.0 |
| 60 | 1.67 | 4.83 | 4.21 | 31.0 |
| 55 | 1.68 | 4.89 | 4.22 | 30.5 |
| 50 | 1.69 | 4.93 | 4.23 | 30.5 |
| 45 | 1.70 | 4.95 | 4.24 | 30.0 |
| 40 | 1.71 | 4.96 | 4.25 | 29.5 |
| 35 | 1.72 | 4.97 | 4.26 | 29.0 |
| 30 | 1.74 | 4.98 | 4.27 | 28.5 |
| 25 | 1.76 | 4.99 | 4.30 | 28.0 |
| 20 | 1.77 | 5.02 | 4.31 | 28.0 |
| 15 | 1.78 | 5.05 | 4.32 | 27.5 |
| 10 | 1.79 | 5.07 | 4.40 | 27.0 |
| 5 | 1.80 | 5.16 | 4.45 | 26.5 |

Table 3.15 I-Backs—College

| Percentile rank | 10-yard dash | 40-yard dash | Pro agility run | Vertical jump |
|---|---|---|---|---|
| 100 | 1.45 | 4.33 | 3.85 | 38.5 |
| 95 | 1.47 | 4.44 | 3.86 | 37.0 |
| 90 | 1.49 | 4.50 | 4.01 | 36.5 |
| 85 | 1.52 | 4.54 | 4.04 | 35.0 |
| 80 | 1.55 | 4.56 | 4.08 | 34.0 |
| 75 | 1.58 | 4.57 | 4.11 | 33.0 |
| 70 | 1.61 | 4.63 | 4.12 | 32.5 |
| 65 | 1.62 | 4.68 | 4.14 | 32.0 |
| 60 | 1.63 | 4.70 | 4.15 | 31.5 |
| 55 | 1.64 | 4.71 | 4.16 | 31.0 |
| 50 | 1.65 | 4.76 | 4.18 | 30.5 |
| 45 | 1.66 | 4.78 | 4.19 | 30.0 |
| 40 | 1.67 | 4.80 | 4.20 | 29.5 |
| 35 | 1.68 | 4.81 | 4.21 | 29.0 |
| 30 | 1.70 | 4.83 | 4.24 | 28.5 |
| 25 | 1.71 | 4.84 | 4.26 | 28.0 |
| 20 | 1.72 | 4.90 | 4.27 | 27.5 |
| 15 | 1.76 | 4.92 | 4.31 | 27.0 |
| 10 | 1.78 | 5.00 | 4.42 | 26.5 |
| 5 | 1.79 | 5.03 | 4.48 | 25.5 |

Table 3.16 Quarterbacks—College

| Percentile rank | 10-yard dash | 40-yard dash | Pro agility run | Vertical jump |
|---|---|---|---|---|
| 100 | 1.50 | 4.40 | 4.00 | 36.0 |
| 95 | 1.52 | 4.42 | 4.05 | 35.5 |
| 90 | 1.54 | 4.45 | 4.10 | 34.5 |
| 85 | 1.56 | 4.58 | 4.13 | 34.0 |
| 80 | 1.57 | 4.68 | 4.14 | 33.5 |
| 75 | 1.58 | 4.69 | 4.15 | 33.0 |
| 70 | 1.59 | 4.71 | 4.16 | 32.5 |
| 65 | 1.60 | 4.73 | 4.17 | 32.0 |
| 60 | 1.62 | 4.74 | 4.18 | 31.5 |
| 55 | 1.63 | 4.75 | 4.19 | 31.0 |
| 50 | 1.64 | 4.78 | 4.20 | 31.0 |
| 45 | 1.65 | 4.79 | 4.27 | 30.5 |
| 40 | 1.66 | 4.80 | 4.29 | 30.5 |
| 35 | 1.67 | 4.82 | 4.30 | 30.0 |
| 30 | 1.69 | 4.84 | 4.31 | 29.5 |
| 25 | 1.70 | 4.85 | 4.34 | 29.0 |
| 20 | 1.71 | 4.86 | 4.37 | 28.0 |
| 15 | 1.73 | 5.00 | 4.39 | 27.5 |
| 10 | 1.74 | 5.10 | 4.48 | 27.0 |
| 5 | 1.75 | 5.20 | 4.53 | 26.5 |

**Table 3.17 Tight Ends—College**

| Percentile rank | 10-yard dash | 40-yard dash | Pro agility run | Vertical jump |
|---|---|---|---|---|
| 100 | 1.53 | 4.65 | 4.04 | 36.5 |
| 95 | 1.58 | 4.70 | 4.06 | 36.0 |
| 90 | 1.60 | 4.75 | 4.09 | 35.0 |
| 85 | 1.65 | 4.78 | 4.12 | 34.0 |
| 80 | 1.69 | 4.79 | 4.16 | 32.0 |
| 75 | 1.70 | 4.91 | 4.17 | 31.5 |
| 70 | 1.71 | 4.92 | 4.24 | 31.0 |
| 65 | 1.72 | 5.00 | 4.26 | 30.5 |
| 60 | 1.73 | 5.01 | 4.28 | 30.0 |
| 55 | 1.74 | 5.02 | 4.29 | 29.5 |
| 50 | 1.75 | 5.05 | 4.32 | 29.5 |
| 45 | 1.76 | 5.07 | 4.33 | 29.5 |
| 40 | 1.77 | 5.10 | 4.34 | 29.0 |
| 35 | 1.78 | 5.11 | 4.35 | 28.5 |
| 30 | 1.79 | 5.12 | 4.36 | 28.5 |
| 25 | 1.80 | 5.16 | 4.37 | 28.0 |
| 20 | 1.81 | 5.17 | 4.38 | 27.5 |
| 15 | 1.82 | 5.19 | 4.40 | 26.0 |
| 10 | 1.83 | 5.21 | 4.42 | 25.5 |
| 5 | 1.85 | 5.23 | 4.59 | 24.5 |

**Table 3.18 Centers—College**

| Percentile rank | 10-yard dash | 40-yard dash | Pro agility run | Vertical jump |
|---|---|---|---|---|
| 100 | 1.68 | 4.90 | 4.24 | 35.5 |
| 95 | 1.72 | 4.96 | 4.25 | 35.0 |
| 90 | 1.75 | 5.08 | 4.34 | 34.5 |
| 85 | 1.78 | 5.10 | 4.36 | 34.0 |
| 80 | 1.80 | 5.15 | 4.39 | 32.5 |
| 75 | 1.81 | 5.19 | 4.41 | 30.5 |
| 70 | 1.82 | 5.22 | 4.46 | 29.5 |
| 65 | 1.84 | 5.24 | 4.47 | 29.0 |
| 60 | 1.85 | 5.25 | 4.49 | 28.5 |
| 55 | 1.86 | 5.27 | 4.51 | 28.0 |
| 50 | 1.87 | 5.30 | 4.53 | 27.0 |
| 45 | 1.88 | 5.33 | 4.56 | 26.5 |
| 40 | 1.89 | 5.43 | 4.62 | 26.0 |
| 35 | 1.91 | 5.47 | 4.66 | 25.5 |
| 30 | 1.92 | 5.48 | 4.67 | 25.0 |
| 25 | 1.94 | 5.52 | 4.70 | 22.0 |
| 20 | 1.95 | 5.63 | 4.72 | 21.0 |
| 15 | 1.97 | 5.70 | 4.75 | 20.0 |
| 10 | 2.03 | 5.85 | 4.81 | 19.5 |
| 5 | 2.09 | 6.02 | 4.84 | 19.0 |

Table 3.19 Offensive Guards—College

| Percentile rank | 10-yard dash | 40-yard dash | Pro agility run | Vertical jump |
|---|---|---|---|---|
| 100 | 1.60 | 4.87 | 4.19 | 34.0 |
| 95 | 1.70 | 4.93 | 4.20 | 33.5 |
| 90 | 1.72 | 4.97 | 4.33 | 33.0 |
| 85 | 1.73 | 5.04 | 4.34 | 32.0 |
| 80 | 1.74 | 5.08 | 4.35 | 31.5 |
| 75 | 1.77 | 5.13 | 4.36 | 30.0 |
| 70 | 1.78 | 5.17 | 4.44 | 29.5 |
| 65 | 1.81 | 5.18 | 4.45 | 28.5 |
| 60 | 1.82 | 5.21 | 4.47 | 28.0 |
| 55 | 1.83 | 5.24 | 4.48 | 27.5 |
| 50 | 1.84 | 5.25 | 4.49 | 26.5 |
| 45 | 1.85 | 5.26 | 4.50 | 26.0 |
| 40 | 1.86 | 5.28 | 4.54 | 25.5 |
| 35 | 1.87 | 5.30 | 4.60 | 25.0 |
| 30 | 1.88 | 5.35 | 4.66 | 24.5 |
| 25 | 1.89 | 5.36 | 4.67 | 24.0 |
| 20 | 1.90 | 5.41 | 4.68 | 23.5 |
| 15 | 1.91 | 5.43 | 4.69 | 23.0 |
| 10 | 1.92 | 5.46 | 5.02 | 22.0 |
| 5 | 1.94 | 5.49 | 5.05 | 20.5 |

Table 3.20 Offensive Tackles—College

| Percentile rank | 10-yard dash | 40-yard dash | Pro agility run | Vertical jump |
|---|---|---|---|---|
| 100 | 1.70 | 4.93 | 4.10 | 39.5 |
| 95 | 1.71 | 4.98 | 4.11 | 34.5 |
| 90 | 1.73 | 5.01 | 4.30 | 32.0 |
| 85 | 1.75 | 5.06 | 4.36 | 30.0 |
| 80 | 1.77 | 5.11 | 4.38 | 29.0 |
| 75 | 1.78 | 5.12 | 4.40 | 28.0 |
| 70 | 1.79 | 5.14 | 4.41 | 27.5 |
| 65 | 1.84 | 5.18 | 4.48 | 27.0 |
| 60 | 1.85 | 5.27 | 4.58 | 26.0 |
| 55 | 1.86 | 5.35 | 4.60 | 25.5 |
| 50 | 1.87 | 5.40 | 4.64 | 25.0 |
| 45 | 1.89 | 5.46 | 4.65 | 24.5 |
| 40 | 1.91 | 5.48 | 4.66 | 24.0 |
| 35 | 1.92 | 5.51 | 4.68 | 23.5 |
| 30 | 1.93 | 5.54 | 4.71 | 23.0 |
| 25 | 2.03 | 5.58 | 4.75 | 22.5 |
| 20 | 2.04 | 5.62 | 4.79 | 22.0 |
| 15 | 2.05 | 5.89 | 4.89 | 21.5 |
| 10 | 2.15 | 6.05 | 4.91 | 21.0 |
| 5 | 2.21 | 6.30 | 4.93 | 19.5 |

Table 3.21 Cornerbacks—College

| Percentile rank | 10-yard dash | 40-yard dash | Pro agility run | Vertical jump |
|---|---|---|---|---|
| 100 | 1.48 | 4.40 | 3.91 | 41.5 |
| 95 | 1.49 | 4.41 | 3.92 | 41.0 |
| 90 | 1.50 | 4.45 | 3.96 | 40.0 |
| 85 | 1.53 | 4.53 | 4.01 | 38.0 |
| 80 | 1.55 | 4.54 | 4.05 | 36.5 |
| 75 | 1.56 | 4.57 | 4.07 | 35.0 |
| 70 | 1.58 | 4.58 | 4.09 | 34.0 |
| 65 | 1.59 | 4.63 | 4.11 | 33.0 |
| 60 | 1.62 | 4.66 | 4.12 | 32.0 |
| 55 | 1.63 | 4.70 | 4.14 | 31.5 |
| 50 | 1.64 | 4.73 | 4.15 | 31.0 |
| 45 | 1.65 | 4.77 | 4.18 | 30.5 |
| 40 | 1.66 | 4.80 | 4.20 | 30.0 |
| 35 | 1.67 | 4.82 | 4.22 | 29.5 |
| 30 | 1.68 | 4.84 | 4.24 | 28.5 |
| 25 | 1.70 | 4.86 | 4.26 | 28.0 |
| 20 | 1.71 | 4.89 | 4.30 | 27.5 |
| 15 | 1.77 | 4.92 | 4.38 | 27.0 |
| 10 | 1.81 | 5.00 | 4.49 | 26.5 |
| 5 | 1.82 | 5.80 | 4.55 | 26.0 |

Table 3.22 Free Safeties—College

| Percentile rank | 10-yard dash | 40-yard dash | Pro agility run | Vertical jump |
|---|---|---|---|---|
| 100 | 1.50 | 4.50 | 4.02 | 37.5 |
| 95 | 1.52 | 4.53 | 4.03 | 37.0 |
| 90 | 1.54 | 4.56 | 4.04 | 36.5 |
| 85 | 1.55 | 4.57 | 4.05 | 35.5 |
| 80 | 1.56 | 4.58 | 4.09 | 34.0 |
| 75 | 1.57 | 4.59 | 4.11 | 33.5 |
| 70 | 1.58 | 4.60 | 4.13 | 31.5 |
| 65 | 1.59 | 4.63 | 4.14 | 30.5 |
| 60 | 1.60 | 4.65 | 4.15 | 30.0 |
| 55 | 1.61 | 4.69 | 4.16 | 30.0 |
| 50 | 1.62 | 4.71 | 4.17 | 30.0 |
| 45 | 1.64 | 4.73 | 4.19 | 29.5 |
| 40 | 1.66 | 4.75 | 4.20 | 29.5 |
| 35 | 1.67 | 4.87 | 4.22 | 29.0 |
| 30 | 1.68 | 4.91 | 4.25 | 29.0 |
| 25 | 1.69 | 4.94 | 4.30 | 28.5 |
| 20 | 1.70 | 4.95 | 4.31 | 28.5 |
| 15 | 1.71 | 4.97 | 4.32 | 28.0 |
| 10 | 1.72 | 5.01 | 4.33 | 28.0 |
| 5 | 1.73 | 5.03 | 4.34 | 28.0 |

Table 3.23 Strong Safeties—College

| Percentile rank | 10-yard dash | 40-yard dash | Pro agility run | Vertical jump |
|---|---|---|---|---|
| 100 | 1.49 | 4.41 | 3.83 | 41.0 |
| 95 | 1.55 | 4.50 | 4.01 | 38.0 |
| 90 | 1.59 | 4.60 | 4.04 | 36.0 |
| 85 | 1.62 | 4.72 | 4.06 | 34.0 |
| 80 | 1.64 | 4.81 | 4.07 | 33.0 |
| 75 | 1.65 | 4.82 | 4.09 | 32.5 |
| 70 | 1.66 | 4.83 | 4.13 | 32.0 |
| 65 | 1.67 | 4.84 | 4.18 | 31.5 |
| 60 | 1.68 | 4.85 | 4.19 | 31.0 |
| 55 | 1.69 | 4.86 | 4.21 | 31.0 |
| 50 | 1.70 | 4.87 | 4.23 | 30.5 |
| 45 | 1.71 | 4.88 | 4.25 | 30.0 |
| 40 | 1.72 | 4.91 | 4.29 | 30.0 |
| 35 | 1.73 | 4.93 | 4.30 | 29.5 |
| 30 | 1.74 | 4.94 | 4.31 | 29.5 |
| 25 | 1.75 | 4.96 | 4.36 | 29.0 |
| 20 | 1.76 | 4.99 | 4.37 | 29.0 |
| 15 | 1.77 | 5.02 | 4.41 | 27.5 |
| 10 | 1.78 | 5.03 | 4.43 | 27.0 |
| 5 | 1.79 | 5.04 | 4.52 | 26.5 |

Table 3.24 Linebackers—College

| Percentile rank | 10-yard dash | 40-yard dash | Pro agility run | Vertical jump |
|---|---|---|---|---|
| 100 | 1.55 | 4.64 | 4.05 | 38.0 |
| 95 | 1.57 | 4.67 | 4.07 | 37.0 |
| 90 | 1.61 | 4.70 | 4.09 | 36.0 |
| 85 | 1.62 | 4.74 | 4.13 | 35.0 |
| 80 | 1.64 | 4.80 | 4.20 | 34.0 |
| 75 | 1.67 | 4.85 | 4.22 | 33.0 |
| 70 | 1.68 | 4.87 | 4.23 | 32.0 |
| 65 | 1.69 | 4.91 | 4.30 | 31.5 |
| 60 | 1.70 | 4.92 | 4.31 | 31.0 |
| 55 | 1.71 | 4.97 | 4.32 | 30.0 |
| 50 | 1.73 | 4.98 | 4.33 | 29.5 |
| 45 | 1.74 | 4.99 | 4.35 | 28.5 |
| 40 | 1.76 | 5.01 | 4.36 | 28.0 |
| 35 | 1.77 | 5.04 | 4.37 | 27.5 |
| 30 | 1.78 | 5.11 | 4.38 | 27.0 |
| 25 | 1.79 | 5.13 | 4.40 | 26.5 |
| 20 | 1.80 | 5.15 | 4.45 | 26.0 |
| 15 | 1.83 | 5.20 | 4.49 | 25.5 |
| 10 | 1.88 | 5.26 | 4.53 | 25.0 |
| 5 | 1.89 | 5.32 | 4.62 | 24.5 |

Table 3.25 Outside Linebackers—College

| Percentile rank | 10-yard dash | 40-yard dash | Pro agility run | Vertical jump |
|---|---|---|---|---|
| 100 | 1.55 | 4.60 | 4.05 | 41.0 |
| 95 | 1.58 | 4.65 | 4.09 | 38.0 |
| 90 | 1.62 | 4.70 | 4.13 | 37.0 |
| 85 | 1.65 | 4.75 | 4.17 | 36.0 |
| 80 | 1.68 | 4.79 | 4.23 | 35.0 |
| 75 | 1.70 | 4.86 | 4.24 | 34.0 |
| 70 | 1.71 | 4.88 | 4.27 | 33.0 |
| 65 | 1.73 | 4.89 | 4.29 | 32.5 |
| 60 | 1.75 | 4.90 | 4.30 | 32.0 |
| 55 | 1.77 | 4.93 | 4.32 | 31.5 |
| 50 | 1.79 | 4.95 | 4.33 | 31.0 |
| 45 | 1.80 | 4.97 | 4.34 | 30.5 |
| 40 | 1.81 | 5.00 | 4.35 | 30.0 |
| 35 | 1.82 | 5.09 | 4.38 | 29.5 |
| 30 | 1.83 | 5.10 | 4.40 | 29.0 |
| 25 | 1.84 | 5.15 | 4.44 | 28.5 |
| 20 | 1.85 | 5.16 | 4.47 | 28.0 |
| 15 | 1.86 | 5.20 | 4.50 | 27.0 |
| 10 | 1.87 | 5.22 | 4.54 | 26.0 |
| 5 | 1.89 | 5.24 | 4.63 | 24.5 |

Table 3.26 Defensive Tackles—College

| Percentile rank | 10-yard dash | 40-yard dash | Pro agility run | Vertical jump |
|---|---|---|---|---|
| 100 | 1.65 | 4.63 | 4.18 | 36.5 |
| 95 | 1.67 | 4.75 | 4.19 | 35.0 |
| 90 | 1.72 | 4.86 | 4.21 | 34.0 |
| 85 | 1.75 | 4.99 | 4.25 | 33.5 |
| 80 | 1.77 | 5.03 | 4.28 | 33.0 |
| 75 | 1.78 | 5.04 | 4.32 | 32.5 |
| 70 | 1.79 | 5.07 | 4.33 | 30.0 |
| 65 | 1.81 | 5.12 | 4.35 | 29.5 |
| 60 | 1.82 | 5.16 | 4.39 | 29.0 |
| 55 | 1.83 | 5.17 | 4.41 | 28.5 |
| 50 | 1.84 | 5.23 | 4.43 | 27.5 |
| 45 | 1.85 | 5.24 | 4.44 | 27.0 |
| 40 | 1.87 | 5.26 | 4.48 | 26.5 |
| 35 | 1.88 | 5.32 | 4.50 | 26.0 |
| 30 | 1.90 | 5.35 | 4.53 | 25.5 |
| 25 | 1.91 | 5.36 | 4.56 | 25.0 |
| 20 | 1.93 | 5.44 | 4.58 | 24.5 |
| 15 | 1.95 | 5.50 | 4.66 | 24.0 |
| 10 | 1.96 | 5.54 | 4.80 | 23.5 |
| 5 | 2.01 | 5.57 | 4.83 | 23.0 |

Table 3.27 Middle Guards—College

| Percentile rank | 10-yard dash | 40-yard dash | Pro agility run | Vertical jump |
|---|---|---|---|---|
| 100 | 1.70 | 4.85 | 4.10 | 35.0 |
| 95 | 1.73 | 4.95 | 4.19 | 33.5 |
| 90 | 1.75 | 5.00 | 4.28 | 32.0 |
| 85 | 1.78 | 5.05 | 4.35 | 31.0 |
| 80 | 1.79 | 5.12 | 4.39 | 30.0 |
| 75 | 1.80 | 5.17 | 4.40 | 29.0 |
| 70 | 1.81 | 5.22 | 4.41 | 28.5 |
| 65 | 1.82 | 5.31 | 4.42 | 27.5 |
| 60 | 1.83 | 5.33 | 4.44 | 27.0 |
| 55 | 1.84 | 5.34 | 4.46 | 26.5 |
| 50 | 1.85 | 5.36 | 4.49 | 26.5 |
| 45 | 1.86 | 5.39 | 4.50 | 26.0 |
| 40 | 1.87 | 5.40 | 4.51 | 26.0 |
| 35 | 1.88 | 5.41 | 4.54 | 25.5 |
| 30 | 1.89 | 5.42 | 4.57 | 25.5 |
| 25 | 1.90 | 5.43 | 4.58 | 25.0 |
| 20 | 1.91 | 5.44 | 4.59 | 24.5 |
| 15 | 1.92 | 5.45 | 4.60 | 24.0 |
| 10 | 1.93 | 5.46 | 4.61 | 24.0 |
| 5 | 1.96 | 5.47 | 4.66 | 23.5 |

agility. He is better off spending more time correcting his agility than his speed and power, which are already in the good and excellent categories.

## KEEPING A TESTING HISTORY

Keep a history of scores recorded each time you test (table 3.29). This record keeping allows you and your athletes to evaluate their progress. Usually most progress is shown in the first year of training. Each succeeding year as an athlete nears his athletic potential he won't make as much progress. The key is that the player needs to continue to show progress, especially in the areas in which he has weaknesses.

## SETTING GOALS

Establishing goals is an essential element of any sports conditioning program. Without goals you cannot develop workouts that give direction and progressively increase in intensity. Without goals you cannot determine how far each player has come and how far he has to go. The

**Table 3.28 Performance Profile**

Name: *Bill Jones*

Running Backs

| Percentile rank | 10-yard dash | 40-yard dash | Pro agility run | Vertical jump |
|---|---|---|---|---|
| 100 | 1.52 | 4.36 | 3.99 | 36.0 |
| 95 | 1.62 | 4.53 | 4.22 | 33.5 |
| 90 | 1.70 | 4.62 | 4.29 | 32.0 |
| 85 | 1.72 | 4.71 | 4.35 | 29.5 |
| 80 | 1.75 | 4.89 | 4.38 | 27.0 |
| 75 | 1.77 | 4.95 | 4.41 | 26.5 |
| 70 | 1.78 | 5.00 | 4.45 | 26.0 |
| 65 | 1.80 | 5.04 | 4.48 | 25.5 |
| 60 | 1.82 | 5.08 | 4.50 | 25.0 |
| 55 | 1.85 | 5.11 | 4.53 | 24.5 |
| 50 | 1.86 | 5.14 | 4.56 | 24.0 |
| 45 | 1.87 | 5.18 | 4.58 | 23.5 |
| 40 | 1.88 | 5.20 | 4.62 | 23.0 |
| 35 | 1.90 | 5.23 | 4.65 | 22.5 |
| 30 | 1.91 | 5.26 | 4.68 | 22.0 |
| 25 | 1.92 | 5.35 | 4.72 | 21.5 |
| 20 | 1.93 | 5.42 | 4.76 | 21.0 |
| 15 | 1.94 | 5.49 | 4.81 | 20.5 |
| 10 | 1.97 | 5.57 | 4.89 | 20.0 |
| 5 | 2.15 | 5.75 | 5.00 | 12.5 |

goal-setting procedure is very simple: Seek to improve each player's performance of each test every time that you test.

Some coaches recommend realistic yet challenging goals. But we have found that this does not work very well for us. Making progress the first year on a conditioning program is pretty easy. But progress after that becomes very difficult. Setting performance goals for tests takes only 1.5 to 5 seconds, but improvements come in hundredths of a second from one test period to the next. This means goals have to be set allowing for hundredths of a second improvement. The first year a normal gain in the vertical jump is two to three inches. A typical vertical jump improvement after four years of training is four inches. So making a half-inch improvement from one test period to another is very good after two years of training.

With improvements coming with so much more difficulty after several years of training, why set numerical goals? Instead make the goal to improve each performance of each test every time that you test. The goal will likely be easy to attain the first few times, but after that it will become more difficult. After a few years it may take two or three test periods before an athlete shows an improvement in the 40-yard dash. He will

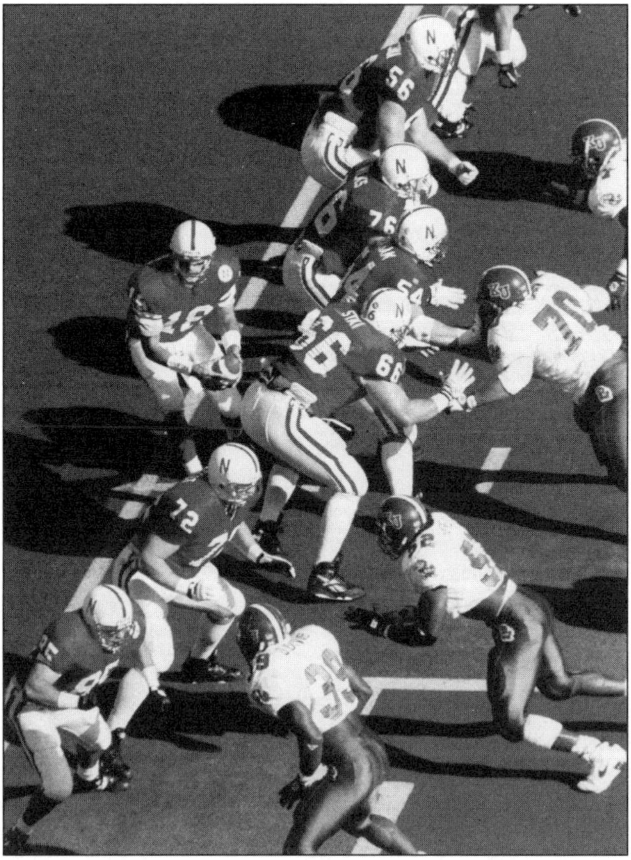

typically show improvement on one or two of the four tests. Remember that if improvement is shown in one test and not the other three, he is still making progress. Sometimes he must take a step backward to take two steps forward. Encourage him to persevere and stick with the program, and he'll see progress.

More realistic yet challenging goals can be set in strength training and body composition. Keep a strength training progress chart (see chapter 9) and testing history (see table 3.29), and you have all the necessary information to set goals. Once goals are achieved, it is necessary to reevaluate each athlete's progress and set new goals. Do not allow the athlete to become satisfied with what he has achieved in the past, or his work habits will deteriorate and performance may decline. This happens many times as a player attains status as a first-stringer and rests on his laurels. Once you set your players' goals and they learn the drills in the following chapters, they can follow through on the programs outlined in chapter 9.

**Table 3.29 Testing History**

Name ______________________ Position ______________________

| Date | Height | Weight | Waist | Vertical jump | 10-yard dash | 40-yard dash | 300-yard shuttle run |
|---|---|---|---|---|---|---|---|
| | | | | | | | |
| | | | | | | | |
| | | | | | | | |
| | | | | | | | |
| | | | | | | | |
| | | | | | | | |
| | | | | | | | |
| | | | | | | | |
| | | | | | | | |
| | | | | | | | |
| | | | | | | | |
| | | | | | | | |
| | | | | | | | |
| | | | | | | | |
| | | | | | | | |
| | | | | | | | |
| | | | | | | | |
| | | | | | | | |

Comments

CHAPTER 4

# FLEXIBILITY TRAINING

Flexibility is the ability to move a joint and surrounding musculature through a full range of motion. Range of motion is specific to each joint; that is, a high degree of flexibility in one joint of the body does not necessarily indicate a similar level of flexibility in another. The lack of an optimal level of flexibility in any muscle group can cause inefficient movements that hinder the desired performance. Warming up and then stretching the muscles not only improves your flexibility, it assists in preparing for workouts and may help prevent injuries. Make proper stretching drills an integral part of the warm-up and cool-down periods of your training program. We discuss warming up and cooling down in more detail with the specific workouts and practice schedules in chapter 9.

It is difficult to determine the amount of flexibility necessary for any athletic event; minimal research exists on the topic. Great flexibility does not guarantee a player that he will have great performance skills. Some players have great football skills, but lack a high degree of flexibility when tested on the sit-and-reach test. The requirements of flexibility vary from activity to activity and tend to be developed specifically as a result of the imposed demands of a particular skill. Therefore, a good guideline for football players is to develop their range of motion to be adequate for allowing performance of position-specific skills without extreme soft tissue resistance.

The dynamic ranges of motion utilized when Barry Sanders makes a cut require tremendous flexibility, but the flexibility required to go through these joint movements cannot be achieved by practicing static stretching exercises. Functional dynamic stretching drills called mobility drills must be incorporated to reach maximum performance.

## WARM-UP ROUTINE

It is important that you always warm up your muscles, ligaments, and tendons by doing all the following warm-up drills (8 to 10 minutes of moderate exercise) before beginning your stretching routine. The drills

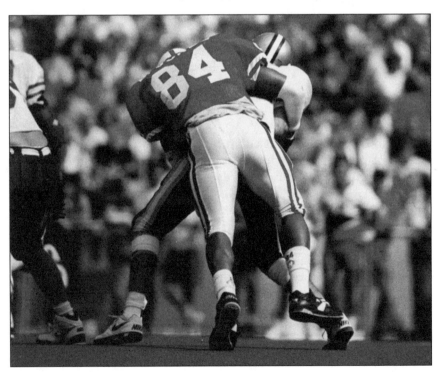

not only warm up the body for the workout, but also help with active flexibility of the hip and leg area. These drills, if done properly, also develop speed mechanics. Do these warm-up drills every day, first thing, before the workout.

## HIGH KNEES

**Purpose:** To develop muscles needed for a fast, long stride and flexibility in the hamstring. All good sprinters have a good high knee action. The higher the knee lift when running, the longer the stride.

**Procedure:**

1. Mark a 10-yard course.
2. Sprint the course, taking quick, short, one-foot steps. Drive your knees high so that your thighs are parallel to the ground.
3. When you lift one leg, be sure the other leg is fully extended.
4. Bend forward slightly at the waist and keep your back straight.

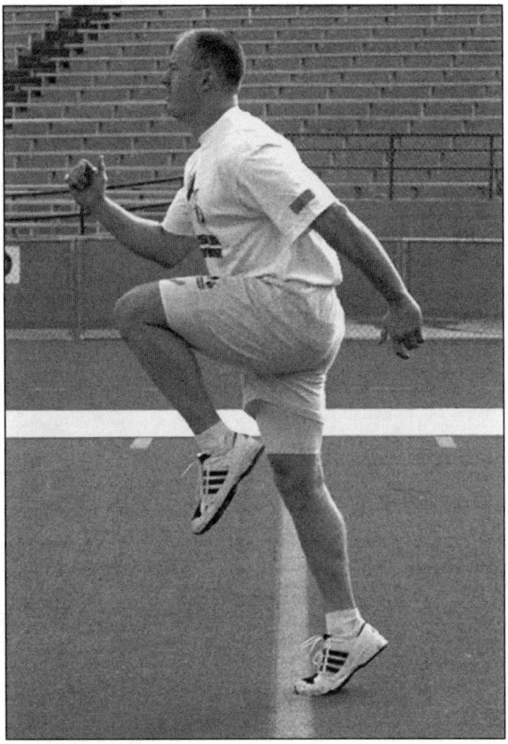

**Volume:** Do two repetitions of 10 yards.

**Rest Interval:** Walk back to the starting line as a rest interval between reps.

**Key Points**

1. Avoid leaning back or taking long steps.
2. Swing arms freely at the shoulders with good arm action.
3. Keep your face and neck relaxed.
4. Achieve at least 30 steps in 10 yards.

# HEEL-UPS

**Purpose:** To develop strength in the hamstring and flexibility in the quadriceps. When the heels come up to the hips in running, the thighs swing through faster, increasing stride frequency and speed.

**Procedure:**

1. Mark a 10-yard course on the field.
2. Start drill by running on your toes and alternately swinging heel of each foot up to buttocks.
3. Keep action quick and smooth; produce the swinging at the knee.

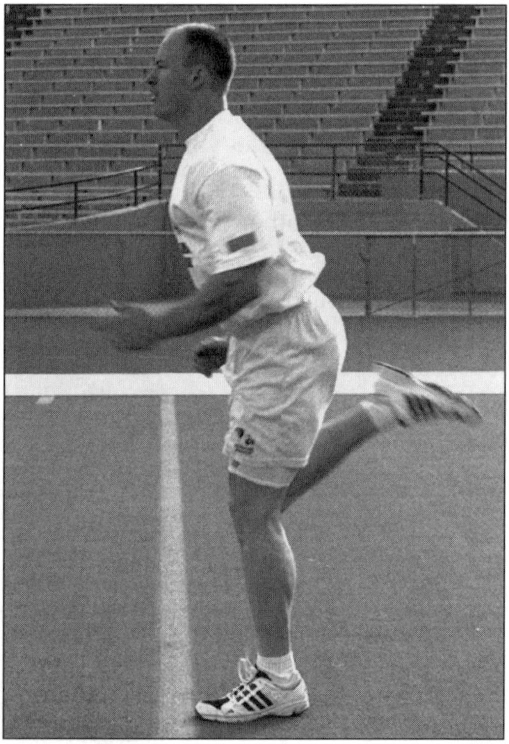

**Volume:** Do two repetitions of 10 yards each.

**Rest Interval:** Walk back to the starting line as a rest interval between reps.

**Key Points:**

1. Maintain good forward lean.
2. Keep knees pointed down toward the ground.
3. Keep arms relaxed at the sides.
4. Avoid moving forward too fast, using the arms, or lifting the knees by flexing at the hips.

## HIGH KNEES WITH HEEL-UPS

**Purpose:** To develop sprinting rhythm and action

**Procedure:**

1. Mark a 20-yard course on the field.
2. Begin drill with 5 yards of high knees.
3. After 5 yards of high knees, combine high knees with heel-ups for 15 yards.
4. Stay on your toes, drive hard off of your back leg, swing your heel up to the buttocks, and pull thigh through to a high knee position.
5. Produce a reflexive, quick, and smooth swinging motion from the knee joint.

**Volume:** Do two repetitions of 20 yards each.

**Rest Interval:** Walk back to the starting line as a rest interval between reps.

# HIGH KNEES WITH FORELEG EXTENSION

**Purpose:** To develop your ability to reach with foreleg during sprinting. *Note:* The movement pattern resembles skipping with the swing leg extending forward explosively.

**Procedure:**

1. Lift right knee high.
2. When right knee reaches highest position the left leg does a little skip.
3. As you skip, extend the right foreleg until it is parallel with the ground.
4. Repeat on the other side.

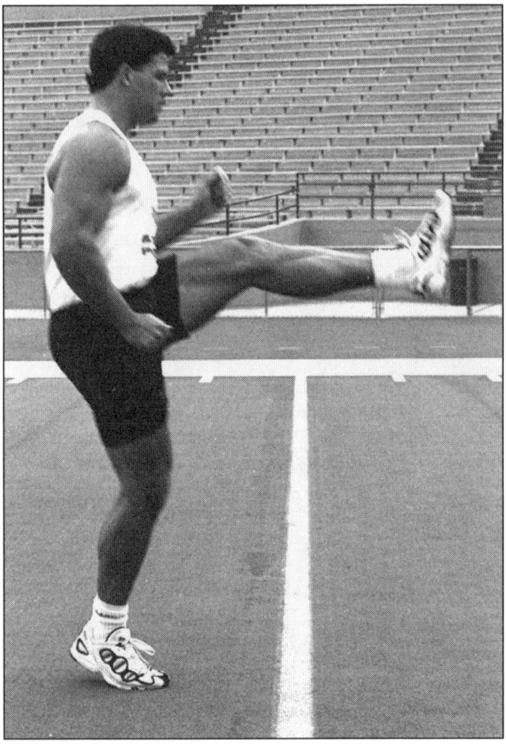

**Volume:** Do two repetitions of 15 yards each.

**Rest Interval:** Walk back to the starting line as a rest interval between reps.

**Key Points:**

1. Maintain proper forward lean. (No drum major strides.)
2. Thighs should get parallel before the knee is straightened.
3. Extend your foreleg out and up forcefully.
4. Avoid incomplete extension of foreleg and unrhythmic movement.

# CARIOCA DRILL

**Purpose:** To develop lateral movement and hip flexibility. Often during a game a player must turn his body and run. It takes good flexibility in the hips to make a quick, smooth turn.

**Procedure:**

1. Get into a good hitting stance with knees flexed and shoulders facing squarely forward.
2. Move laterally to your left, crossing the right foot over in front of the left, and then bring the right foot behind on the next step. (If moving right, reverse the procedure.)
3. While moving, remain in your hitting stance, keep your shoulders squared, and get good hip rotation.
4. Do this movement pattern for 20 yards and then change direction.

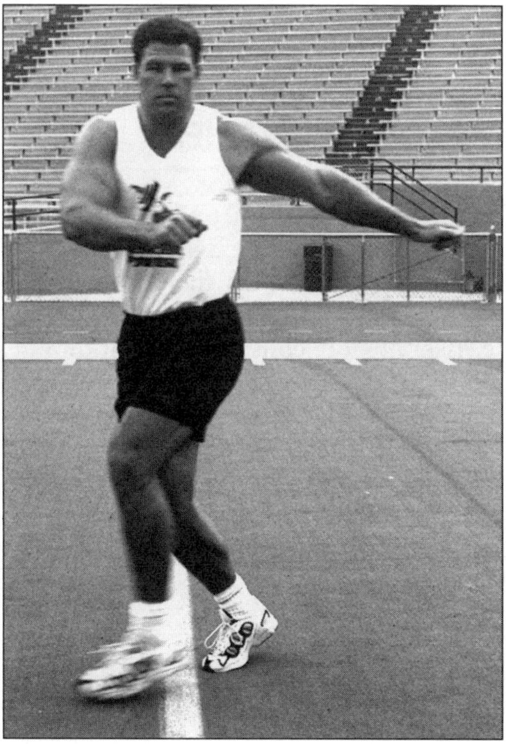

**Volume:** Do two repetitions of 20 yards each.

**Rest Interval:** Walk back to the starting line as a rest interval between reps.

**Key Points:**

1. Start in a hitting stance (power stance).
2. Twist hips around as far as possible, while keeping shoulders squared.
3. Take the biggest steps possible.
4. Avoid moving too fast so you don't lose your hip rotation.

## 40-YARD BUILDUPS

**Purpose:** To develop proper sprinting technique and the ability to accelerate

**Procedure:**

1. Begin running at the goal line and build up speed for 30 yards.
2. Stride remaining 10 yards.

**Volume:** Do two repetitions of 40-yard pickups.

**Rest Interval:** Walk back to the starting line as a rest interval between reps.

**Key Points:**

1. Demonstrate proper arm action.
2. Lift knees high and bring heels up into the hips.
3. Start the run slowly and gradually build up.

## PARTNER STRETCHES

Partner static stretching precedes the warm-up routine. Ideally, stretching routines should be designed to each athlete's needs. The partner stretches below stretch the major muscle groups our medical staff, players, and strength staff at the University of Nebraska consider necessary before continuing a workout. It should take you 8 to 10 minutes to complete the six partner stretches. Hold each stretch for approximately 10 seconds.

In partner stretching, the stretcher should not stretch his partner to the point of pain, but should slowly and smoothly stretch to the point of tightness or before muscular discomfort occurs in the muscles being stretched. For safety purposes, emphasize proper form and be sure no motion is forced.

# 1: LYING HAMSTRING STRETCH

**Focus:** Hamstring muscles

**Procedure:**

1. Lie on your back with legs straight and toes pointing up.
2. Allow your partner to lift your right leg and to apply pressure with his hand while holding your left leg down. He will do this until you feel a comfortable stretch in the hamstring.
3. Hold the stretch for 10 seconds. Repeat with other leg.

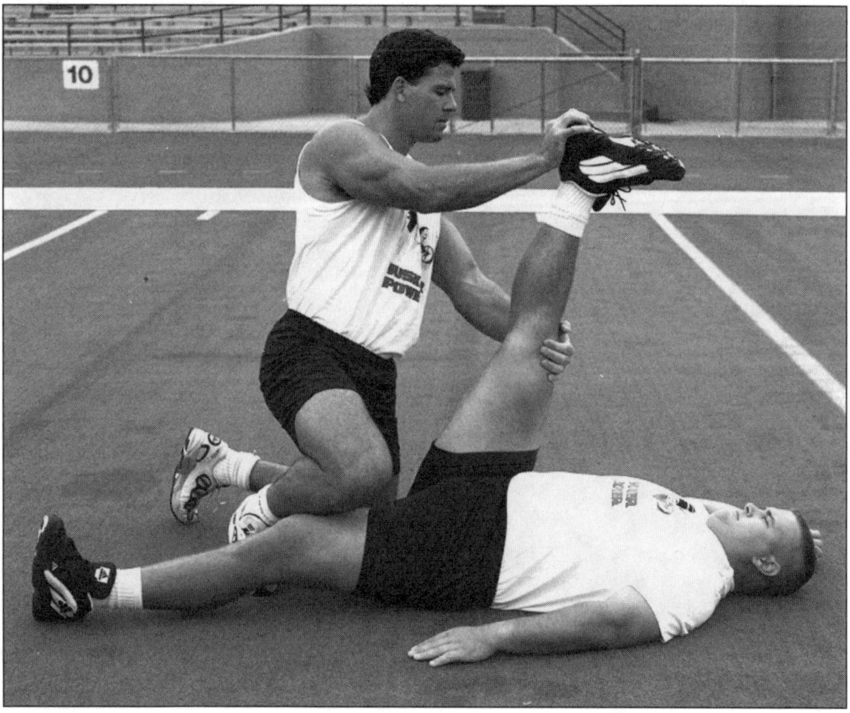

# 2: KNEE TO CHEST STRETCH

**Focus:** Gluteals, groin, hamstrings

**Procedure:**

1. From stretch #1, partner bends your right leg at the knee and pushes it toward your chest while keeping your left leg straight.
2. Partner applies pressure by leaning forward, guiding the knee to your chest while holding down the left leg.
3. Hold the stretch for 10 seconds. Repeat with other leg.

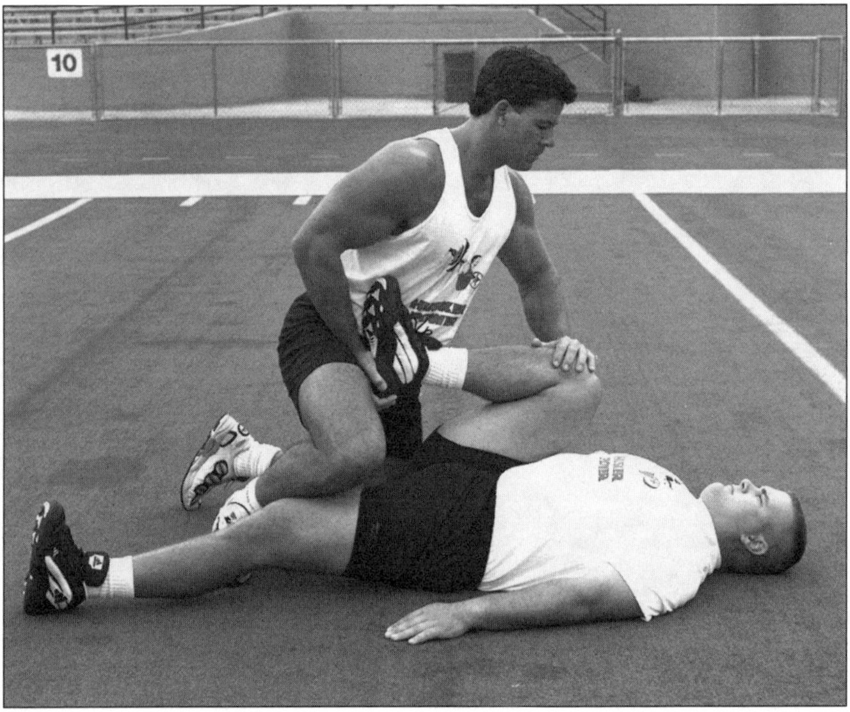

## 3: LYING SPINAL TWIST

**Focus:** Lower back erectors, lateral region of the gluteal muscles

**Procedure:**

1. From stretch #2, partner pulls your bent leg (right) over your straight leg (left), applying pressure to your bent knee and opposite shoulder.
2. Partner makes sure you keep your shoulders flat against the floor.
3. Hold stretch for 10 seconds. Repeat with other leg.

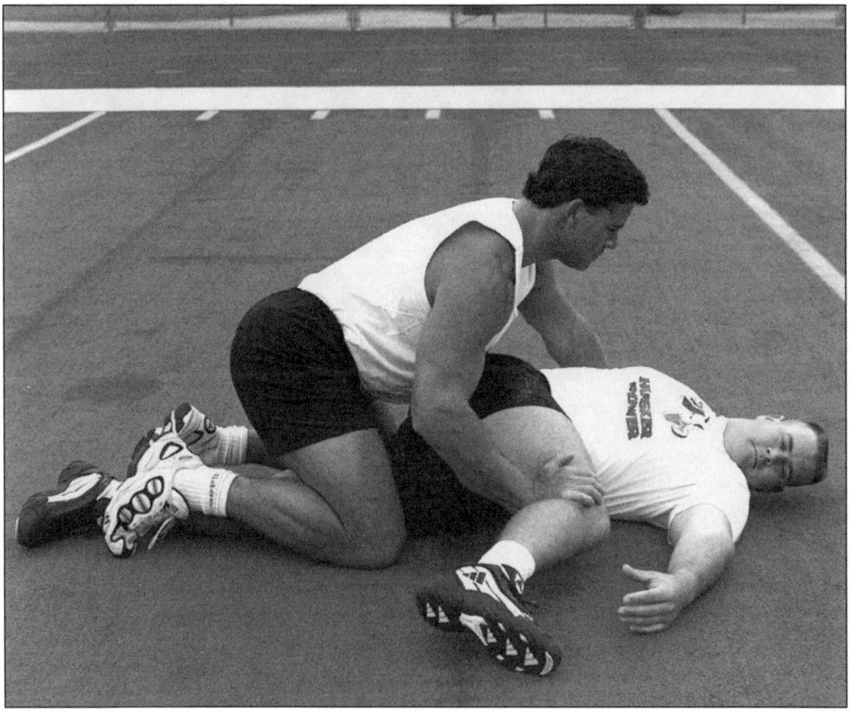

# 4: QUAD STRETCH

**Focus:** Quadriceps

**Procedure:**

1. Lie on your stomach in an extended position.
2. Partner bends one of your legs at the knee and guides your heel to your buttocks while applying pressure to your lower back.
3. Hold stretch for 10 seconds. Repeat with other leg.

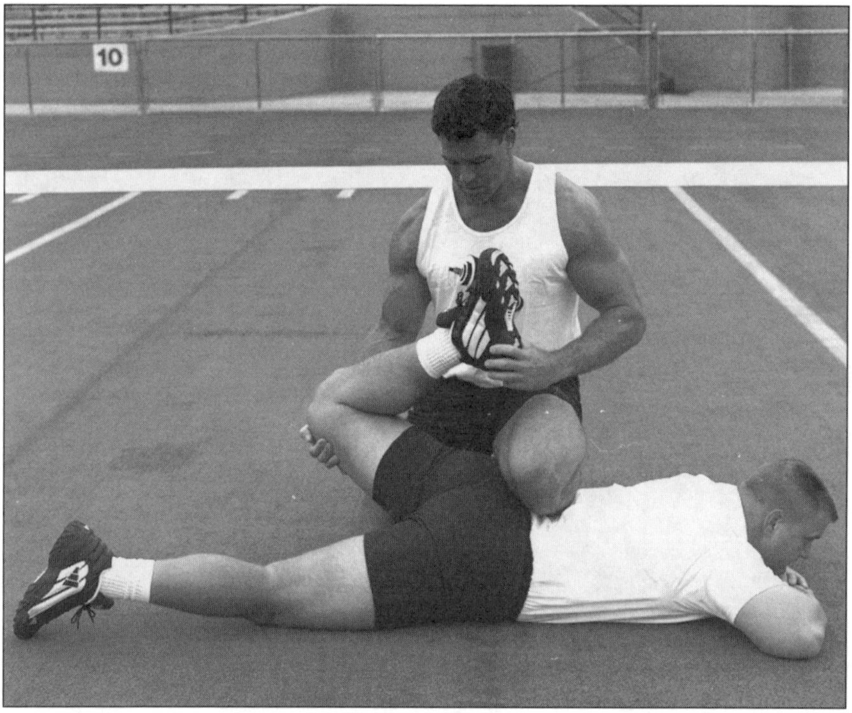

# 5: HIP FLEXOR STRETCH

**Focus:** Hip flexors

**Procedure:**

1. From stretch #4, partner lifts the leg up and back at the knee while applying pressure to your lower back.
2. Hold stretch for 10 seconds. Repeat with other leg.

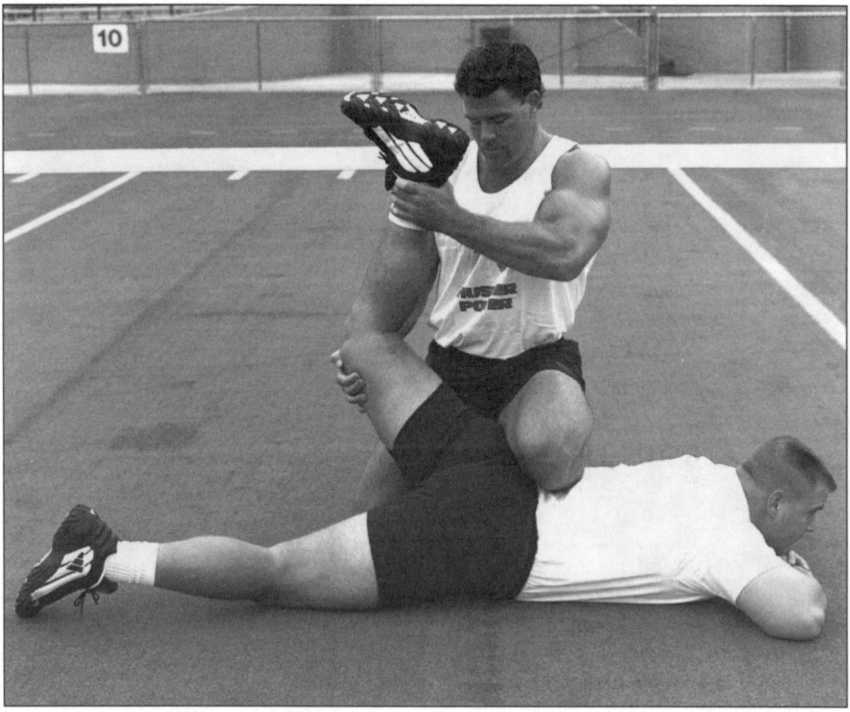

# 6: SEATED SPLIT-LEGGED STRETCH

**Focus:** Groin, hamstrings

**Procedure:**

1. Sit with legs straight, straddled, and toes pointing up.
2. Partner applies pressure in the middle of your back, allowing you to stretch forward (to the center) as far as possible.
3. Relax in sitting position before having partner assist in stretching to the right toe and left toe.
4. Keep your head up and back straight while performing this stretch.
5. Hold stretch for 10 seconds each time.

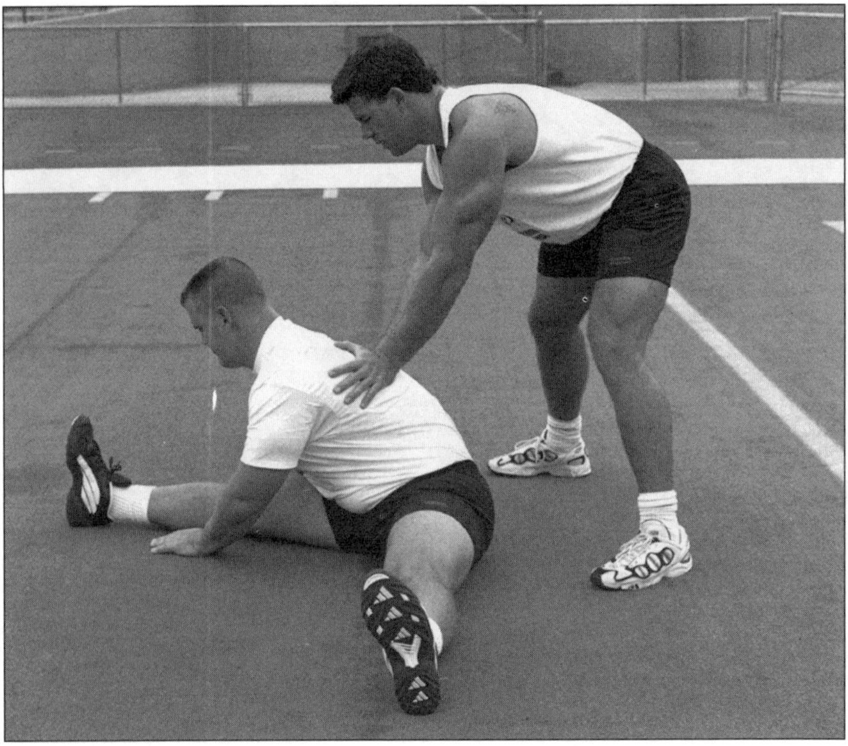

# MOBILITY DRILLS

For our purpose, we use the term mobility drills to denote functional dynamic stretching exercises. The dynamic movements of the mobility drills presented here aim to

- warm the internal temperature of the muscles,
- gently stretch and strengthen muscles of the body in positions that specific muscles require,
- stimulate the nervous system (motoneurons of contracting muscles) of the body for readiness for physical activity, and
- teach motor skills related to football skills.

Mobility drills (dynamic stretches) and ballistic stretching exercises are not the same. Ballistic stretching utilizes repetitive bouncing movements to increase your range of motion, while mobility drills involve moving body parts through entire ranges of motion without jerking or bouncing movements. Every mobility drill starts each movement slowly, then progressively increases the range of motion and the speed of movement through the entire drill.

The goal of mobility drills is not to isolate but to integrate the muscles into dynamic functional movement patterns (multiplane movements: rotational, diagonal, flexion, and extension), since this is how the muscles are used in making plays under game conditions. To achieve this integration, it is necessary to condition and prepare the whole body as a link system with all parts working together. We discuss mobility drills in more detail with the specific workouts and practice schedules in chapter 9.

We use the following drills at the University of Nebraska after a regular workout. Do these drills using regulation track hurdles that can be adjusted to each athlete's physical capabilities and progression of skill level. Depending upon your purpose, imagination, and equipment available, you can perform other variations of these drills.

The overall purpose of these drills is to improve torso, trunk, and hip flexibility through dynamic athletic-type movements. These drills activate and strengthen the synergistic, stabilizing muscles of the hip and groin area.

Set up for the following two drills by placing 6 to 10 hurdles in a conventional parallel position, with the distance of the rocker arm of the hurdle determining the space between successive crossbars. Each drill starts by walking slowly over or under the hurdles, then progressively increases in the range of motion and the speed of movement through the entire drill.

# FORWARD STEP: UP AND OVER ALTERNATE LEG LEAD

**Purpose:** To improve torso, trunk, and hip flexibility

**Procedure:**

1. Place your hands on hips and ensure that shoulders, hips, and feet are squared to the crossbars before beginning exercise.
2. Begin by leading with and lifting the right knee/foot up and over the first crossbar.
3. Continue by leading with and lifting the trailing leg up and over the next crossbar.
4. Continue alternating and overcoming successive crossbars until all hurdles are overcome.

**Volume:** Two repetitions

**Rest Interval:** Walk back to first hurdle to start second repetition.

**Key Points:**

1. Land each foot in a forward-facing position.
2. When lifting each leg, attempt a straight up and over motion, rather than an excessive outward, swinging motion.
3. Hold upper torso erect whenever possible, rather than leaning forward.
4. Focus eyes 15 yards ahead, rather than down at each crossbar.
5. Maintain a rhythmic pattern of stepping over the hurdles.
6. Start with slow, deliberate movements and build to faster speeds as proficiency increases.

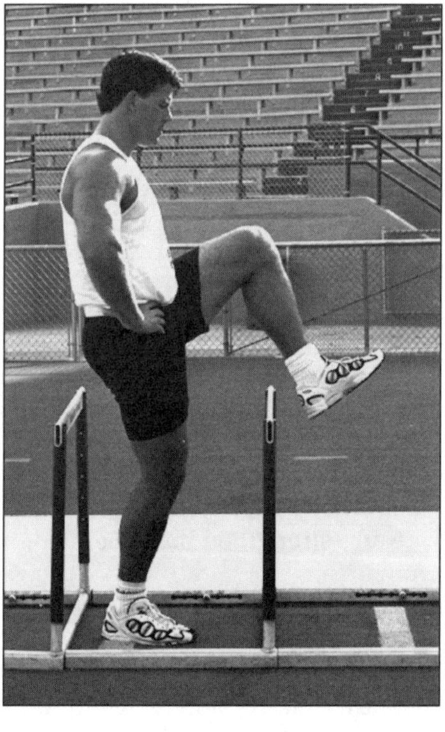

# LATERAL STEP: UP AND OVER LEFT AND RIGHT LEG LEAD

**Purpose:** To improve torso, trunk, and hip flexibility

**Procedure:**

1. Place hands on your hips and insure that shoulders, hips, and feet are squared but perpendicular to the hurdles before beginning exercise.
2. Begin by leading with and lifting the left knee / foot up and over the first crossbar.
3. Continue by leading with and lifting the trailing leg up and over the same crossbar.
4. Continue alternating and overcoming each crossbar until all hurdles are overcome.
5. Repeat exercise leading with right leg.

**Volume:** Do six hurdles up and back.

**Key Points:**

1. Land each foot in a forward-facing position.
2. Attempt lifting each leg with a straight up and over motion without rotating the hips and torso.
3. Hold upper torso erect, rather than leaning forward.
4. Focus eyes 15 yards ahead, rather than down at each crossbar.
5. Maintain a rhythmic pattern of stepping over the hurdles, starting with slow, deliberate movements and building to faster speeds as proficiency increases.
6. Ensure that the first foot is far enough away from the hurdle to allow space for the trailing foot.

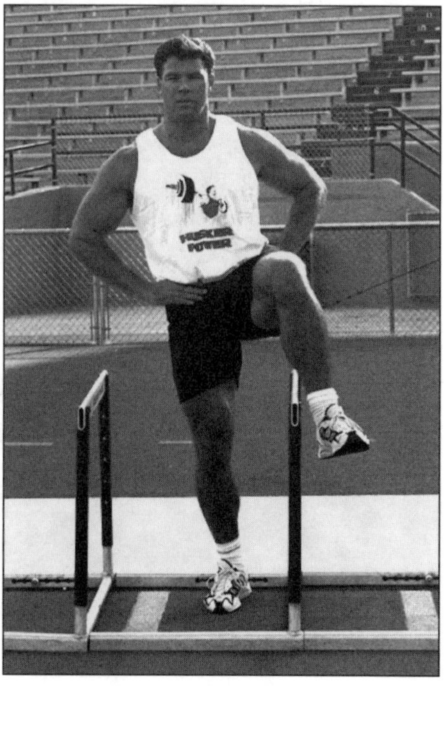

# FACING FORWARD: WEAVE IN AND OUT UNDERNEATH HURDLES

**Purpose:** To improve torso, trunk, and hip flexibility

**Procedure:**

1. Place hurdles side by side to form a straight line of all crossbars, with rocker arms alternating from the left and right.
2. Place hands in football blocking position.
3. Ensure that shoulders, hips, and feet are squared but perpendicular to the hurdles before beginning exercise.
4. Begin exercise by crouching in a low squat position and leading left leg under and through the first crossbar.
5. Remain in low position and step under crossbar with your trailing leg.
6. Remain in low position and step forward with your left leg to the next crossbar.

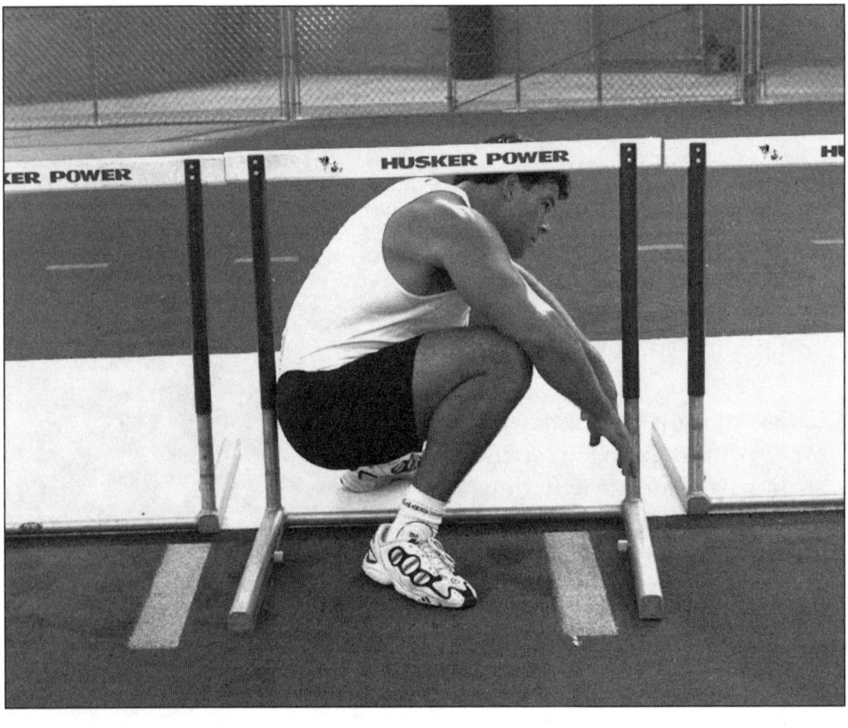

7. Continue by leading with and lifting the right leg under and through the next crossbar.
8. Continue alternating left and right legs in this manner until all hurdles are overcome.

**Volume:** Do six hurdles up and back.

**Key Points:**

1. Land each foot in a forward-facing position.
2. When lifting each leg, attempt a straight under and through motion without rotating the hips and torso.
3. Keep hands in football blocking position and keep hips below shoulders in low squat position.
4. Hold upper torso erect, rather than leaning forward.
5. Focus eyes 15 yards ahead, rather than down at each crossbar.
6. Maintain a rhythmic stepping pattern through the hurdles, starting with slow, deliberate movements and building to faster speeds as proficiency increases.
7. Ensure that the first foot is placed far enough away from the hurdle to allow space for trailing foot.

CHAPTER 5

# LIFTING TECHNIQUES

This chapter describes correct lifting techniques for the strength exercises used in this book. Proper technique is necessary for maximum performance enhancement and injury prevention. Keep in mind, technique before strength. That is, always make sure your lifting form is correct before increasing the weight (intensity) of the lift.

## LIFTING GUIDELINES

Before you begin any lifting program it is important to understand how to get the most out of each lift to make you a better player while preventing injuries. In addition to the training principles of mass and acceleration, stabilization, and coordination discussed in chapter 2, which apply to effective strength training, the following five factors are important for proper lifting.

## Warming Up

When a muscle is cold, a sudden contraction can result in muscle damage. Therefore, before lifting always warm up your muscles properly by performing the same lifting movements with a lighter weight. Thus, you cannot warm up properly for heavy bench presses by performing squats. If you are bench pressing, warm up by performing a few sets of bench presses with a resistance well below the weight you intend to use for a maximum attempt.

## Having Spotters

When performing exercises involving free weights, especially the squat, it is best to have two spotters working with you. Spotters should keep their hands under the bar without touching it and should be alert at all times. They can also load the weights for you, greatly reducing your workout time. Moreover, when three athletes are working together the time it takes to rotate athletes and change the weights provides about the right amount of rest between each set.

## Lifting Through the Full Range of Motion

Execute all exercises outlined in this chapter through their full range of motion if you want to receive the full benefits of strength training. Partial movements are unwise because after a period of time they reduce the joints' range of motion; this makes you less flexible and increases your chances of pulling or straining a muscle. Perform each exercise exactly as described.

## Breathing Properly

Correct breathing helps you get the most benefit from exercises. Holding your breath stabilizes the chest muscles, allowing you to exert greater force on the weight. Always inhale at the starting position of the exercise. Hold your breath until the repetition is nearly complete, then forcibly exhale.

## Controlling the Resistance

When lowering the weight during slow-movement exercises, control the bar to keep the tension on the muscle groups being used. This will lengthen the muscle fibers similar to the stretching of a rubber band. If you drop the weight so that the bar bounces at the bottom of the movement, no tension has been built up in the muscle. When reversing the direction of the bar, take advantage of this elastic energy by lifting the bar as explosively as possible. This takes advantage of the stretch-shortening cycle described in chapter 2. When using exercise machines do not allow the resistance to bang the machine.

# STABILIZATION AND SYNERGISM

In chapter 2 we said that anything that substitutes as a stabilizer, other than the muscles of the body, limits effective stabilization and synergism. Belts and wraps are also counterproductive to maximum stability development within the body because they act as stabilizers in place of the appropriate muscle groups. Belts and wraps limit the synergetic

### Is Bench Pressing for Football Players?

Many coaches and athletes incorporate the bench press as a major exercise to develop the upper body. The bench press is a good lift for developing muscular size and strength and should be included in your program, but it is not very effective for preventing shoulder injuries. When an offensive lineman is blocking, the muscles of the shoulder girdle stabilize the actions of the arm and chest muscles. The bench press does not allow the muscles of the shoulder girdle to stabilize the pressing action of the chest—the bench stabilizes the action. Dips and push-ups done with resistance are better exercises. These exercises are ground based and require the shoulder girdle to act as a stabilizer so the chest and arms can exert force. The bench press is more effective in developing the chest muscles, but you can probably prevent shoulder injuries if you supplement bench pressing with Jammer exercises, dips, and push-ups.

muscles' ability to regulate and coordinate the movement pattern of the resistance. If the muscles surrounding the joints aren't trained as stabilizers and synergists, the joint structure becomes the weak link and you aren't effectively preventing potential joint injuries. Therefore, only use belts and wraps when going for a maximum attempt on a lift; only then are they absolutely necessary to protect a current injury or to prevent a new one.

## EXERCISE SELECTION

Strength training exercises for football must apply principles of ground-based activities, multiple joint actions, multiple plane movements, stabilization, synergism, the stretch-shortening cycle, and acceleration (refer to chapter 2) to develop explosive blocking and tackling skills. Our program includes explosive and strength exercises complemented by exercises done on the ground-based Jammer and hip sled and specialty exercises that isolate muscle groups to promote muscle growth and strengthen injuries. Table 5.1 lists the exercises in the program.

**Table 5.1 Strength Training Exercises**

| Explosive | Complementary | Base strength | Specialty |
|---|---|---|---|
| Clean shrug | Jammer extension | Clean dead lift | Leg extension |
| Rack clean | Jammer rotation | Squat | Leg curl |
| Hang clean | Jammer press | Front squat | Back extension |
| Box snatch | | Snatch squat | Lat pulldown |
| Hang snatch | | Standing shoulder press | Bench press |
| Power press | | Romanian dead lift | Incline press |
| | | Good morning | Seated shoulder press |
| | | Low lat pull | Shoulder raises |
| | | Trunk twist | Front raise |
| | | | Lateral raise |
| | | | Bent-over raise |
| | | | Barbell curl |
| | | | Triceps extension |
| | | | Neck machine |
| | | | Crunch |

# EXPLOSIVE EXERCISES

Explosive exercises are exercises done at high speeds, allowing lifting movements to take place in approximately two-tenths of a second. In chapter 2 we discussed that during powerful movements the triple extension takes that amount of time to complete; the execution of a block or tackle takes slightly less. Olympic lifting movements combine the use of heavy weights and high velocities to generate the greatest power of any exercise movement. The hang clean or power press each takes roughly two-tenths of a second to perform, with weight that approaches or exceeds the body weight of opponents encountered on the football field. To be fresh for the explosive lifts you should do them on Monday and Thursday, before the base strength exercises on Tuesday and Friday.

The major exercises of our strength program are the Olympic lifts—the power clean and power snatch. They are ground-based, multiple joint, multiple plane exercises that must be done explosively. The clean uses a shoulder-width grip. The bar is pulled in one continuous motion and is caught on the shoulders. The snatch uses a wide grip. The bar is pulled in one continuous motion and is caught overhead. The basic pulling techniques are similar for both lifts. The six fundamental positions for the pulling actions of both lifts are illustrated below.

It is difficult to observe and analyze these lifts during normal execution because of the continuous motion, so it is a good idea to videotape the execution of the lifts and play them back in slow motion. Once the bar reaches a certain position the video can be put on freeze-frame and the fundamental positions can be analyzed.

## START POSITION (POSITION 1)

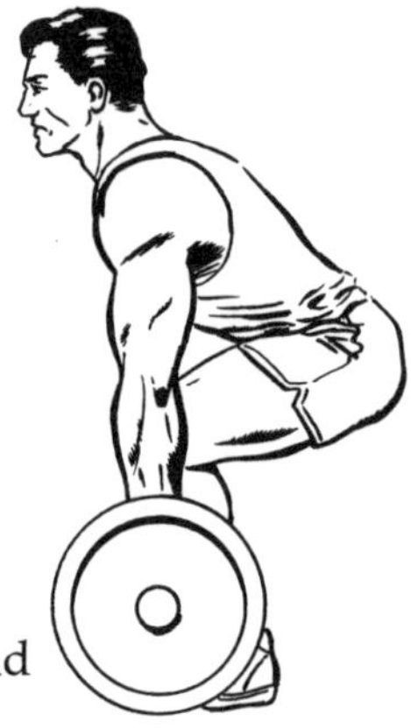

1. Place feet hip-width apart, flat on floor.
2. Bend legs with the lower leg touching the bar and hips slightly higher than knees.
3. Use an overhand grip with hands placed shoulder-width apart.
4. Extend arms with elbows pointed out.
5. Inhale to fill chest with air and hold it high.
6. Keep back flat.
7. Position shoulders just ahead of bar and set head in a comfortable position.

## FIRST PULL (POSITION 2)

1. Extend your legs elevating the bar to just above the knees, keeping the angle of your back constant.
2. Do not jerk the bar off the floor; pull it smoothly and under control.
3. Keep the bar close to your legs and your arms extended with elbows pointed out.

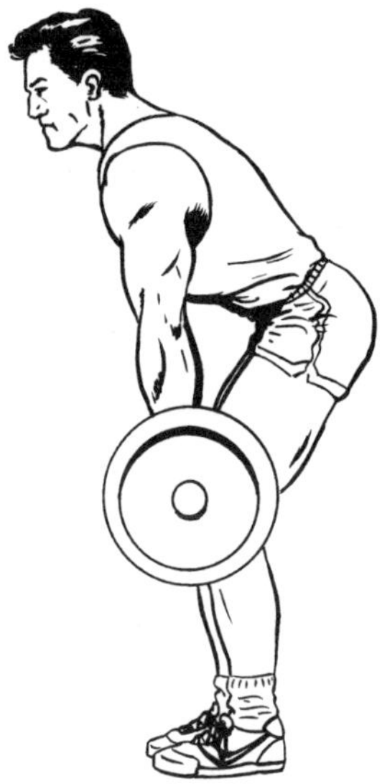

## SECOND PULL (POSITION 3)

1. Extend your hips up and forward explosively.
2. If you keep your arms straight (elbows pointed out) your knees will automatically flex or rebend as the hips extend. This movement, known as the double knee bend or scooping action, puts the lifter at position 3.
3. The bar should ride up the thighs.

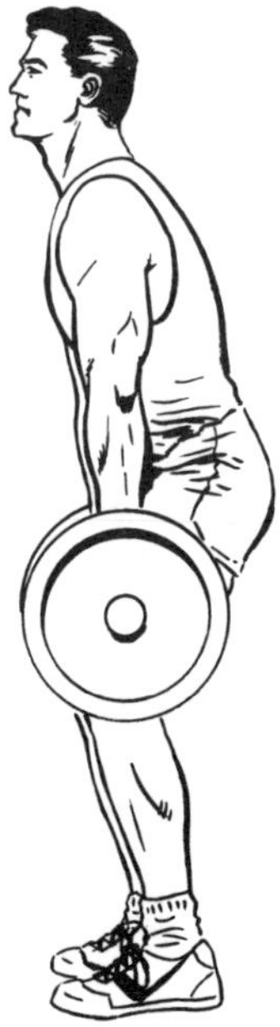

## EXPLOSIVE PHASE (POSITION 4)

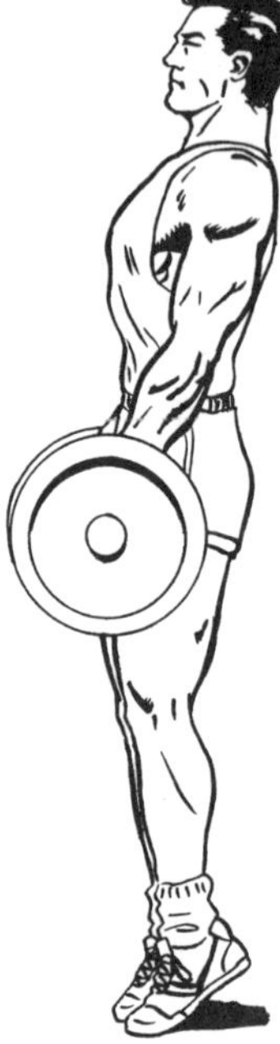

1. Extend onto the balls of your feet while simultaneously shrugging your shoulders. Your ankles, knees, and hips should extend simultaneously, accelerating the bar upward. This is known as the triple extension.
2. Keep the bar close to your body and your arms extended with elbows pointing out.

## RECEIVING THE BAR—CLEAN (POSITION 5)

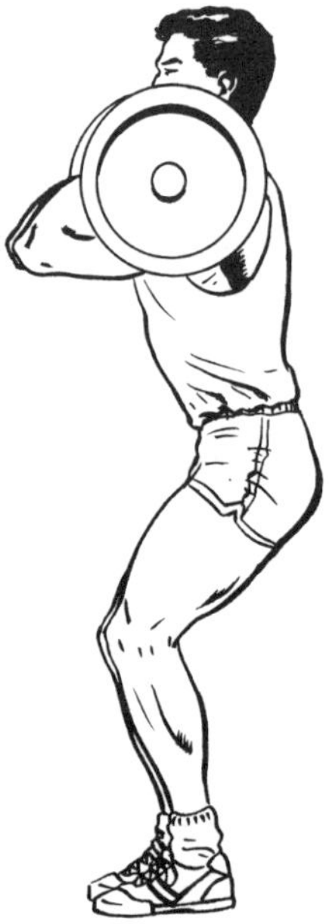

1. Pull yourself down and under the bar.
2. Elevate the feet and move them out into a squatting stance.
3. Rotate elbows down and then up ahead of the bar.
4. Catch bar on the front portion of the shoulders.
5. Flex your knees and hips to absorb the weight of the bar.
6. Once the catch is made, stand erect with feet flat on the ground and shoulders directly over the balls of the feet.

## RECEIVING THE BAR—SNATCH (POSITION 6)

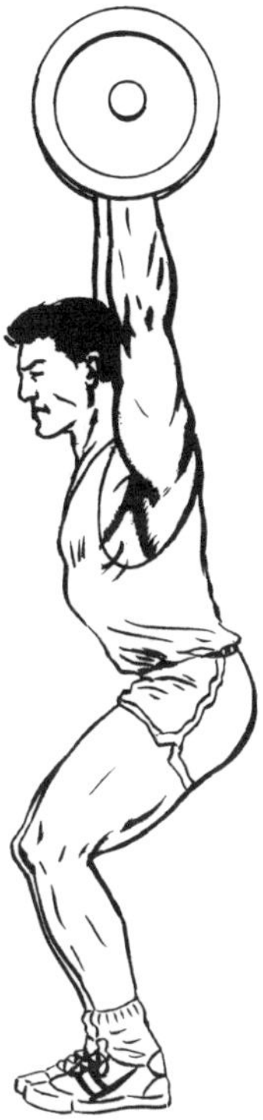

1. Pull yourself down and under the bar by elevating the feet and moving them into a squatting stance.
2. Rotate elbows down as the bar passes the chest.
3. Extend the arms and catch the bar overhead.
4. Flex the knees and hips to absorb the weight of the bar.
5. Once the catch is made, stand erect.

A common problem in executing the clean and snatch is pulling with the arms before the body is completely extended. Make sure you extend onto the balls of your feet and shrug your shoulders, then pull yourself down and under the bar as quickly as possible. Elevate your feet off the platform to help accelerate your body under the bar. As your feet are in the air, move them into a squat stance to catch the bar. Be careful not to spread your feet too wide. Some other tips:

- As the bar lands on your shoulders, throw your elbows up hard (clean).
- As the bar is caught overhead, press up and out hard on the bar (snatch).
- Keep your chest up and back straight.

Now that you understand the correct technique for the clean and snatch we can build off of these basics with some related exercises.

# CLEAN SHRUG

**Purpose:** To allow the lifter to execute the triple extension without involving the arms. This movement must be mastered for success in the power clean.

**Start Position:** Place feet hip-width apart and slightly pointed out; flex hips and bend knees. Extend arms completely with elbows pointing out, making sure shoulders are directly above the bar (see position 3 of the power clean). Position the bar on boxes or in power rack so shoulders, bar, and insteps of the feet are aligned.

**Procedure:**

1. Extend your hips and knees explosively.
2. Extend up onto the balls of the feet while simultaneously shrugging the shoulders.

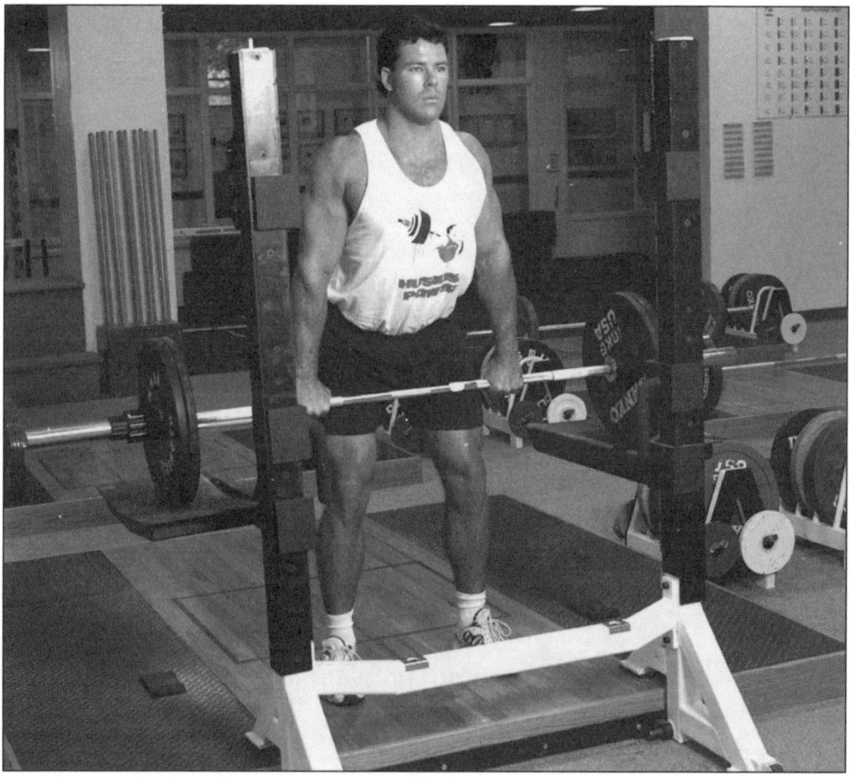

**Key Point:** Keep the bar in constant contact with the thighs, and keep your arms completely extended during the entire movement.

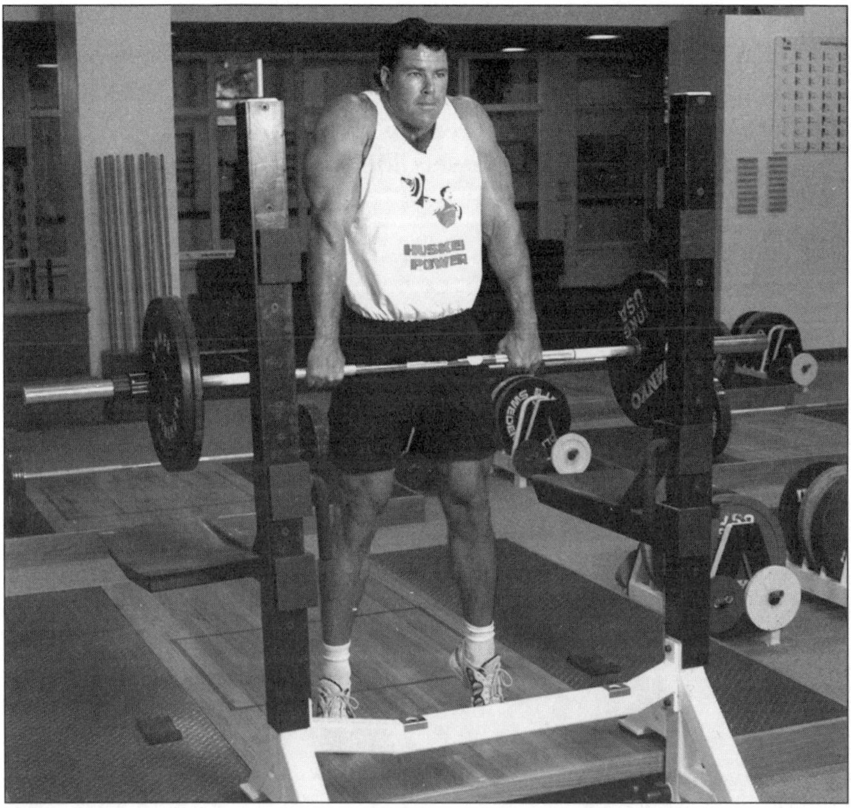

# RACK CLEAN

**Purpose:** To develop the explosive phase of the pull and to learn how to get under the bar quickly

**Start Position:** Keep feet hip-width apart and slightly pointed out; flex hips slightly and bend knees. Extend arms completely, with elbows pointing out and shoulders directly above the bar. Position the bar on boxes or in power rack so your shoulders, bar, and insteps are aligned (see position 3).

**Procedure:**

1. Extend your hips and knees explosively.
2. Extend onto the balls of your feet while simultaneously shrugging your shoulders.
3. Pull yourself down and under the bar; elevate your feet and move them into a squatting stance.

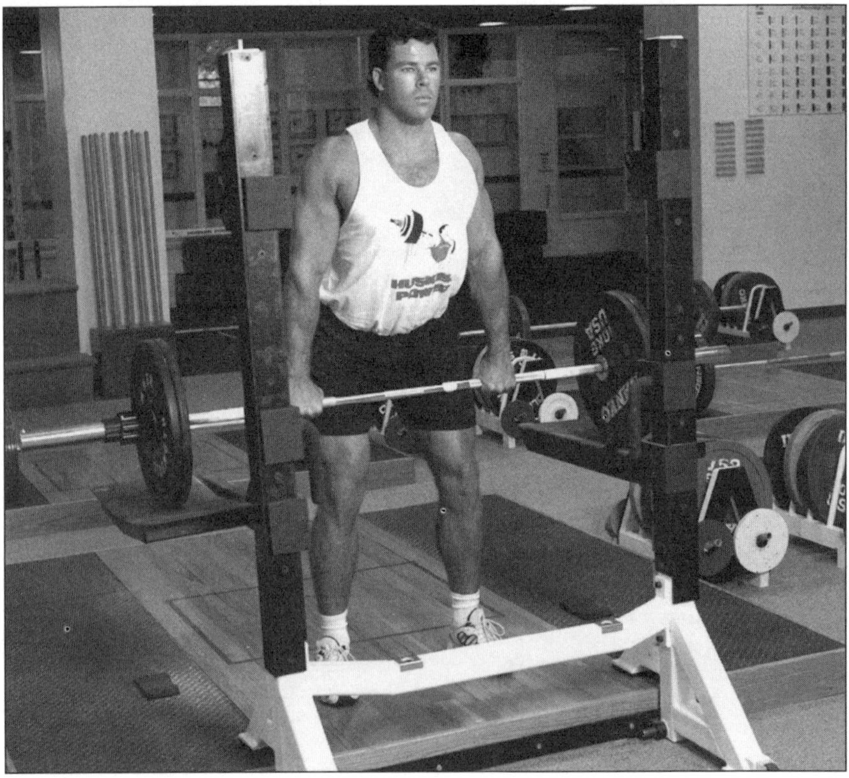

4. Rotate elbows down and then up ahead of the bar; catch bar on front portion of your shoulders.
5. Flex your knees and hips to absorb the weight of the bar.

**Key Point:** A common problem is pulling with the arms before the body is completely extended. Extend up onto the balls of your feet and shrug your shoulders. Then pull yourself down and under the bar as quickly as possible.

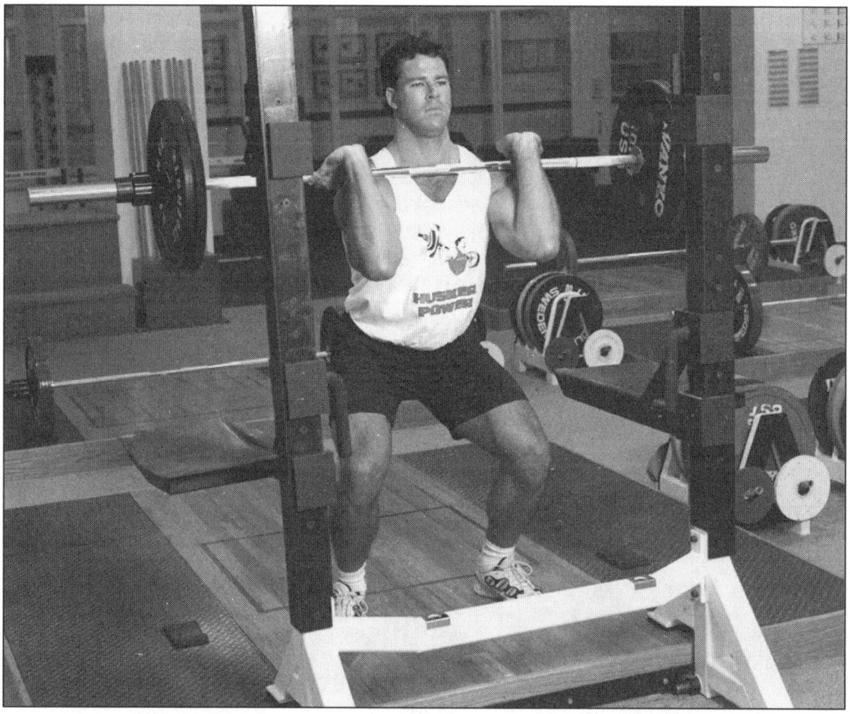

# HANG CLEAN

**Purpose:** To develop explosive power in the hips and legs

**Start Position:** Stand erect holding the bar with an overhand grip slightly wider than shoulder width and extend arms completely. Keep your feet hip-width apart (use the legs to lift the bar off the ground).

**Procedure:**

1. Lower the bar to the top of the knees by flexing at the hips (position 2) and knees.
2. Position shoulders ahead of the bar.
3. Extend the hips up and forward explosively (position 3).
4. Extend up onto the balls of the feet while simultaneously shrugging the shoulders (position 4).
5. Pull yourself down and under the bar.

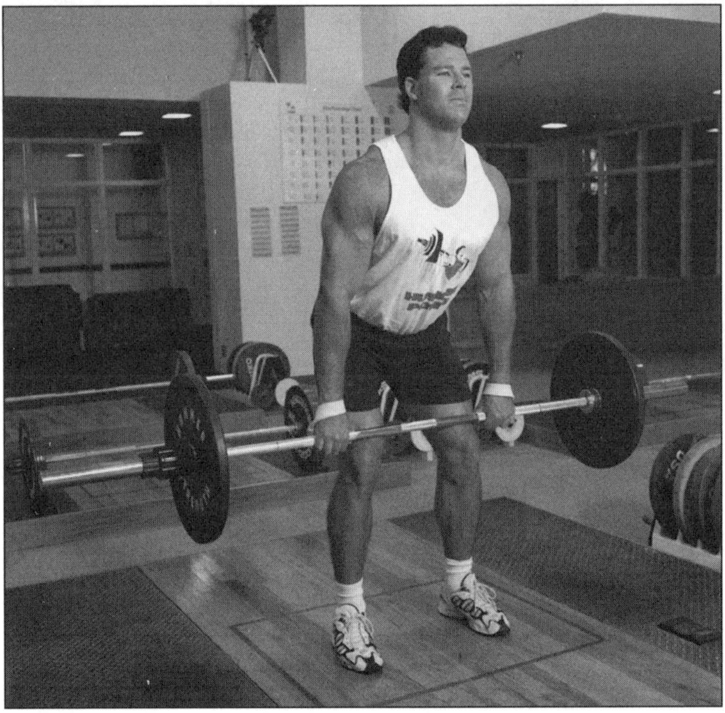

6. Rotate elbows down and then up ahead of the bar.
7. Elevate the feet and move them into a squatting stance.
8. Catch bar on the front portion of the shoulders, flexing knees and hips to absorb the weight of the bar (position 5).

**Key Point:** When lowering the bar don't hesitate at the top of the knees; extend the hips right away. This allows you to take advantage of the stretch-shortening cycle.

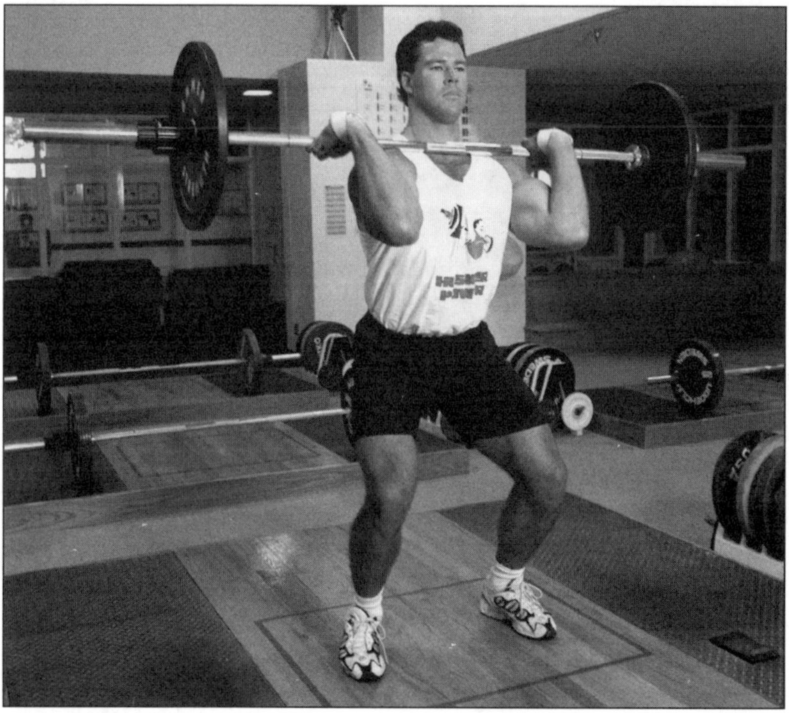

## Determining Width of Snatch Grip

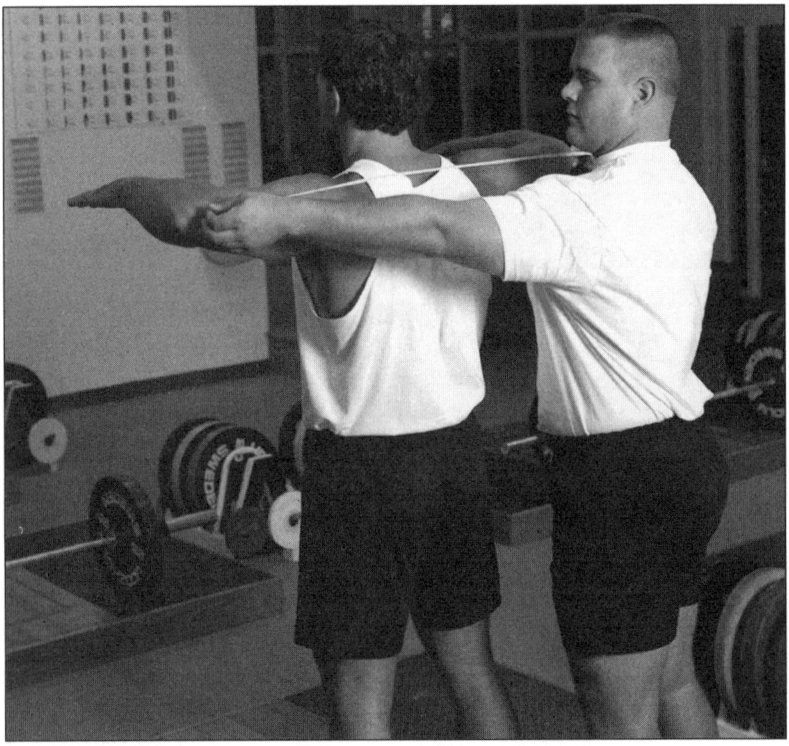

**Purpose:** To determine your proper grip for all snatch movements. A wider grip can be used so the bar does not have to be pulled as high to receive the bar overhead.

**Procedure:**

1. Hold your arms out to your sides parallel to the ground and flex your elbows at 90 degrees.
2. Have someone measure from one elbow to the other to get the distance of the grip between your hands.

# BOX SNATCH

**Purpose:** To develop the explosive phase of the pull and to learn how to get under the bar quickly

**Start Position:** Keep your feet hip-width apart and slightly pointed out, and flex your hips and knees. Using a snatch grip, extend arms, point elbows out, and place shoulders directly above the bar. Position the bar on boxes or in power rack so that the shoulders, bar, and insteps of the feet are aligned (see position 3).

**Procedure:**

1. Extend your hips and knees explosively.
2. Extend onto the balls of the feet while simultaneously shrugging the shoulders.
3. Pull yourself down and under the bar.
4. Elevate the feet and move them out into a squatting stance.

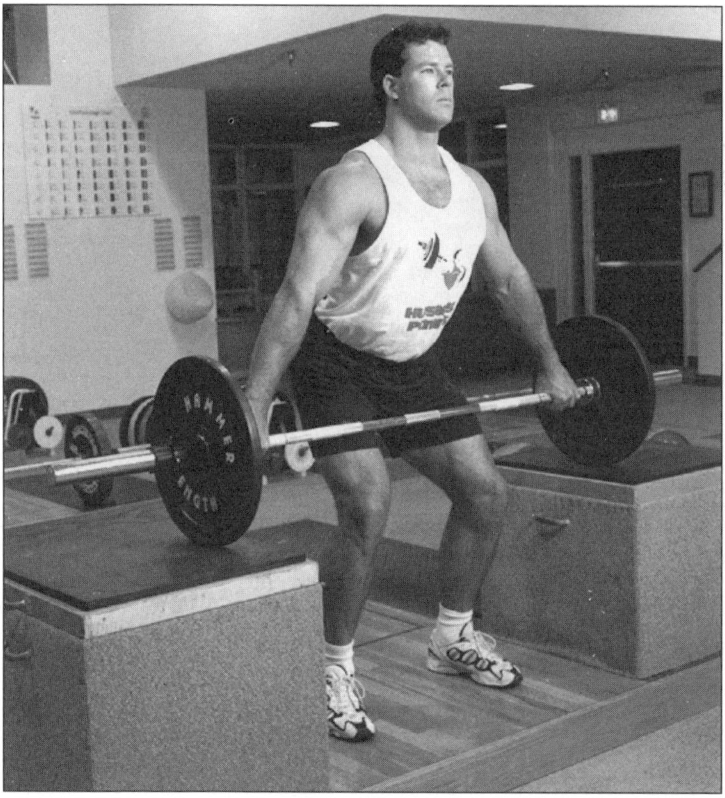

5. Extend the arms and catch the bar overhead (snatch position 6), flexing the knees and hips to absorb the weight of the bar.
6. Once the catch is made, stand erect.

**Key Point:** A common problem is pulling with your arms before your body is completely extended. Make sure you extend up onto the balls of the feet and shrug your shoulders, then pull yourself down and under the bar as quickly as possible.

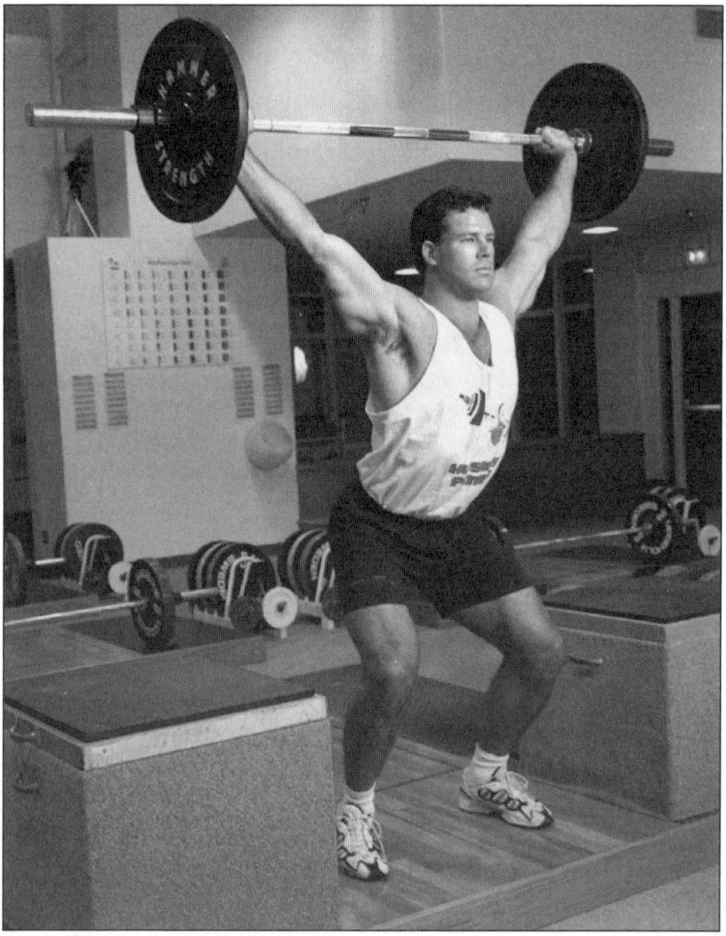

# HANG SNATCH

**Purpose:** To develop explosive power in the hips and legs

**Start Position:** Use a snatch grip and extend arms completely with elbows pointed out. Use your legs to lift the bar off the ground. Slowly extend your legs and stand erect with the bar resting on the top part of your thighs.

**Procedure:**

1. Lower the bar to your mid-thigh by flexing your hips (position 2) and knees.
2. Position shoulders ahead of the bar and extend your hips and knees explosively.
3. Extend up onto the balls of the feet while simultaneously shrugging the shoulders.

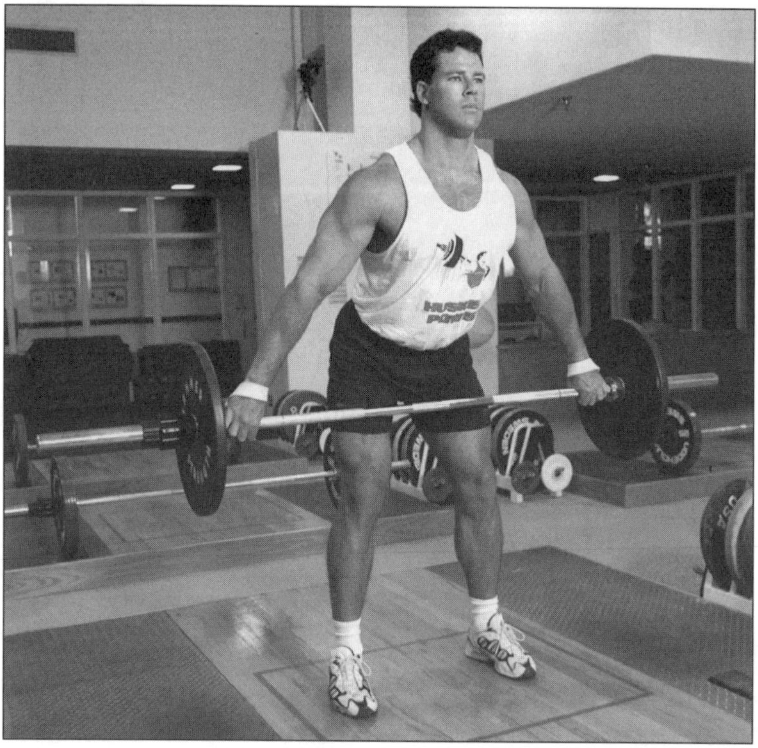

4. Pull yourself down and under the bar.
5. Elevate the feet and move them out into a squatting stance.
6. Extend the arms and catch the bar overhead (snatch position 6), flexing the knees and hips to absorb the weight of the bar.
7. Once the catch is made, stand erect.

**Key Point:** When the bar is lowered, don't hesitate at the top of the knees; extend your hips right away to take advantage of the stretch-shortening cycle.

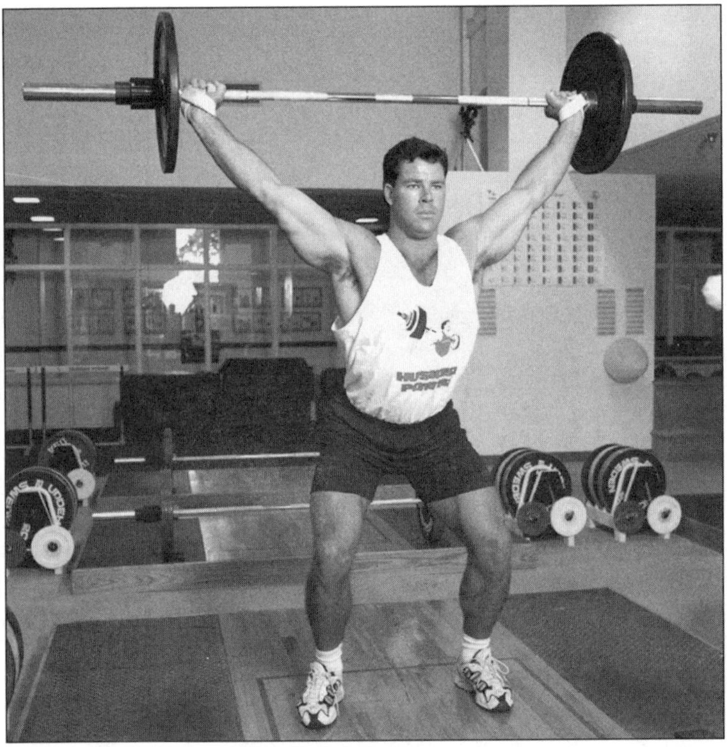

# POWER PRESS

**Purpose:** To develop power in the hips and legs, and to strengthen the shoulder muscles

**Start Position:** Place a bar behind your neck on the shoulders. Stand erect with feet shoulder-width apart, and grip the bar a little wider than shoulder-width apart.

**Procedure:**

1. Dip to a quarter squat position.
2. Extend explosively onto the balls of the feet.
3. Press the bar by extending the arms completely.

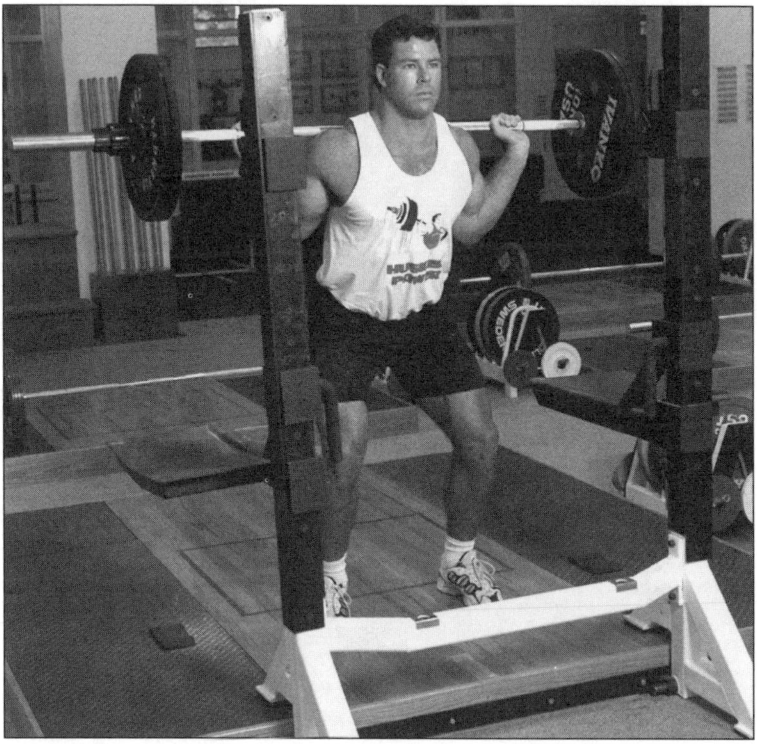

**Key Point:** Do not drop under the bar on this exercise. The drive from the legs will carry the bar about halfway up. Complete the lift by pressing the bar up with the legs straight.

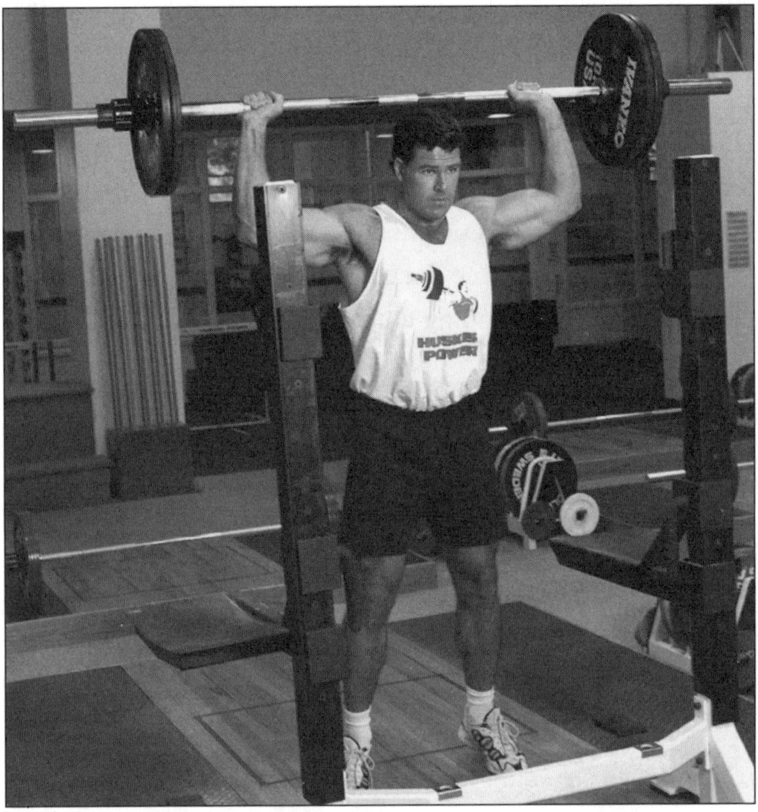

## COMPLEMENTARY EXERCISES

Complement the explosive exercises with exercise machines to train multiple plane movements at high speeds. Changing direction with cutting maneuvers during football plays requires the hip and knee joints not only to extend, but also to rotate or twist. All of the explosive exercises we have outlined are done with free weights using movements caused by extension of the hips, knees, and ankles, with minimum rotation at the hips. Many of the following complementary exercises involve using the Jammer machine, which allows simultaneous explosive rotation and extension movements. The major explosive exercises do not include unilateral movement exercises—exercises that utilize the triple extension with one leg at a time. Football uses unilateral movements frequently, and the Jammer allows these movements. The Jammer is a savior during the in-season when hand and wrist injuries make it difficult to do some of the major explosive exercises.

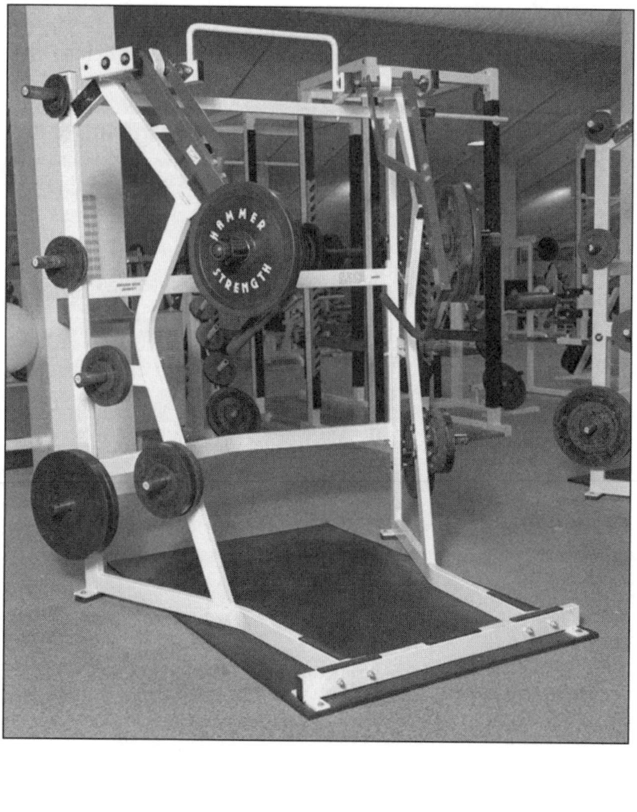

## Ground-Based Jammer

There is an unlimited variety of explosive and slow-movement exercises that can be done with the Jammer. The following exercises deal with the explosive movements. Keep these guidelines in mind when doing any explosive exercises on the Jammer:

1. Determine the correct starting position by noting where your body is positioned at the end of the movement. Start with a light weight to determine where your body finishes. If your body finishes the movement in a straight alignment, then your starting position is correct. If your body doesn't finish in a straight alignment, reposition your feet either forward or backward. Typically, taller athletes need to place their feet farther back than shorter athletes.
2. Flex your hips, knees, and ankles, and make sure your elbows are at your sides before applying force to the Jammer.
3. Extend your hips to start any exercise movement.
4. Finish the exercise with your body positioned in a straight alignment.
5. Lower the weight with control; do not let the lever arm bang.

# JAMMER EXTENSION

**Purpose:** To develop total body power by utilizing a ground-based, multiple-joint movement

**Start Position:** Grasp the handles with your hands as close as possible and your shoulders directly behind your hands. Place your elbows at your sides. Position your feet shoulder-width apart with your heels off the ground, and flex your knees and hips.

**Procedure:**

1. Rock backward, then move forward to the starting position to gain momentum.
2. Explode into the handles by extending at the hips.
3. Follow through by extending your knees, shoulders, ankles, and elbows simultaneously.

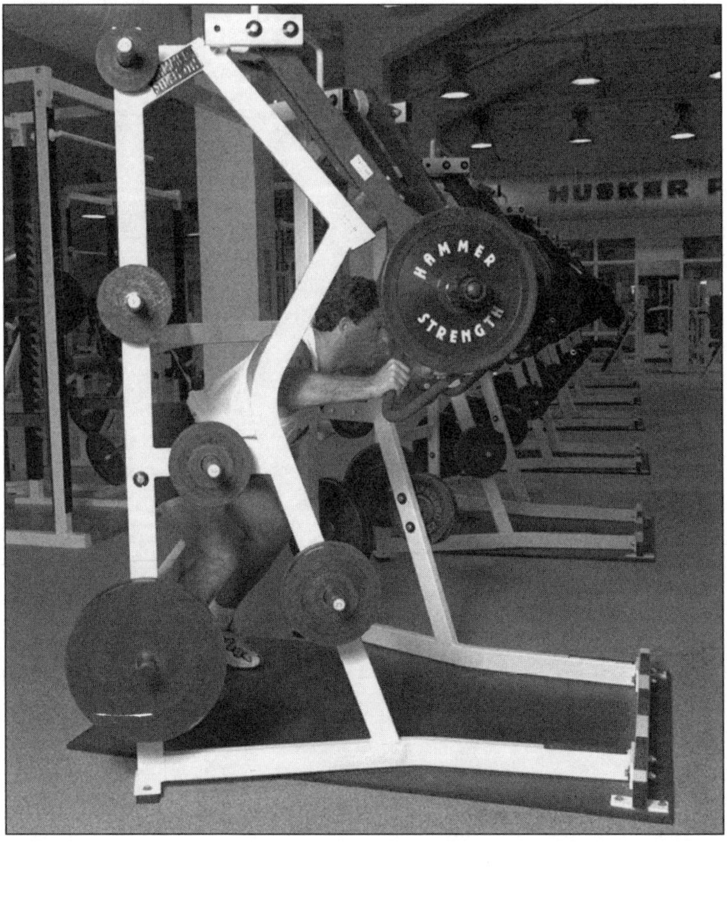

**Key Points:**

1. When rocking backward keep your shoulders below your hands to help maintain the proper hip and knee flexion.
2. Before you extend your hips make sure your shoulders are close to your hands and the elbows are beside your torso.
3. At the end of the exercise be sure your body is aligned straight from your feet to your hands.

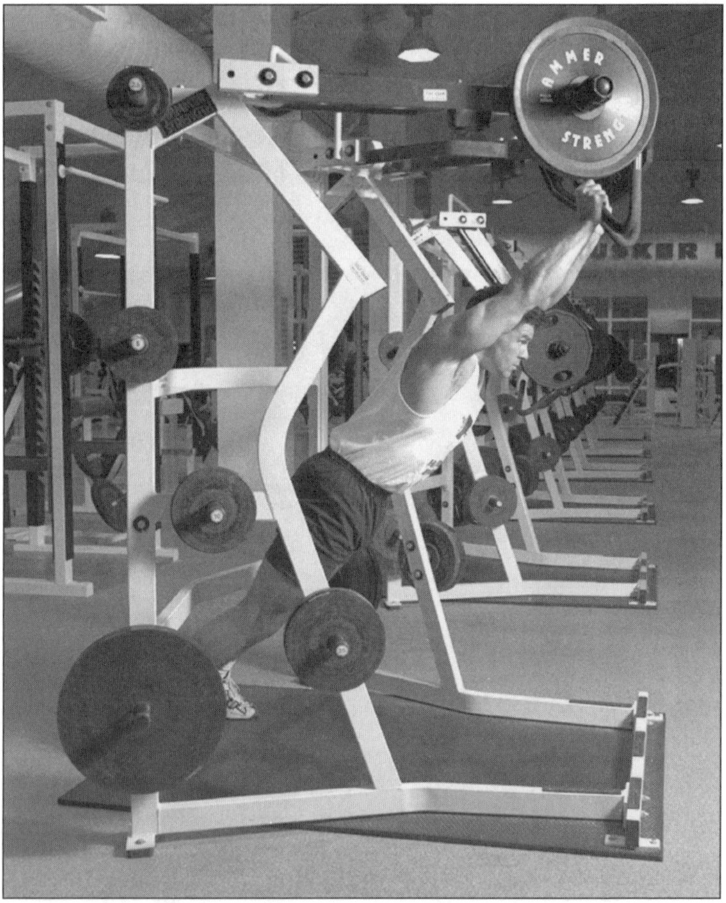

# JAMMER ROTATION

**Purpose:** To develop rotational power in the hips, legs, and torso (but not to simulate rotational sport skills)

**Start Position:** (The following description assumes you are facing the left side of the machine so that your body rotates to the left.) Face the right arm of the machine and grasp the handle with your left hand placed below your right hand. Stand with your feet perpendicular to the lever arm, hip-width apart, and lower your body so your chest is at the height of your hands.

**Procedure:**

1. Drive with your left leg and arm while simultaneously rotating your body 90 degrees.
2. Simultaneously step forward slightly to the side with your right foot.
3. Extend onto the toes of your left foot as it rotates.

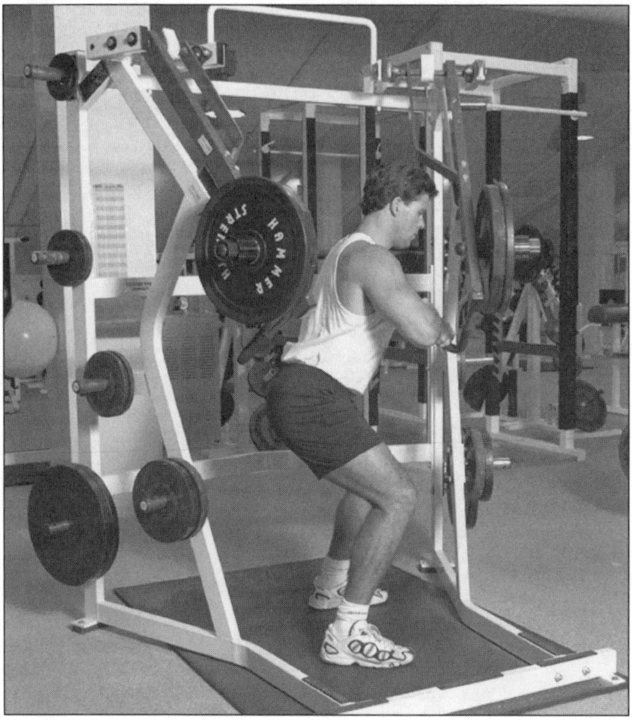

4. Land flat on your right foot with your right leg bent at the knee.
5. Finish with your body aligned in a straight line from your left foot to your left hand, and your feet, hips, and shoulders in a square alignment.

**Key Points:**

1. Your body weight should feel like it is on the front foot at the finish.
2. The right hand can leave the handle as the body rotates, leading with the right elbow.

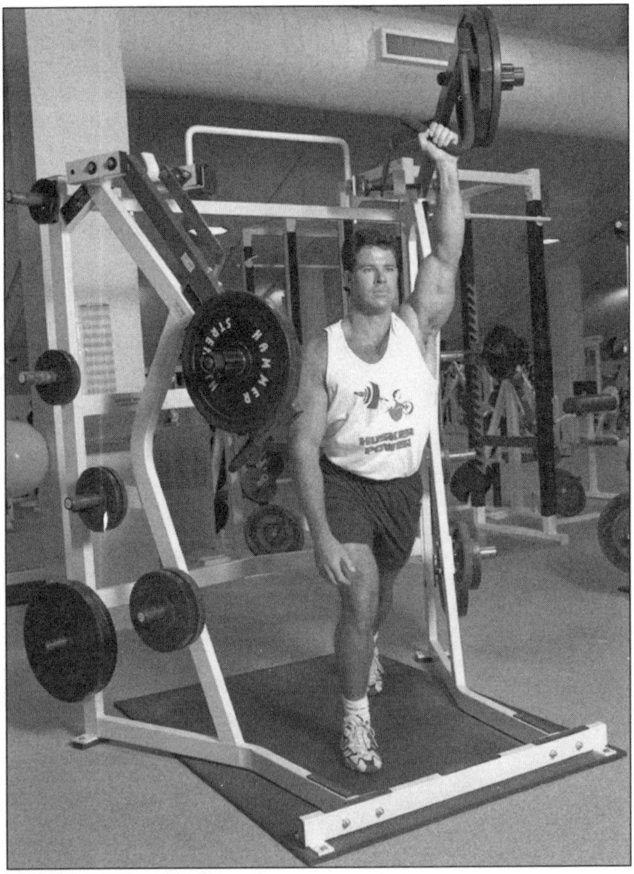

# JAMMER PRESS

**Purpose:** To develop the chest, shoulders, and triceps. The shoulder girdle muscles are also called into play as stabilizers.

**Start Position:** Grasp the handles with hands as close together as possible, and position the shoulders directly behind the hands. Do not allow the shoulders to be positioned higher than the hands. Place your elbows at your side. Position your feet shoulder-width apart, flat on the ground. If your feet are directly below the shoulders, the chest is the prime mover. The more your feet are placed behind your shoulders, the more your shoulders are called upon to serve as prime movers. Flex your knees and hips.

**Procedure:**

1. Press the handles by extending the arms.
2. Keep your hips, knees, and ankles flexed.

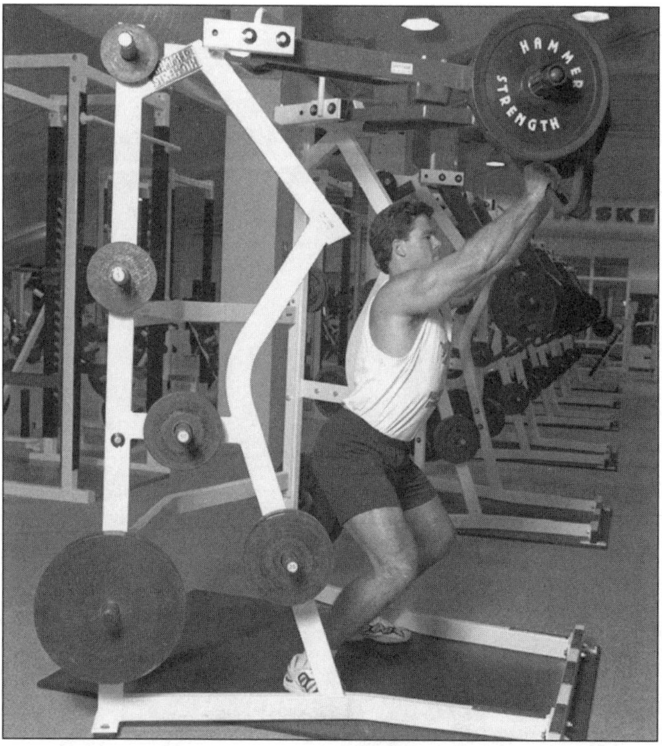

# BASE STRENGTH EXERCISES

The base strength exercises allow multiple joint and ground-based movements at slow speeds.

## CLEAN DEAD LIFT

**Purpose:** To learn how to lift the bar off the ground properly, and to develop the leg, hip, back, and trapezius muscles. Use this lift as a warm-up or as a strength movement.

**Start Position:** Same as position 1 (see page 108).

**Procedure:**

1. Slowly extend legs, elevating the bar to just above the knees (see position 2).
2. Extend hips forward and up.

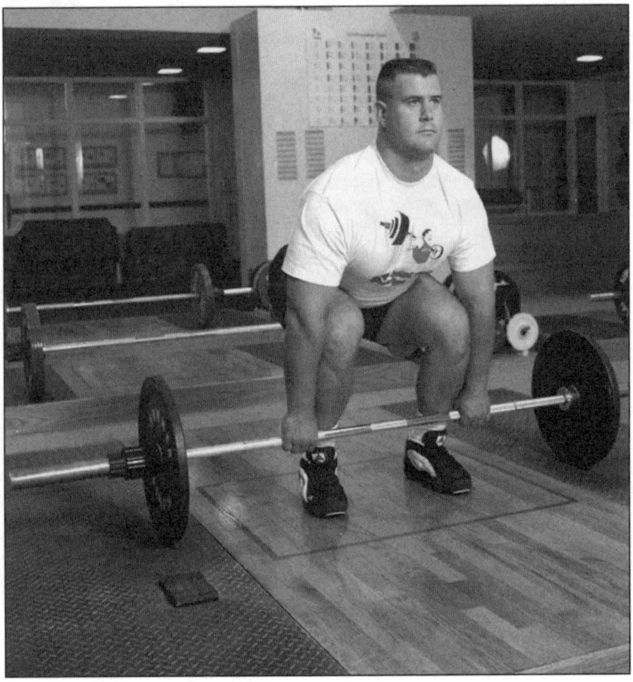

3. Extend up onto the balls of your feet while simultaneously shrugging the shoulders.
4. Align shoulders, hips, and knees as the lift is completed (see position 4).

**Key Points:**

1. Keep the movement of the bar from floor to knees continuous and close to the legs. The shoulders, hips, and bar should move together as a controlled unit.
2. Accelerate the bar as it passes the knees and have the bar ride up the thighs. (Do not bounce the bar off the thighs.)
3. Keep your arms extended with elbows pointed out, and keep your back flat with lower back slightly arched.

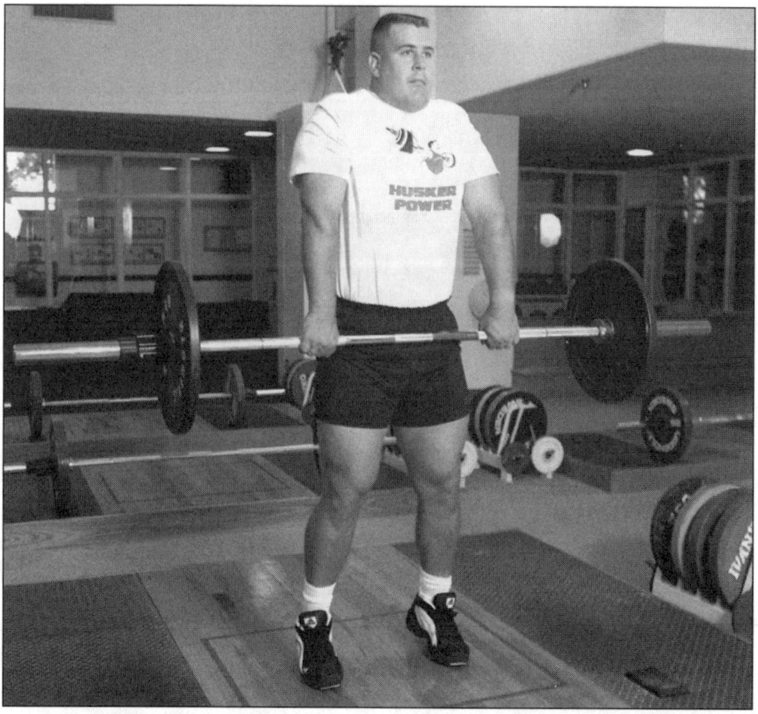

# SQUAT

**Purpose:** To develop the quadriceps, thigh adductors, gluteus maximus, and hamstrings. When done correctly, full squats build up the muscles, ligaments, and tendons surrounding the knee. Keeping the torso erect isometrically contracts the spinal erectors, also developing them to a large degree.

**Start Position:** With the bar chest high on the racks, position hands slightly wider than shoulder width. Step under the bar, keeping feet parallel, knees slightly bent, and hips vertically aligned with your shoulders. Place bar comfortably across the top of the shoulders at the base of the neck or one inch below the top of the shoulders across the traps. Pull your shoulder blades together tightly and lift the bar out of the rack by extending the knees. Step backward, using as few steps as possible, with feet parallel. Point toes out somewhat and keep heels slightly wider than the hips.

**Procedure:**

1. Focus your eyes on the wall with head slightly up; take a deep breath and hold it.

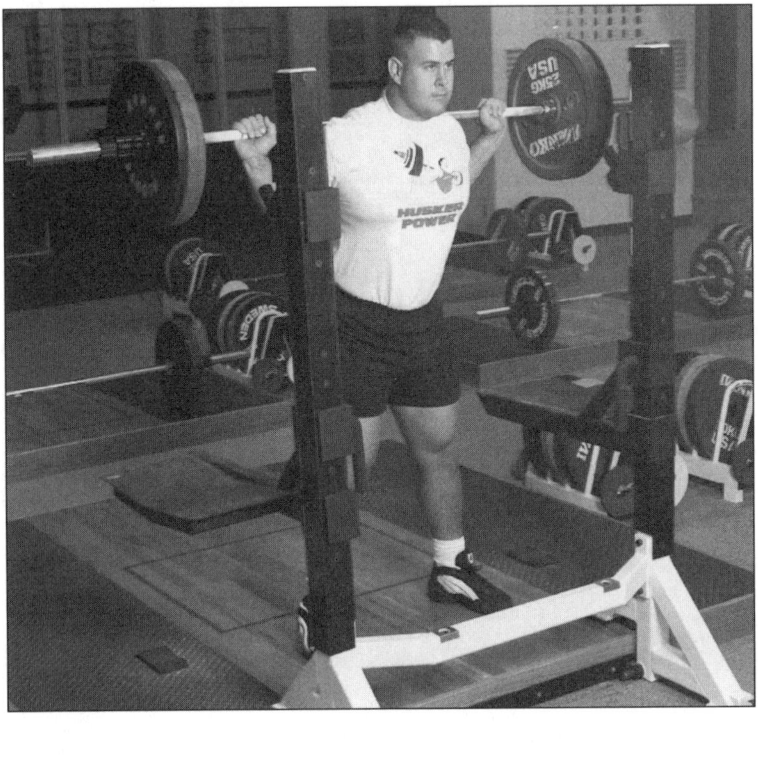

2. In a slow and controlled motion, lower the bar by bending your hips and knees and keeping your knees pointed out in alignment with the feet.
3. The instant your thighs are parallel to the floor, explode up from the bottom.
4. Keep your back flat, weight on your heels, and shoulder blades drawn together. Don't throw your head back.
5. Fully extend your knees and hips and exhale as you near the completion of the lift.

**Key Points:**

1. Don't try to bounce out of the bottom of this lift. If you try to recover to an upright position after bouncing, you will raise your hips too quickly, causing your back to round out and take the stress of the lift. It is imperative to descend slowly and under control.
2. Keep your shoulder blades together. If they relax, your lower back will round out. The closer together you place your hands on the bar, the tighter you can pull your shoulder blades.
3. Picking a spot on the wall in front of you to focus on helps keep your body stable.
4. Squat inside the rack, or use two or three spotters.

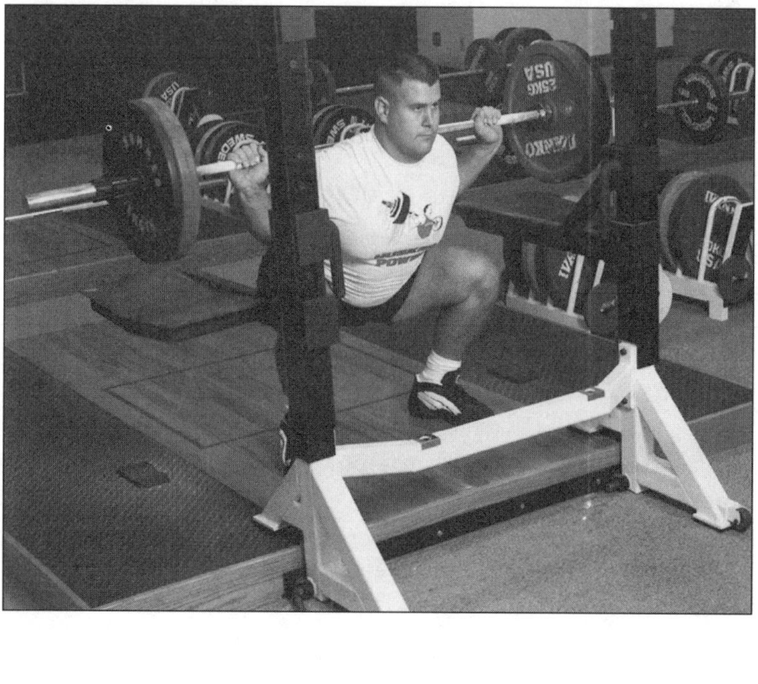

# FRONT SQUAT

**Purpose:** To develop the quadriceps, thigh adductors, gluteus maximus, and hamstrings. When done correctly, full squats build the muscles, ligaments, and tendons surrounding the knee. This exercise is great for athletes who have problems keeping erect during back squats. If an erect position is not maintained during this lift, the bar will tumble forward.

**Start Position:** Place the bar chest high on the racks. Step under the bar and position feet parallel with knees slightly bent. Place the bar comfortably on the front of your shoulders in one of two positions:

- **Clean style:** Place hands on the bar slightly wider than shoulder width and rotate elbows up so they are in front of the bar.
- **Cross-arm style:** Cross arms in front of shoulder and place hands on top of bar with elbows high.

Align hips vertically with the shoulders and lift bar out of rack by extending the knees. Step backward using as few steps as possible.

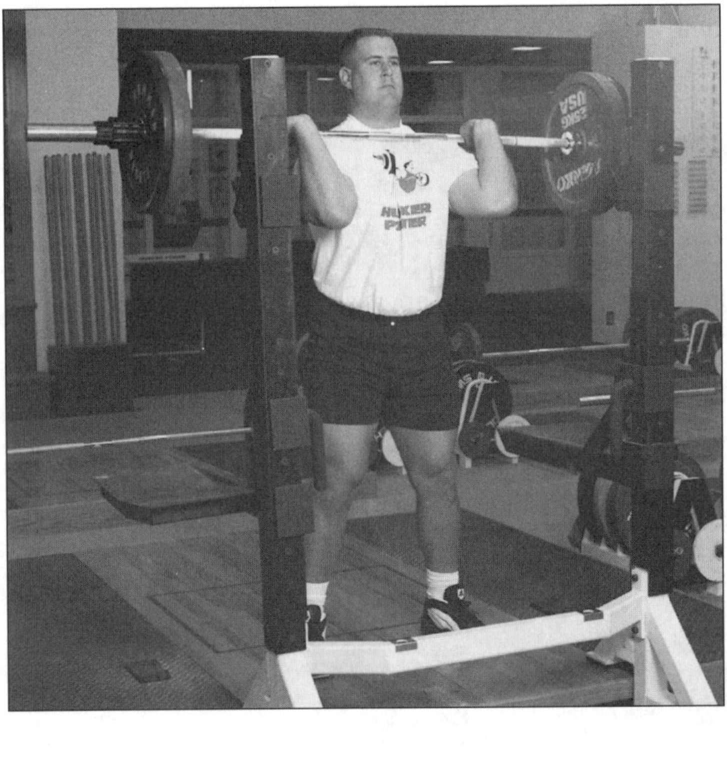

Position feet so they are parallel, toes pointed out slightly, and heels slightly wider than the hips.

**Procedure:**

1. Focus eyes on the wall looking straight ahead, take a deep breath, and hold it.
2. In a slow and controlled motion, lower the bar by bending at the hips and knees. (Keep your knees pointed out and aligned with the feet.)
3. The instant the thighs reach parallel, explode out of the bottom of the lift.
4. Keep your back flat and your weight back on your heels, and do not throw your head back.
5. Fully extend the knees and hips and exhale as you complete the lift.

**Key Points:**

1. Don't try to bounce out of the bottom.
2. Pick a spot on the wall in front of you to focus on throughout the lift. This helps control the bar by keeping your body stable.
3. Squat inside the rack, or use two or three spotters.

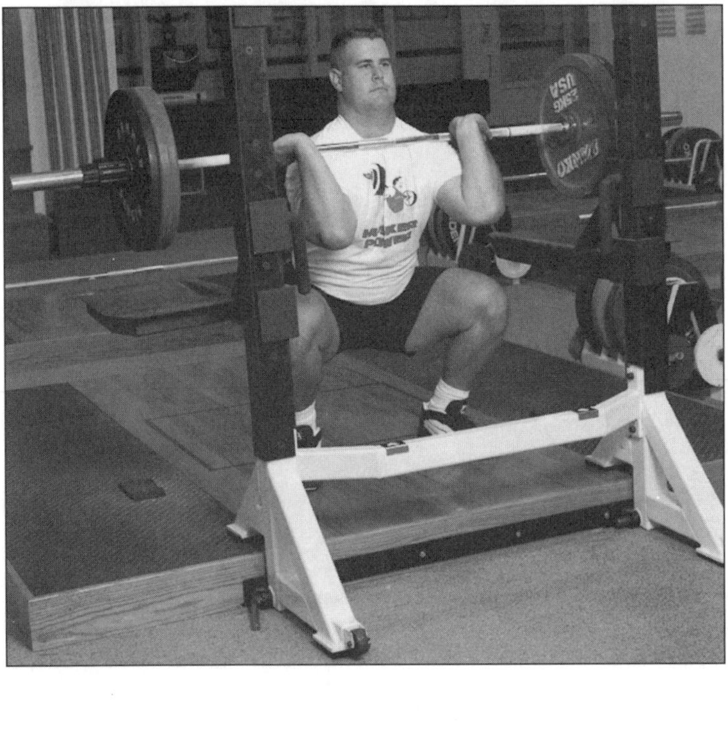

# SNATCH SQUAT

**Purpose:** To strengthen the catching phase of the snatch and to develop hip mobility and balance

**Start Position:** Snatch the barbell overhead and stand with feet shoulder-width apart.

**Procedure:**

1. Focus your eyes on the wall with head slightly up; take a deep breath and hold it.
2. In a slow and controlled motion, lower the bar by bending your hips and knees and keeping your knees pointed out in alignment with the feet.
3. The instant your thighs are parallel to the floor, explode up from the lift.

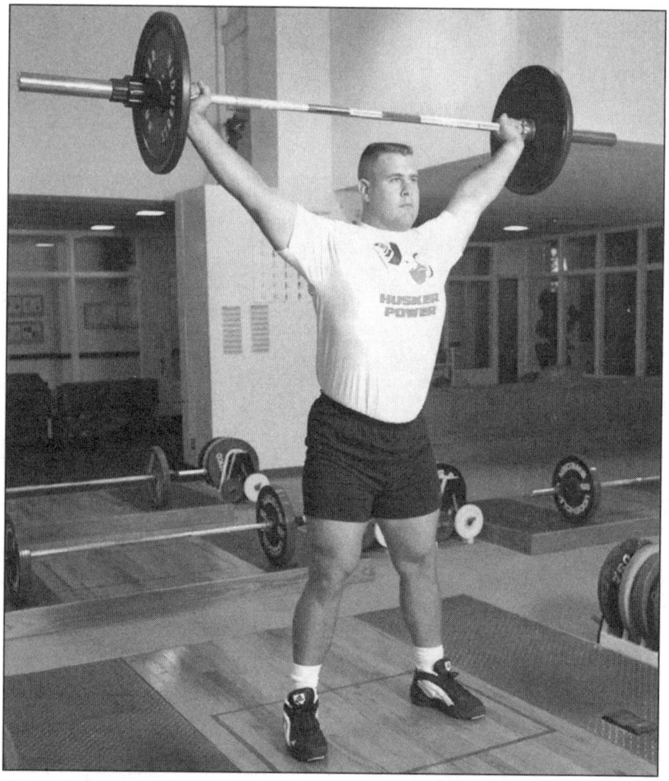

4. Keep your back flat, weight on your heels, and shoulder blades drawn together. Don't throw your head back.
5. Fully extend your knees and hips and exhale as you near the completion of the lift.

**Key Points:**

1. Press out hard on the bar during the entire movement.
2. Keep the chest up and back straight during the entire movement.
3. As you lower into the squat position keep the bar positioned behind the head.

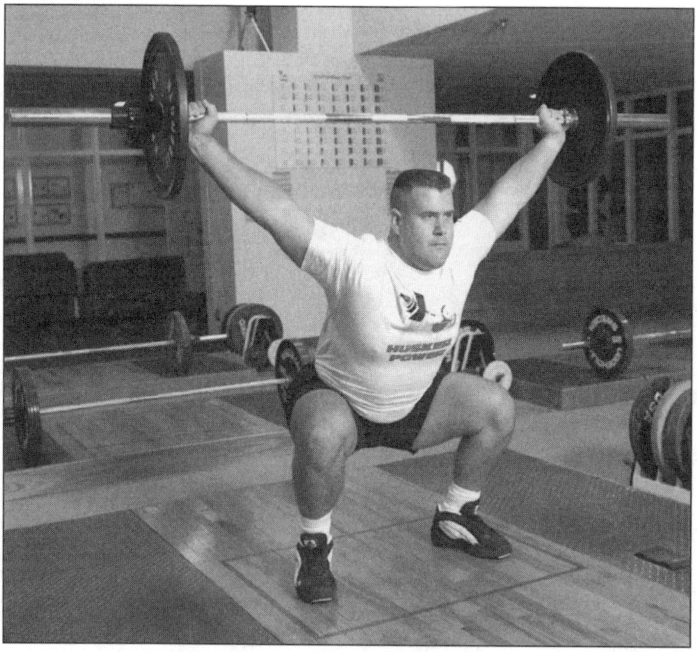

# STANDING SHOULDER PRESS

**Purpose:** To strengthen the muscles of the shoulder girdle and teach the lifter to use the whole body in stabilizing the weight overhead. This exercise is used as an introductory lift for the power press.

**Start Position:** Grip the bar a little wider than shoulder-width apart. Place the bar behind the neck on the shoulders, and stand erect with feet shoulder-width apart.

**Procedure:**

1. Press the bar overhead by extending the arms.
2. Lower the bar to starting position.

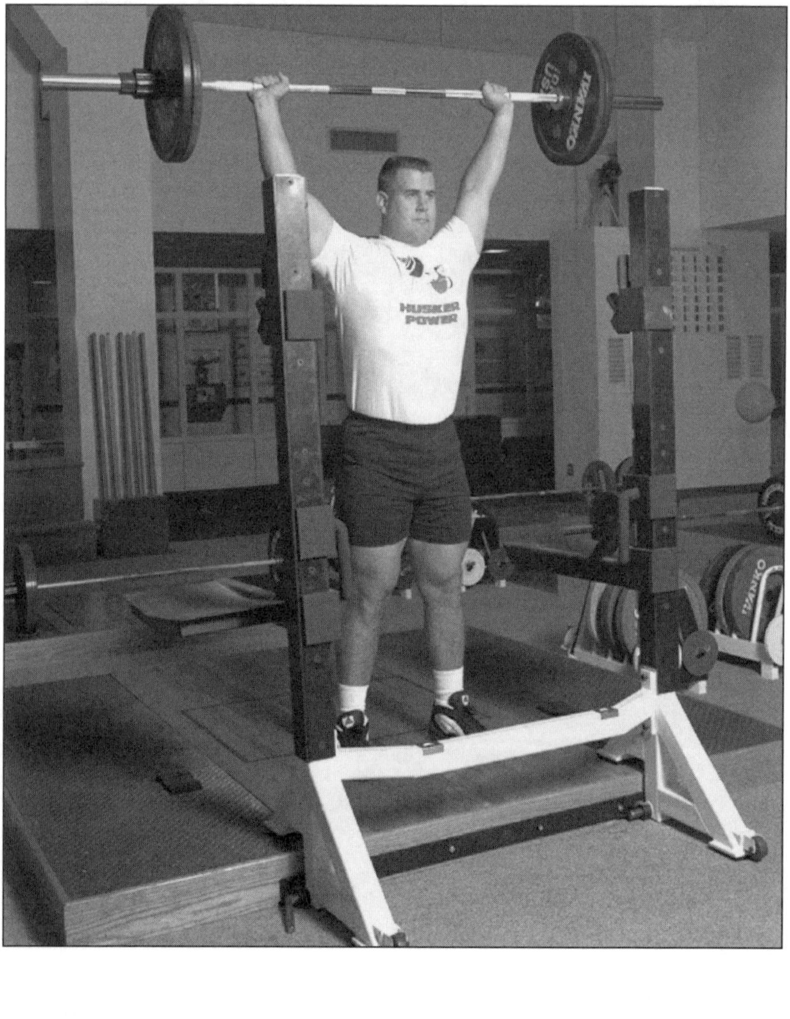

**Key Points:**

1. Keep the shoulders over the hips during the entire range of motion.
2. To help absorb the weight when lowering the bar, simultaneously bend the knees as the bar hits the shoulders.

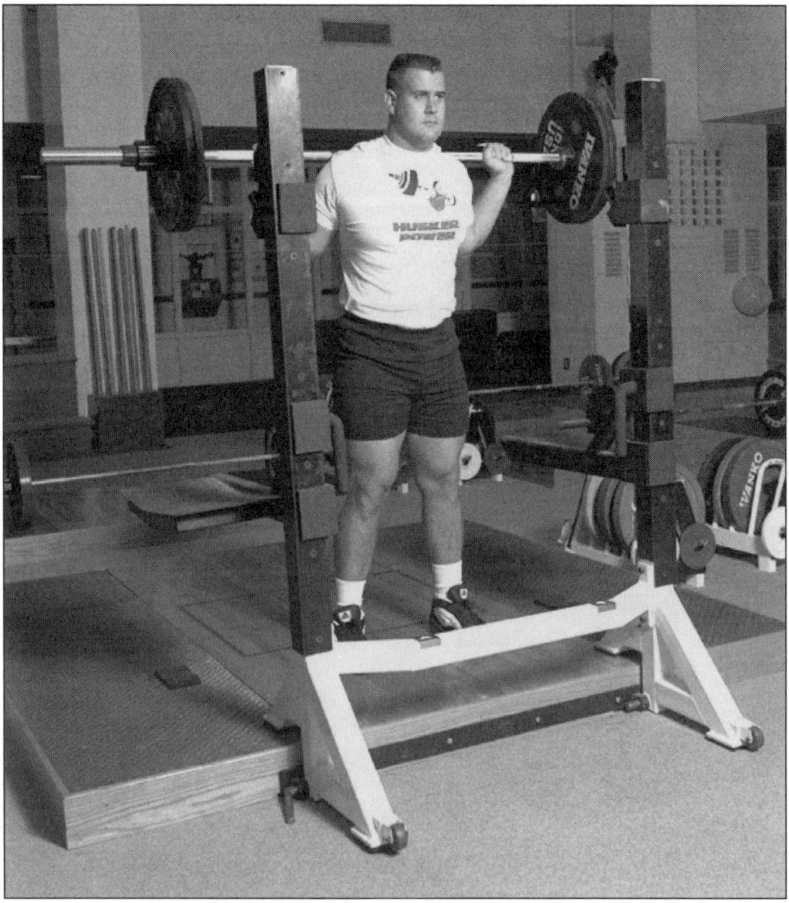

# ROMANIAN DEAD LIFT (RDL)

**Purpose:** To strengthen and develop the hamstrings and lower back. A much lighter weight is used than in the dead lift.

**Start Position:** This exercise can be done with a bar or a hammer dead lift machine. Place feet hip-width apart. Bend knees with the lower leg touching bar. Grasp the bar using an overhand grip with arms extended and hands shoulder-width apart. Stand upright with the bar by extending the legs and hips, and let the bar rest on the thighs. Fill the chest with air and hold high. Bend the knees slightly.

**Procedure:**

1. In a slow and controlled motion, lower the bar to a point just below the knees by bending at the hips. Do not touch the ground.
2. Reverse directions and pull bar back to starting position.

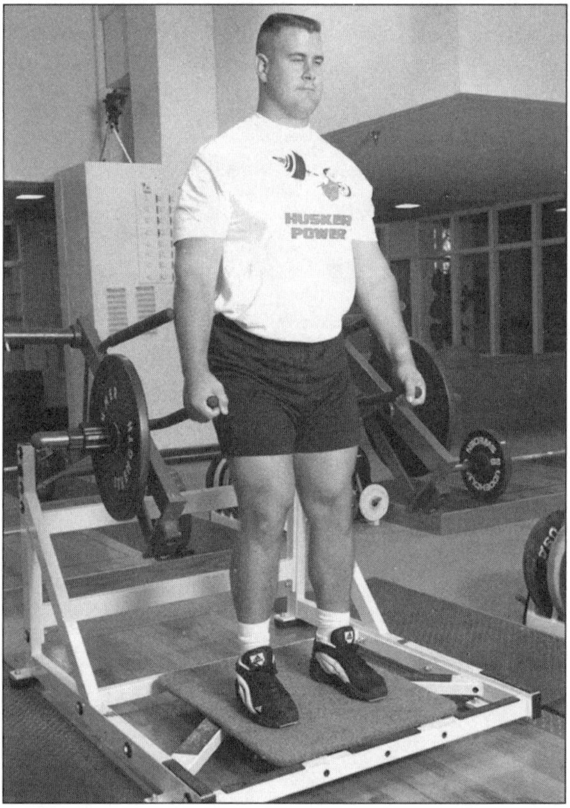

**Key Points:**

1. Keep the shoulder blades pulled together and lower back slightly arched as the bar is slowly and smoothly lowered.
2. Feel the stretch in the hamstrings as the bar is lowered. If the bar touches the ground, the tension will be taken off the hamstrings.

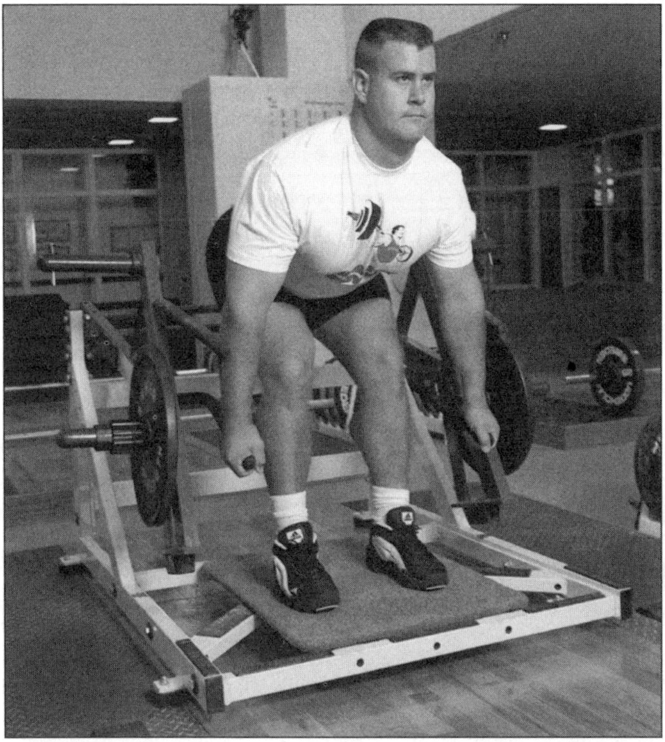

# GOOD MORNING

**Purpose:** To develop the upper hamstrings, gluteus maximus, and erector stabilizers. This exercise is used as an introductory lift for the hang clean.

**Start Position:** Grip the bar a little wider than shoulder-width apart and place the bar behind the neck on the shoulders. Stand erect with feet hip-width apart and toes pointed straight or slightly angled out. Do not place the feet as you would in the squat. Place them as if you were going to perform a vertical jump (hip-width apart).

**Procedure:**

1. Fill your chest with air and hold high.
2. Unlock the knees and bend forward, lowering the bar.
3. The hips move backward as the bar is lowered. Lower the bar until the hips cannot go back any farther.
4. Raise the bar by extending the hips forward to start position.

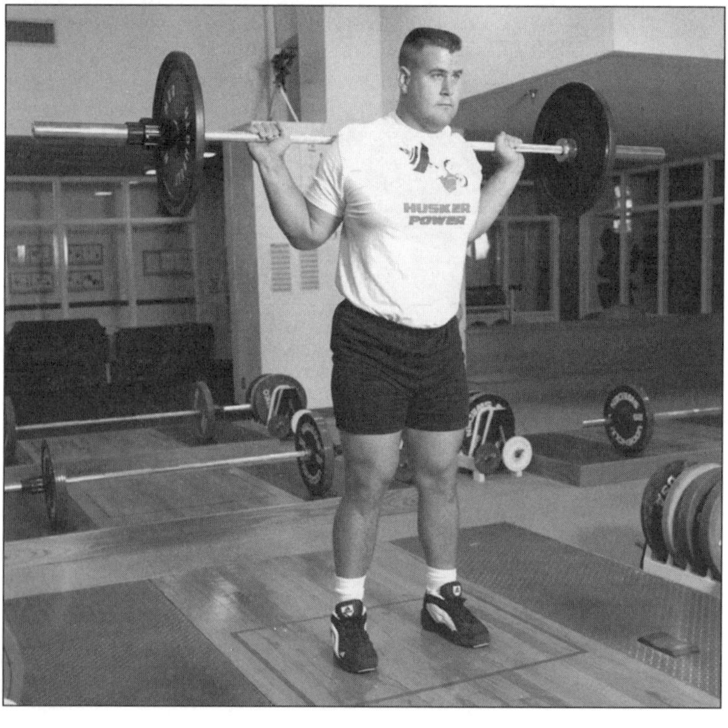

**Key Points:**

1. Keep your back flat and your lower back slightly arched at all times.
2. Move the bar vertically, with little horizontal movement, throughout the lift.

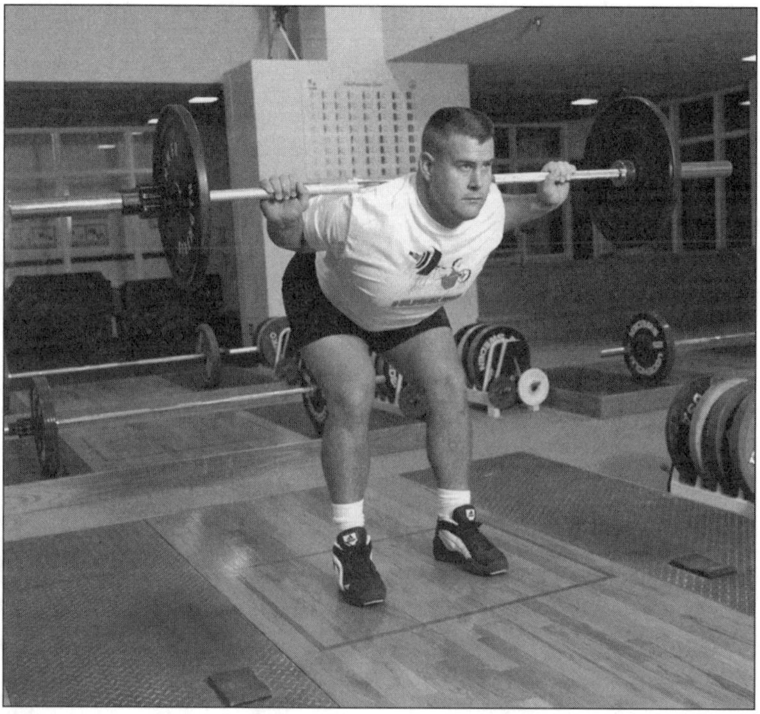

# LOW LAT PULL

**Purpose:** To develop the muscles of the upper back

**Start Position:** Grasp handle with overhand grip and hands 6 to 12 inches apart. Extend arms and sit with feet shoulder-width apart and knees slightly flexed. Lean the torso forward slightly, keeping the back flat.

**Procedure:**

1. Pull bar to the lower chest.
2. Slowly return bar to arm's length and repeat.

**Key Points:**

1. Do this exercise slowly and smoothly. Do not lean forward or backward during the movement.
2. When pulling the handle to the chest, squeeze your shoulder blades together. When returning the handle feel the stretch in the back and shoulders. Visualize the muscles of the back stretching and squeezing during the movement.

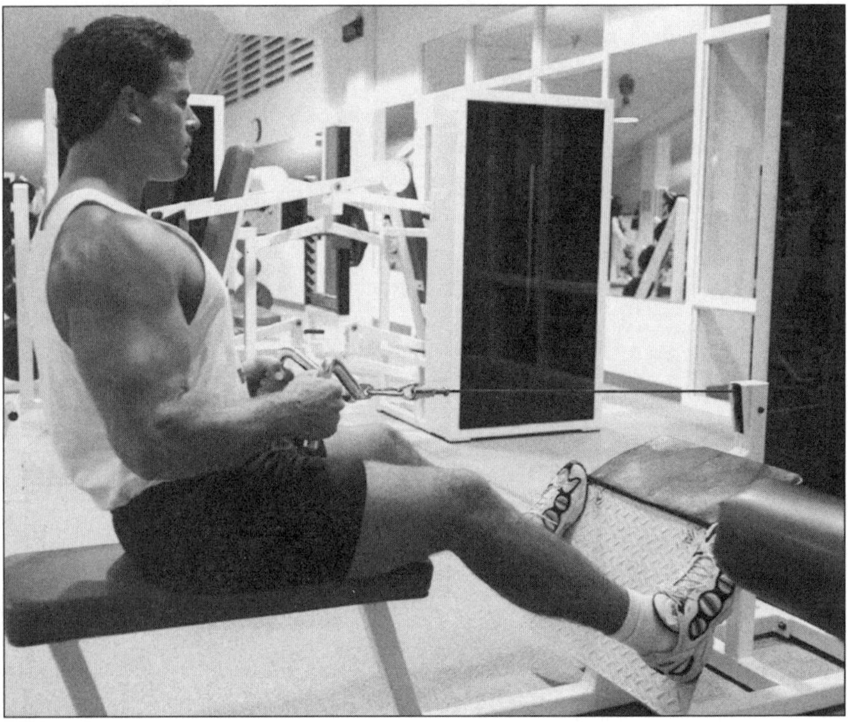

# TRUNK TWIST

**Purpose:** To develop and strengthen the rotary torso muscles of the trunk

**Start Position:** Grip a barbell plate at the three and nine o'clock positions. Line up the shoulders, hips, and feet in a squared position. Lift the plate to the front of the body so that the arms are horizontal.

**Procedure:**

1. Twist as far as possible to the left.
2. Twist back as far as possible to the right.

**Key Points:**

1. Keep the arms horizontal during the entire movement.
2. Keep the feet squared, and rotate from the waist up.
3. Do the twisting motion slowly and under control.

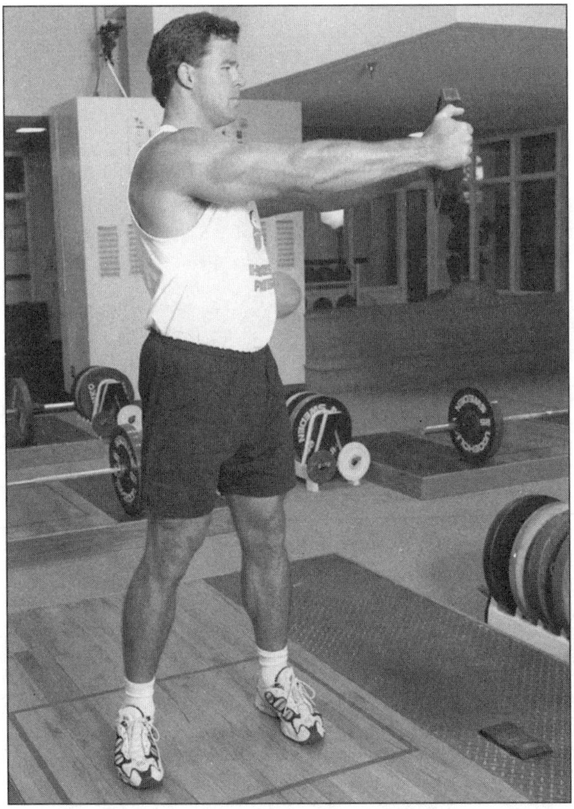

# SPECIALTY EXERCISES

During certain times of the year specialty exercises are added to the lifting program to meet a variety of special needs such as problems with injuries, correcting muscle imbalances, or developing muscular size in an isolated muscle group. The specialty exercises include multiple joint and single joint movements. Specialty exercises, whether done with free weights or machines, are always done at slow speeds. Add specialty exercises during the base phase when the major objective of the program is developing lean body mass. Beginner lifters utilize most of the specialty exercises to develop the muscle and strength necessary to advance to higher-level exercises. Or if a minor injury prevents you from doing a major exercise, a specialty exercise may allow you to maintain strength and power until you can do the major exercises again. The following specialty exercises focus on the legs, back, chest, shoulders, arms, neck, and abdominals.

## LEG EXTENSION

**Purpose:** To isolate and develop the quadriceps

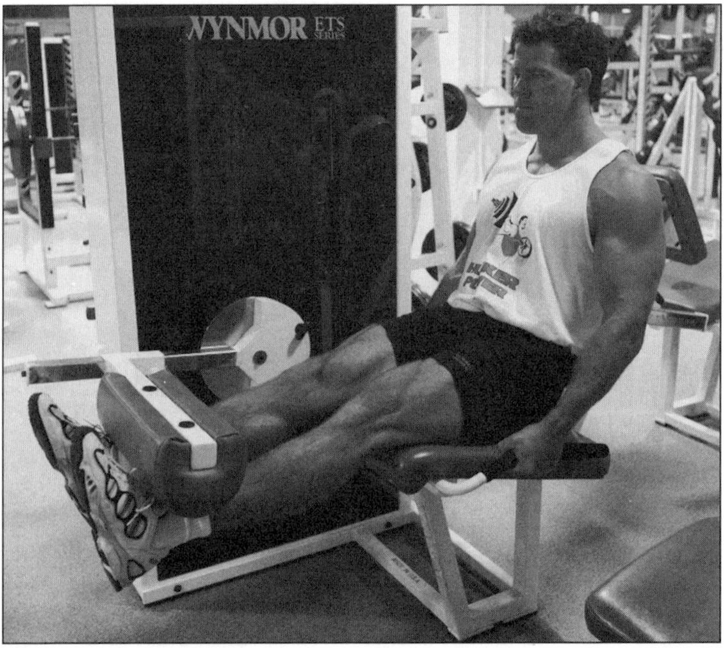

**Start Position:** Sit on a leg extension machine and hook the front of your ankles behind the roller pad. Grasp handles or the seat to keep hips down. Keep knee joints aligned with axis of machine and back flat against back rest.

**Procedure:**

1. Extend your lower legs until the knees are locked out.
2. Lower the weight slowly back to the starting position.

## LEG CURL

**Purpose:** To isolate and develop the hamstrings

**Start Position:** Lie face down on the leg curl machine bench with your knees slightly off the edge. Hook ankles under the roller pad and align knee joints with axis of machine.

**Procedure:**

1. Raise your lower legs as far as possible toward the hips.
2. Lower the weight slowly to the starting position.

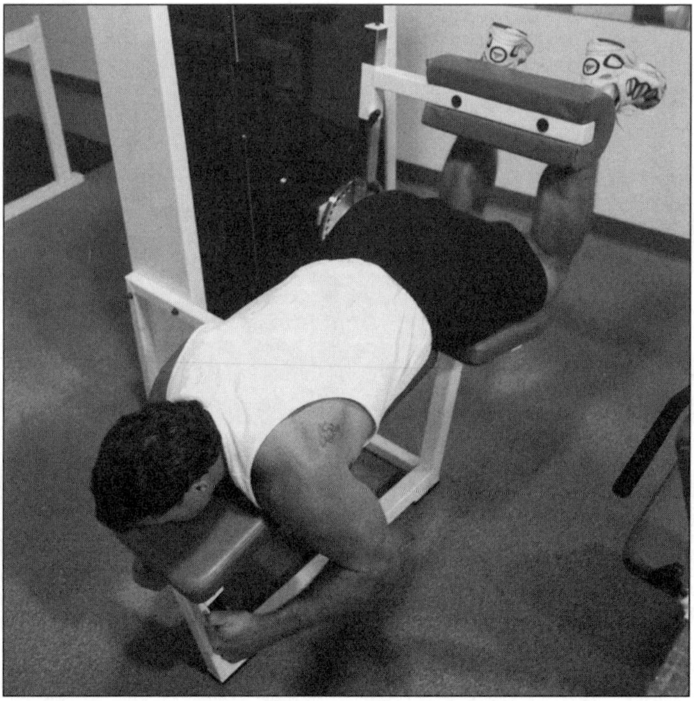

# BACK EXTENSION

**Purpose:** To strengthen the lower back (spinal erectors)

**Start Position:** Lie face down on a bench and anchor your ankles. By bending at the hips, position your hip joints at the edge of the bench so the torso hangs over the bench. Fold hands behind head and pull the shoulder blades together.

**Procedure:**

1. Raise torso until parallel with the floor.
2. Lower body to the starting position and repeat.

**Key Points:**

1. Do this exercise with slow, smooth movements.
2. To keep the torso rigid, keep the shoulder blades drawn together for the entire movement.
3. Avoid hyperextending your lower back.

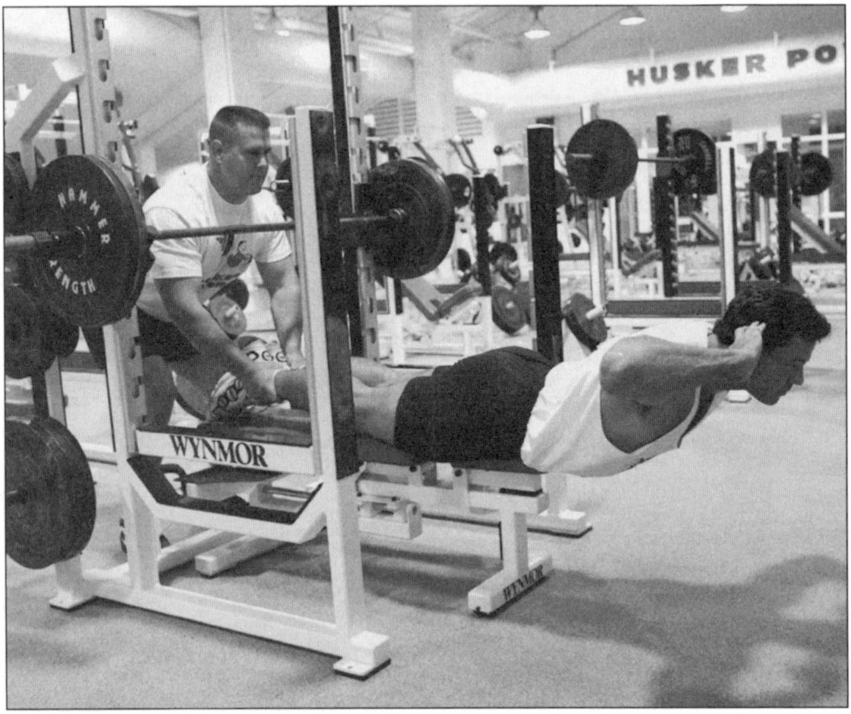

# LAT PULLDOWN

**Purpose:** To develop the muscles of the upper back

**Start Position:** Sit on a stool and anchor thighs under pads. Grip bar with an overhand grip wider than shoulder width, and allow the weight to pull upward on the shoulders and upper back.

**Procedure:**

1. Pull the bar down to the base of the neck.
2. In a controlled motion, return the bar to the starting position and repeat.

**Key Points:**

1. When returning bar to starting position, let your arms fully extend and feel the stretch in your upper back.
2. Keep your back vertical. Do this exercise in a slow, controlled manner.

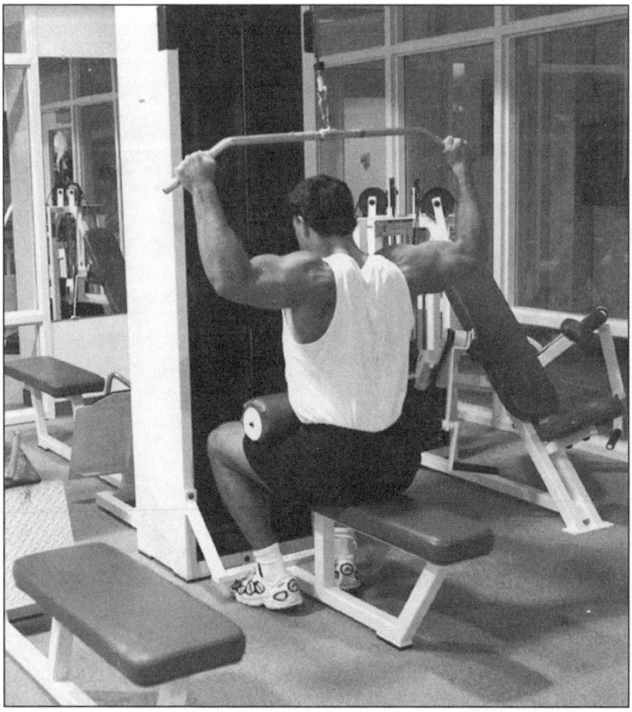

# BENCH PRESS

**Purpose:** To develop the pectoral muscles, anterior deltoids, and triceps

**Start Position:** Lie face up on a bench; make sure feet are flat on the ground and back is slightly arched. Pull your shoulder blades inward as you push your chest upward. Grip the bar slightly wider than shoulder width and position yourself so the bar lines up with the top of your head. Take the bar from the rack with the aid of a spotter and position the bar over your chest.

**Procedure:**

1. Take a deep breath, hold your chest high, and lower the bar to your chest in a slow, controlled movement.
2. Allow the bar to just touch the chest at about nipple level.
3. Drive the bar explosively off the chest so that the movement of the bar is up and slightly back.
4. Exhale as you lock the bar out to full arm's length.

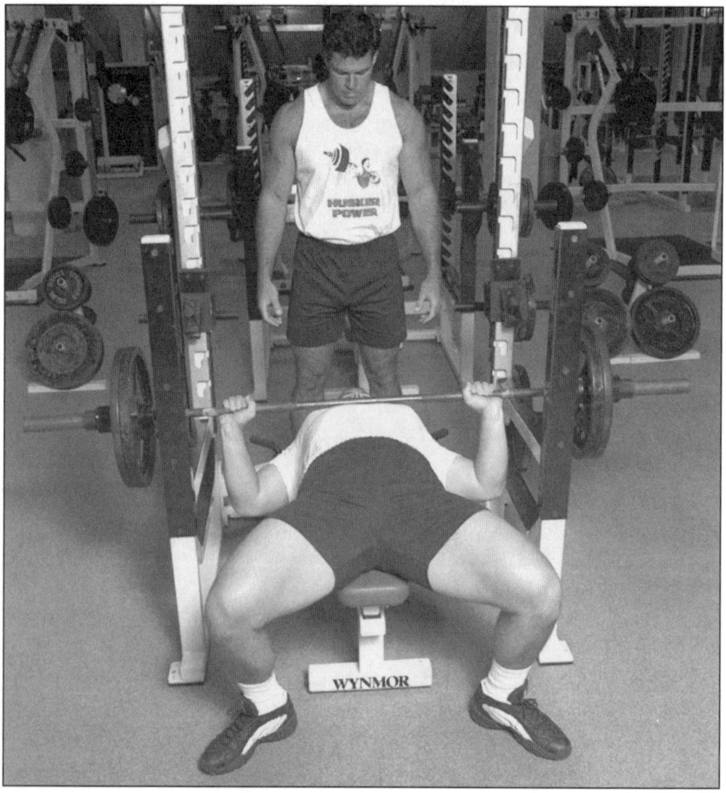

**Key Points:**

1. Grip the bar so that when it touches the chest the elbow joint is at approximately a 90-degree angle. A wider grip doesn't develop the chest and arm muscles as used in football, which is played with the arms in close to the midline of the body.
2. The spotter and lifter must work in a coordinated effort when guiding the bar into a lifting position and getting it racked. The spotter should have his hands under the bar and be alert.
3. It is a good idea to wrap the thumbs around the bar. We have witnessed several lifters lose the bar and drop it on their chests because of an improper grip.

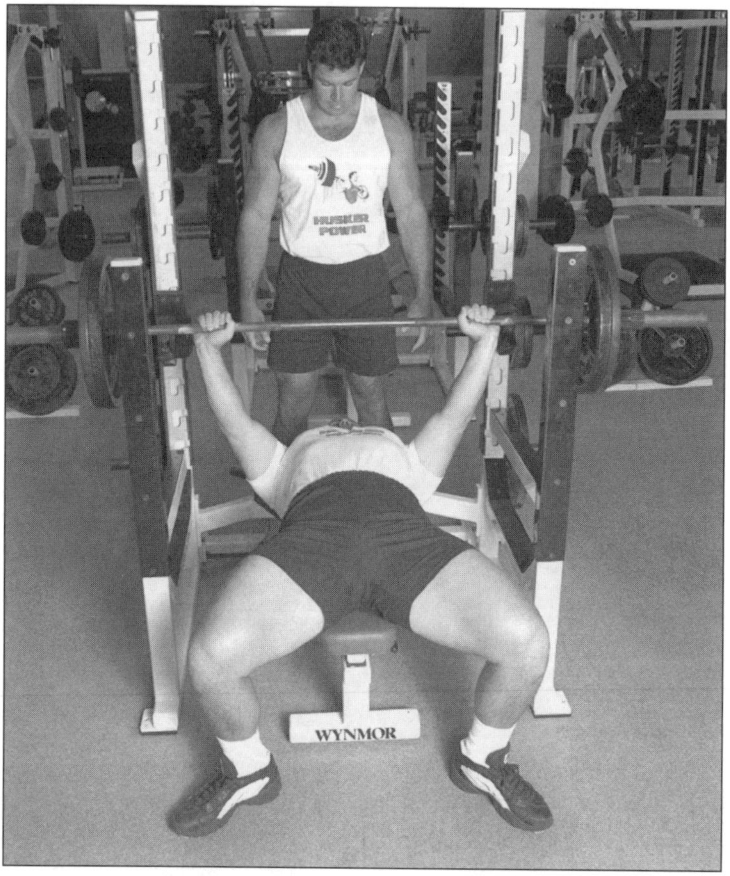

# INCLINE PRESS

**Purpose:** To develop the upper pectoral muscles, the anterior deltoids, and triceps

**Start Position:** Place feet flat on the ground and slightly arch back as you sit on the bench. Pull your shoulder blades inward as you push the chest upward, and grip the bar slightly wider than shoulder width. (Be sure to wrap thumbs around the bar.) Position yourself so the bar lines up with the top of your head. Take the bar from the rack with the aid of a spotter and position bar over chest.

**Procedure:**

1. Take a deep breath and hold chest high as you lower the bar in a slow, controlled motion.

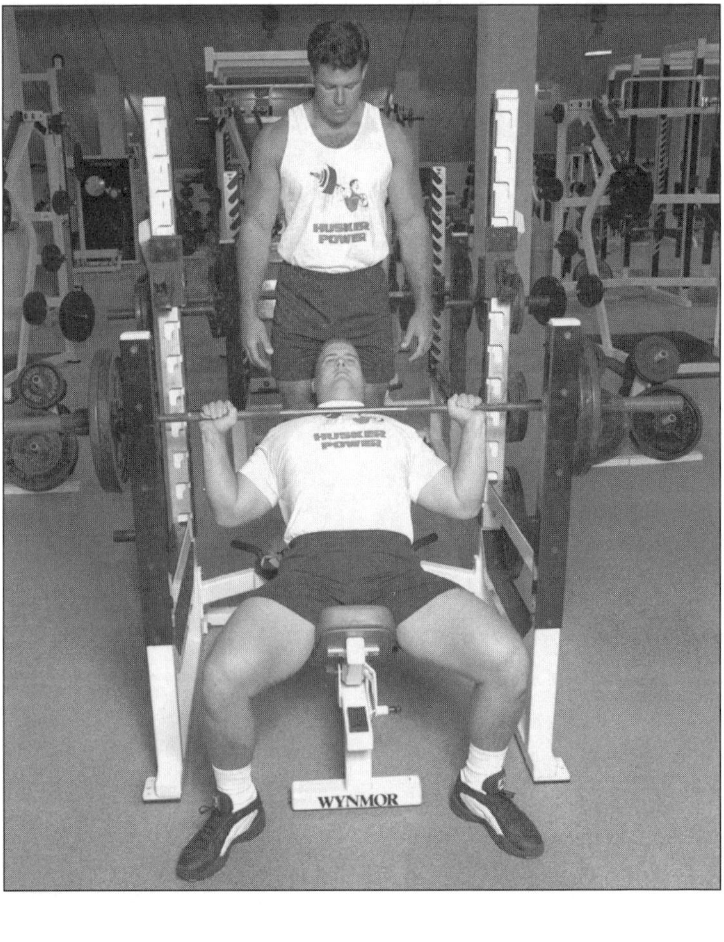

2. Allow the bar to just touch the upper chest at the base of the neck before driving it explosively off the chest. The movement of the bar should be up and slightly back.
3. Exhale as you lock the bar out to full arm's length.

**Key Points:**

1. Grip the bar so that when it touches the chest the elbow joint is approximately at a 90-degree angle. A wider grip doesn't develop the chest and arm muscles as used in football, which is played with the arms in close to the midline of the body.
2. The spotter and lifter must work in a coordinated effort when guiding the bar into a lifting position and getting it racked. The spotter should have his hands under the bar and be alert.
3. It is a good idea to wrap the thumbs around the bar.

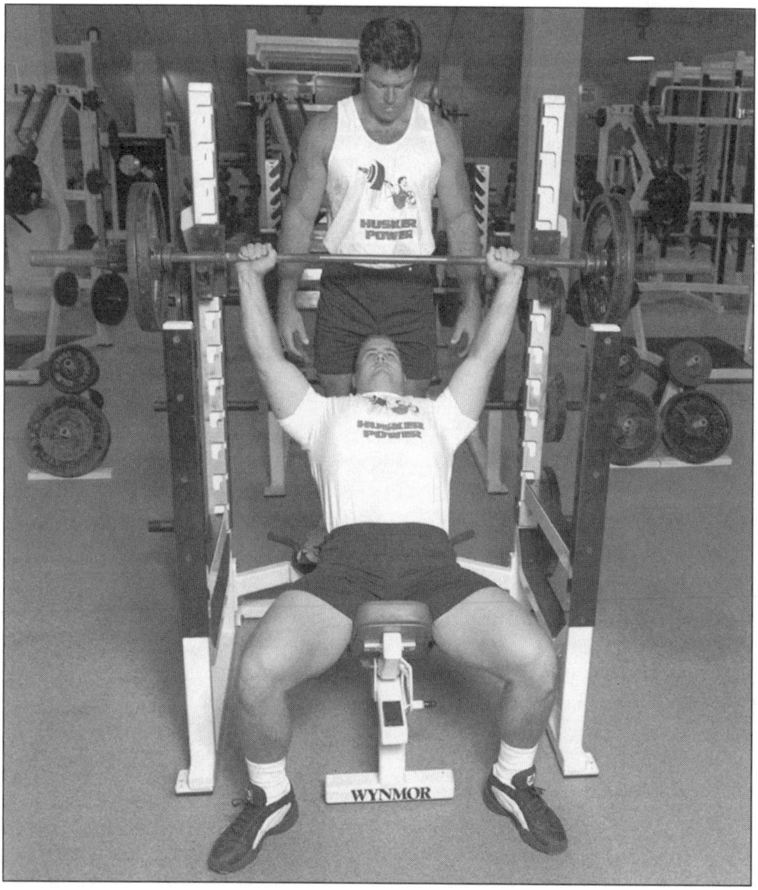

# SEATED SHOULDER PRESS

**Purpose:** To develop the anterior deltoids and the triceps

**Start Position:** Place bar on front of the shoulders and sit on seat with back flat. Use an overhand grip with the hands shoulder-width apart.

**Procedure:**

1. Press the bar overhead by extending the arms.
2. Lower the bar to starting position.

**Key Points:**

1. This exercise can also be done with bar behind the head.
2. Some seats have a back support, but this is not necessary.
3. Use a shoulder press stand or the bench press upright to support the weight.

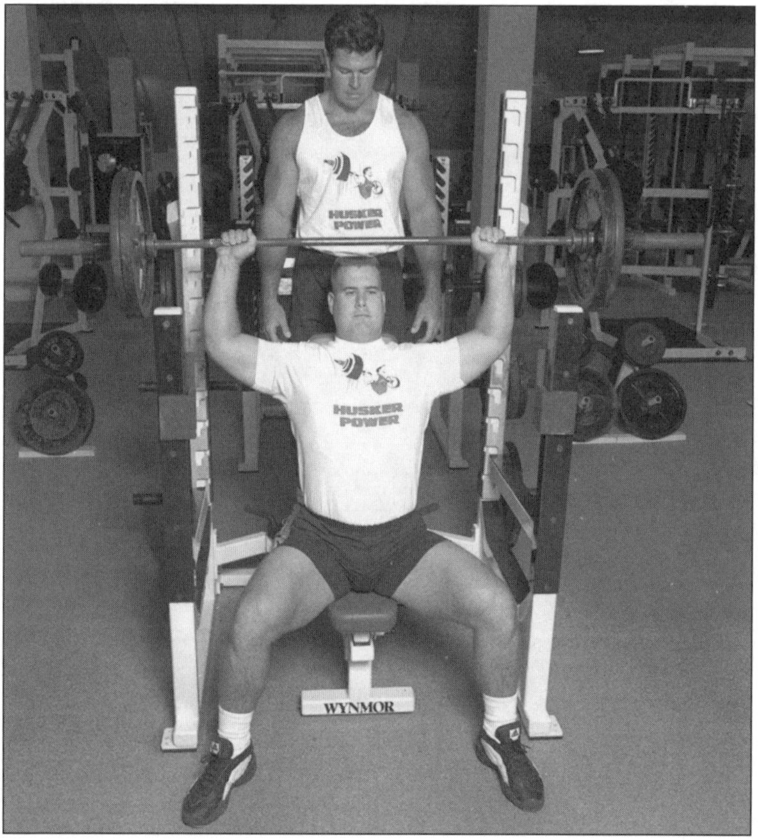

## SHOULDER RAISES

Shoulder raises are a group of three exercises that can be done together in any combination or done separately. All start in the same position, standing with arms extended to the side of thighs, holding dumbbells in an overhand grip. Keep your feet about hip-width apart.

## FRONT RAISE

**Purpose:** To isolate and develop the anterior or front deltoid muscles

**Procedure:**

1. Raise both dumbbells upward and forward until they are at shoulder level.
2. Lower dumbbells and repeat.

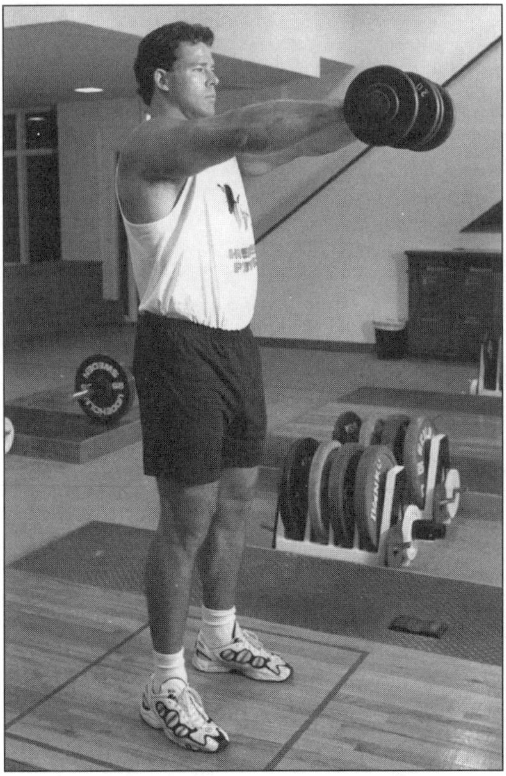

# LATERAL RAISE

**Purpose:** To isolate and develop the lateral or medial deltoid muscles

**Procedure:**

1. Raise both dumbbells upward and sideways until they are at shoulder level.
2. Lower dumbbells and repeat.

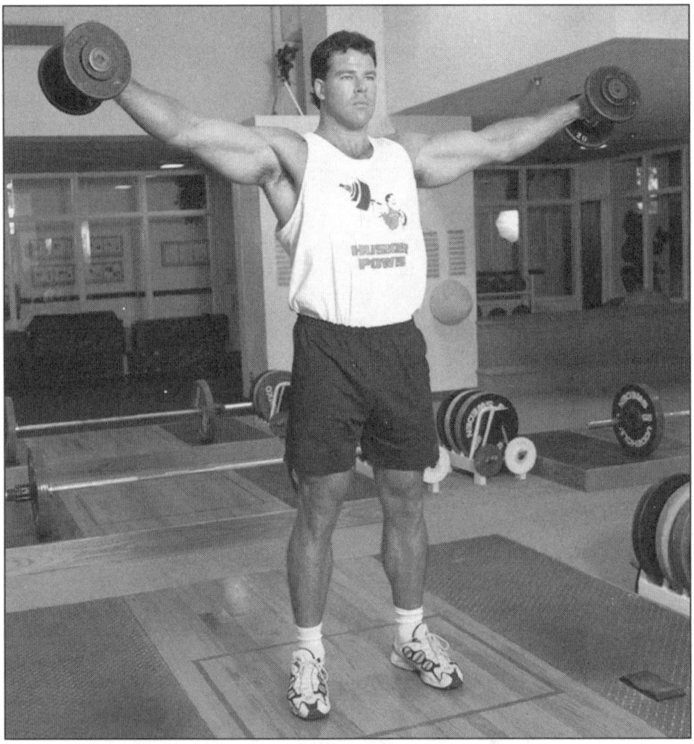

# BENT-OVER RAISE

**Purpose:** To isolate and develop the anterior or posterior deltoid muscles

**Start Position:** Same start position, then bend at hips until the back is parallel with the ground.

**Procedure:**

1. Raise both dumbbells upward and back until they are at shoulder level.
2. Lower dumbbells and repeat.

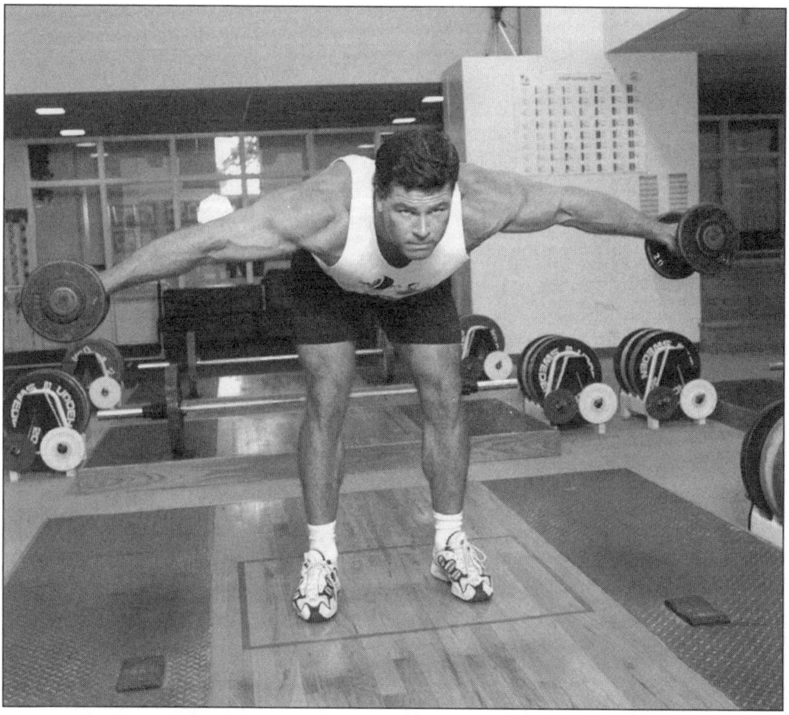

# BARBELL CURL

**Purpose:** To develop the biceps

**Start Position:** Grip a barbell (or handles of a low pulley machine) with an underhand grip slightly wider than shoulder width and extend arms. Position feet shoulder-width apart.

**Procedure:**

1. Pull the bar slowly to the shoulders by bending at the elbows.
2. Lower bar in a controlled manner to the start position.
3. Keep elbows positioned at the sides throughout the movement.

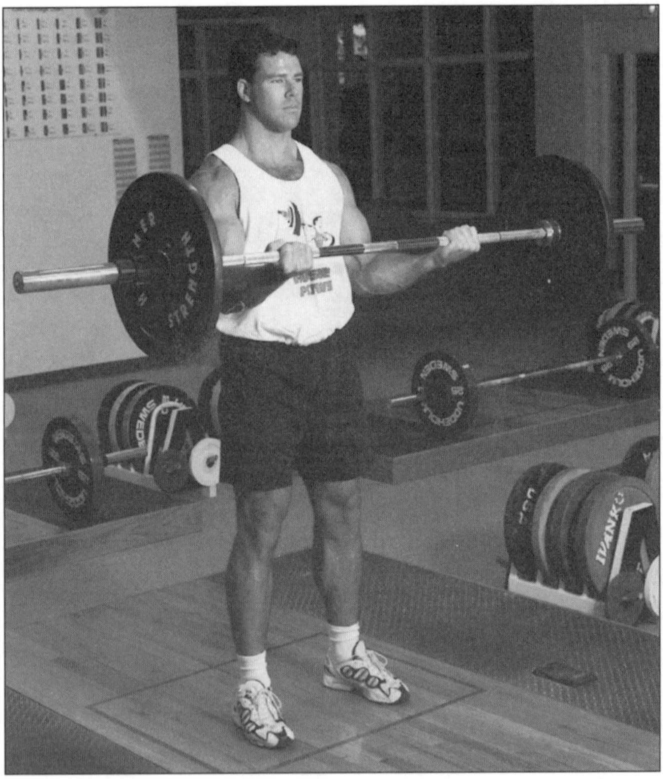

# TRICEPS EXTENSION

**Purpose:** To develop the triceps

**Start Position:** This exercise can be performed with either a barbell with weights or a low pulley handle. Lie on your back on a bench and use an overhand grip on the low pulley handle with hands four to six inches apart. Lift the low pulley handle head and hold at arm's length.

**Procedure:**

1. Lower low pulley handle, under control, to the forehead by flexing at the elbows.
2. Raise the handle by extending the arms. Keep your elbows in the same position throughout movement by keeping upper arm perpendicular to the ground.

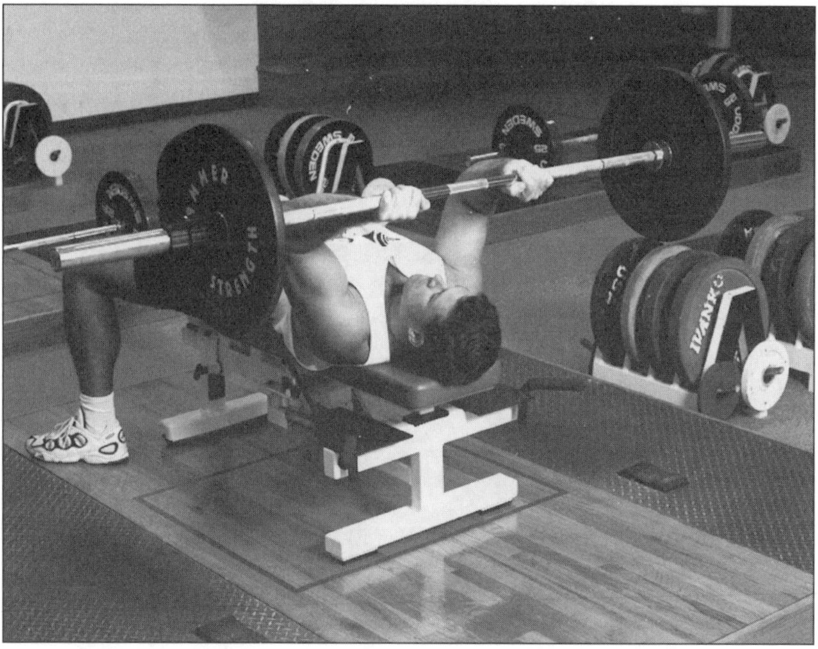

# NECK MACHINE (FORWARD AND BACKWARD)

**Purpose:** To strengthen the neck muscles

**Start Position:** Stand with knees bent so that head is in alignment with pads. Place hands on thighs.

**Procedure:**

1. Flex your head backward as far as you can.
2. Lower the weight until the weights just barely touch.
3. Repeat the movement slowly and smoothly.
4. Do both backward and forward.

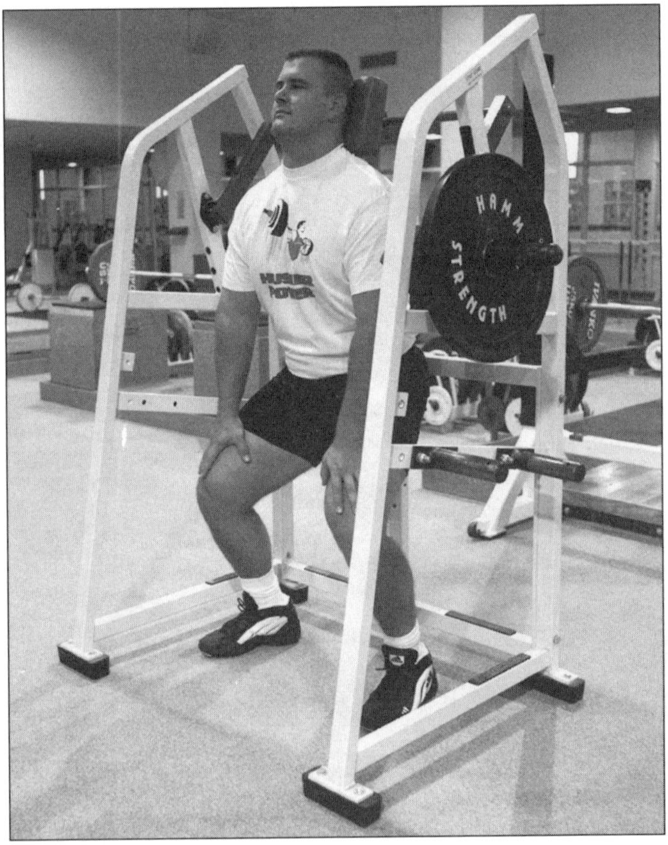

# CRUNCH

**Purpose:** To develop the abdominal muscles

**Start Position (To the Center):** Lie on the floor face up. Bend your knees with feet on the ground and clasp your hands behind the head.

**Procedure:**

1. Place your chin on your chest.
2. Lift your head four to six inches off the ground and hold for one second.
3. Pull your upper body 12 to 18 inches toward your knees using your abdominal muscles; hold for one second.
4. Return slowly to starting position, pause, and repeat.

**Start Position (To the Side):** Lie face up on the floor and spread your legs. Place both hands on your right leg and lift it six inches off the ground.

**Procedure:**

1. Slide your hands up your leg until they reach the knee.
2. Return to starting position and repeat. After required reps, switch to the left side.

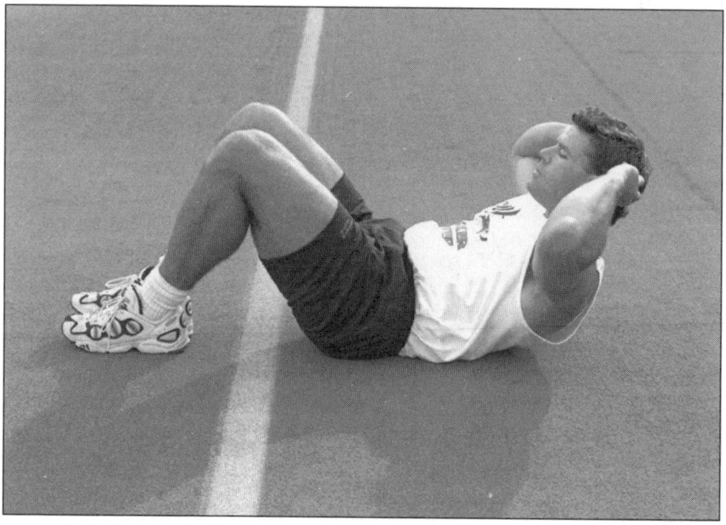

**Key Points:**

1. Keep your legs spread and feet raised six inches for entire movement.
2. Reach for the outside of the knee as you curl yourself up.

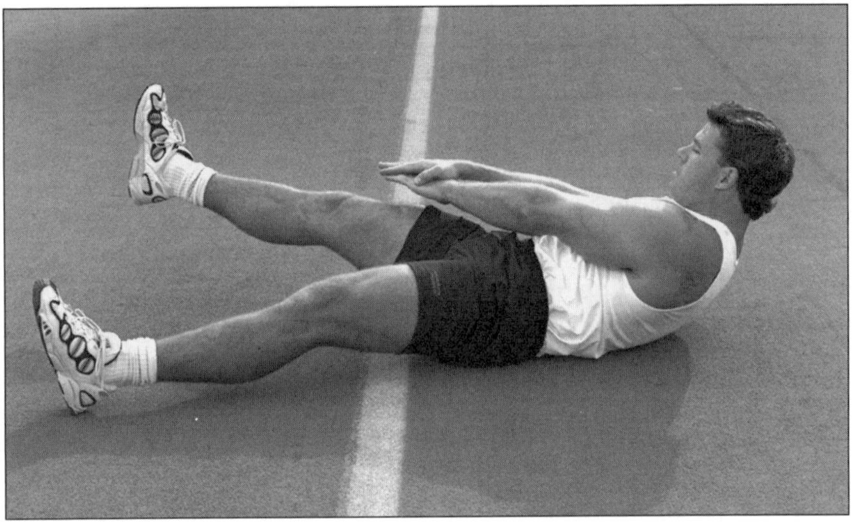

CHAPTER 6

# SPEED DRILLS

In chapter 1 we defined speed as the ability to cover a certain distance from point A to point B in the shortest time possible. We said that speed consists of two components: acceleration and top speed. Acceleration is determined by how much time it takes a player to reach his top speed. Top speed is determined by the maximum possible yards per second a player can run. As we stated in chapter 1, acceleration is more important than top speed in the game of football. Therefore, the speed drills described in this chapter are geared toward developing acceleration.

Many coaches and athletes feel speed is simply inherited, and regardless of what they do they cannot improve it. This perception is true to a certain extent. If you run a 5.5-second 40-yard dash, you most likely won't be able to get your time down to 4.5 seconds. But it is possible to lower your 40-yard time by .3 to as much as .5 second. This has been demonstrated many times by using the following drills within the program outlined in chapter 9. Not only do players get faster, they also put on 20 to 40 pounds of solid muscular body weight when interval speed training is done in conjunction with strength training.

## DEVELOPING YOUR SPEED

Developing speed doesn't simply happen in two to three weeks. It takes a disciplined effort day after day, week after week, year after year. Don't become discouraged; you will get faster if you put forth the effort over a period of time. There are basically two ways to improve speed: by improving technique and running mechanics and by strengthening your legs. While chapter 5 focuses on lifts that strengthen your legs, as your legs get stronger these speed drills will convert this new strength using proper neuromuscular recruitment patterns specific to increased sprinting speed. Most players don't have good running mechanics; thus if they improve their technique, they'll get faster. Moreover, the stronger your legs are, the more force they apply against the ground (see chapter 2), and the faster you run. You cannot reach your full speed potential by simply running sprints. A number of training elements must be fused together in order to achieve maximum speed potential.

Speed is the product of stride length and stride frequency. *Stride length* is the distance you cover with each step as you run. *Stride frequency* is the number of steps that you take per second. Your speed can be improved by increasing your stride length and/or stride frequency. Most experts on speed training agree that improving stride length attains the best results. Stride length is improved by increasing the forces produced by the muscular contraction of the leg and hip muscles against the ground. Strength training and power drills enable you to contract your muscles more forcefully. Stride frequency can be enhanced by concentrating on warm-up drills before each workout on a year-round basis. These drills, detailed in this chapter, are designed to develop mechanically efficient sprinting form. Combine sprint running with strength training (chapter 5) and active flexibility drills (chapter 4) to improve technique to develop an effective program to develop maximum speed.

Some coaches consider plyometrics a good way to improve power. However, only light plyometrics are included in our workout schedule because experience teaches us that when heavy plyometrics or any shock training (such as depth jumping) are done in combination with strength training, the result is often overtraining, injuries (especially shin splints), and loss of speed.

## WARMING UP FOR SPEED DRILLS

You would not want to start any of these drills with cold muscles. A hamstring pull—which can set you back for three or four weeks—is very possible unless you warm up properly. Be sure to do the warm-up drills and stretching routine described in chapter 4 before doing any of the speed drills. The speed drills are to be done with as much intensity as possible, but do the first few repetitions of the workout at about 75 percent intensity and gradually increase the intensity of the drills.

## SPRINT TECHNIQUE

In chapter 1 we discussed that sprinting consists of acceleration and top speed mechanics. Acceleration mechanics consists of the starting stance and the first six to eight strides coming out of the start with a good forward lean. Top speed mechanics consists of proper arm and leg actions with the body in an upright posture during the drive and recovery phases.

### Acceleration Mechanics

In order to get the most benefit out of these speed drills, you need to start with good sprinting form. With this in mind, here are some basic tips to help you do these drills with the best possible sprinting technique.

#### Starting Stance

This will teach you how to get into a good starting stance, a necessity for doing most of the drills. This is the same stance that you use to start the 10- and 40-yard sprints when testing.

1. Place your front foot three to six inches behind the starting line.
2. Place your hand, high on fingertips, opposite your front foot and directly on the starting line, with your thumb and forefinger parallel to the line.
3. Place your other hand to the hip of the forward leg with your elbow up.
4. Be sure your back foot is 6 to 12 inches behind the heel of the forward foot.

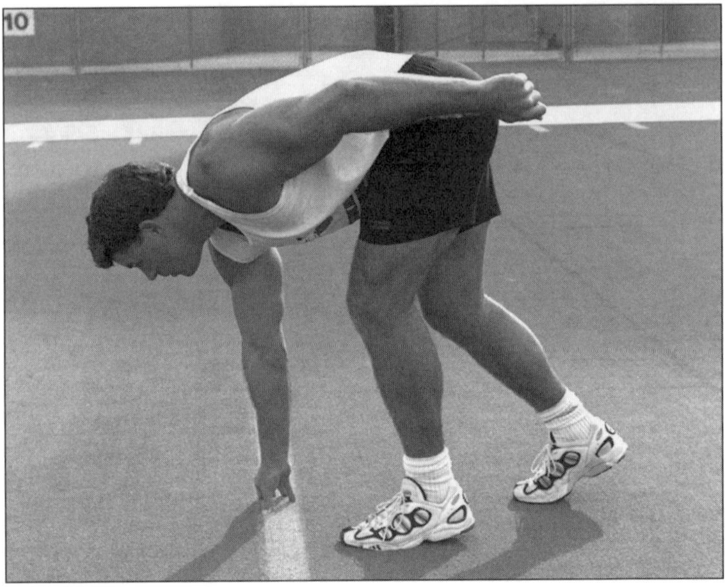

5. Raise your hips slightly above shoulder height and lean forward so the shoulders are slightly ahead of the starting line.
6. Shift the majority of your body weight onto the front leg and hand.
7. Focus eyes two to three feet in front of starting line.

### Acceleration Phase

The forward lean during the acceleration phase puts the body in a pushing position (figure 6.1). This is because the action of the legs occurs behind the center of gravity, thus emphasizing the triple extension (extending the ankles, knees, and hips).

1. Drive off the *balls of the feet* extending completely at the ankles, knees, and hips.
2. Drive your arms vigorously.

## Top Speed Mechanics

The following are some sprinting techniques to be conscious of when doing the speed drills described later in this chapter. During one stride the leg cycles through two different phases: the drive phase (triple extension when the foot pushes against the ground) and the recovery

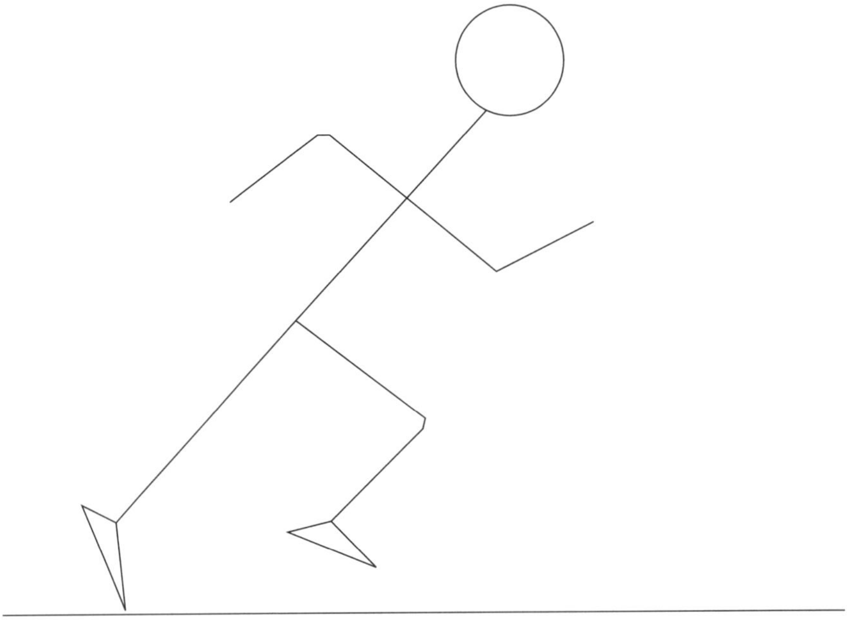

**Figure 6.1**

phase (when the foot leaves the ground and the thigh swings forward from the hip). The basic thing to remember when sprinting at top speed is to learn how to run relaxed. Your muscles cannot respond if you are tense. Most injuries occur when you tense your body trying to shift gears into a higher speed. Learn to relax your hands, shoulders, neck, and face when sprinting.

## Arm Action

Proper arm action does more than anything else to improve sprinting technique. The lower body sprinting action mirrors arm action; thus, if you have problems with your arm action you will have problems with your leg action. The arms act as the motor and the legs are the wheels reacting to the arms. The harder your arms drive, the more force the legs apply against the ground.

1. On the backswing, swing your hands just below the waist, with elbows at approximately a 120-degree angle.
2. Drive elbows back so they rise above the shoulders, with the elbows closing to 90 degrees.

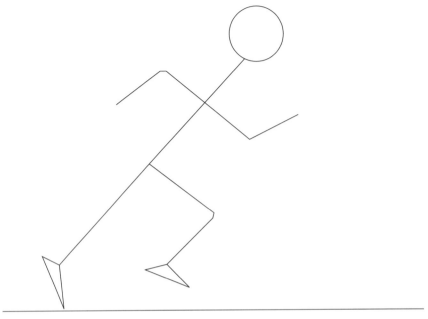

3. On forward swing, bring hands up to the mouth, as if eating an ice cream cone. Keep the angle of your arms tight and your body relaxed.
4. It is important to keep the shoulders squared so that the arms swing independently of them.

## Drive Phase

Though the ankles, knees, and hips are extended, it is important not to attempt to push against the ground during top speed. Quickly and lightly push off the ground for maximum drive (figure 6.2)

1. Land on the balls of the feet, extending completely at the ankles, knees, and hips. Don't try to drive off the toes.
2. Be light and quick with your feet using a pawing-like action.

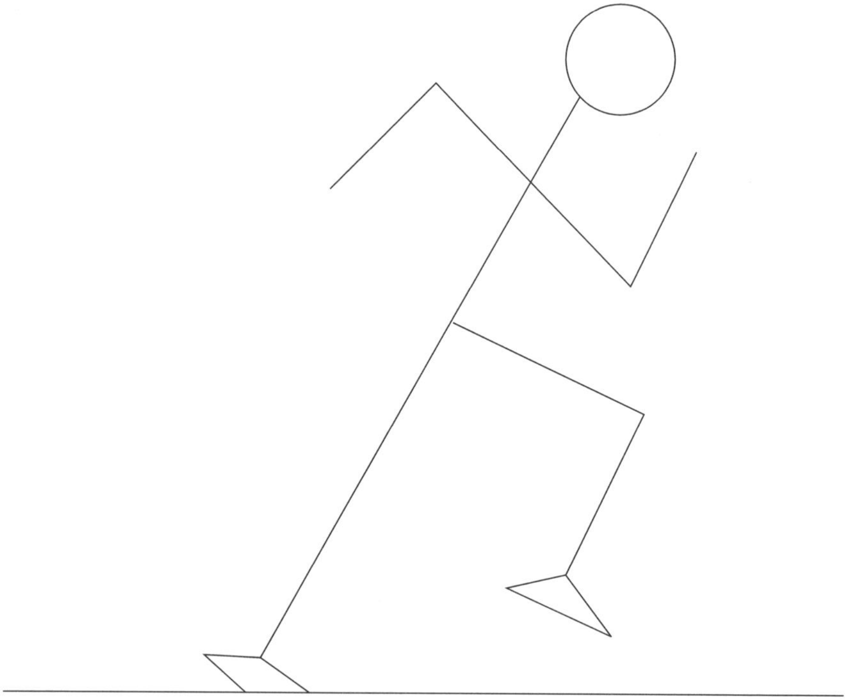

**Figure 6.2**

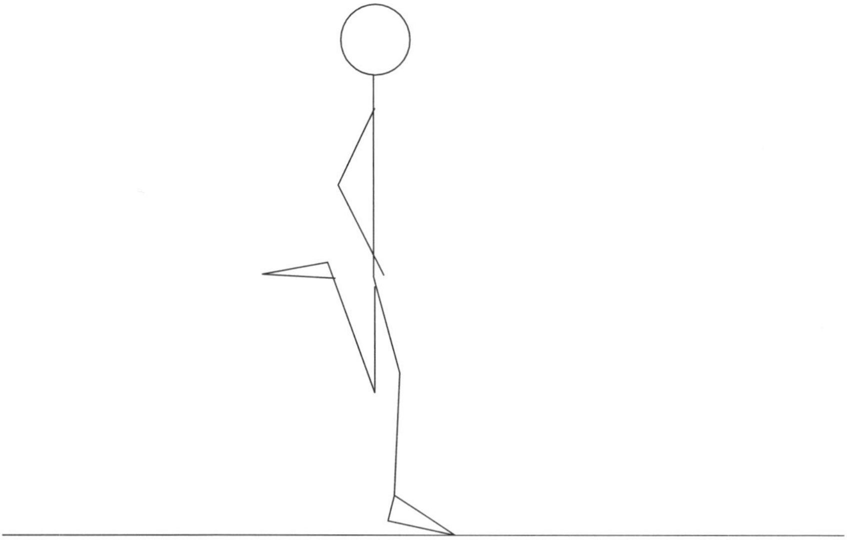

Figure 6.3

## Recovery Phase

Relax as the thigh swings forward and naturally let the foot strike the ground in preparation for the drive phase (figure 6.3)

1. Swing heel up to hips by flexing at the knee joint. The higher the heel comes up to the hips, the shorter the arc becomes when the thigh swings forward.
2. The thigh swings forward and up naturally. Just keep relaxed and let it happen.
3. The lower leg extends as the foot reaches for the ground. Again, let it happen naturally.

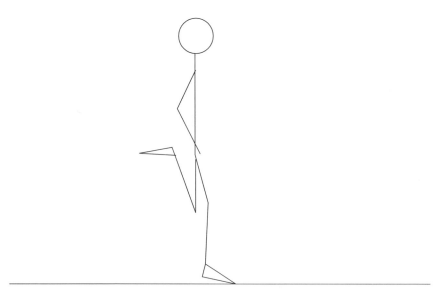

# SPEED DRILLS

While the drills in this chapter will help increase your speed, their primary purpose is to condition you by using interval training principles described in chapter 9. The intention of these drills is not to turn you into a track sprinter, but to develop you into a better football player.

## FORM STARTS

**Purpose:** To develop explosive running starts

**Procedure:**

1. Forcefully pull back leg forward with a quick and long first step.
2. Straighten front leg explosively by extending at ankle, knee, and hip.
3. Forcefully bring elbow of your support arm up and back.
4. Drive hand on the hip straight forward.
5. Move hips forward.
6. Keep head down, relaxing neck, face, jaw, and hands.
7. Accelerate for 10 yards.

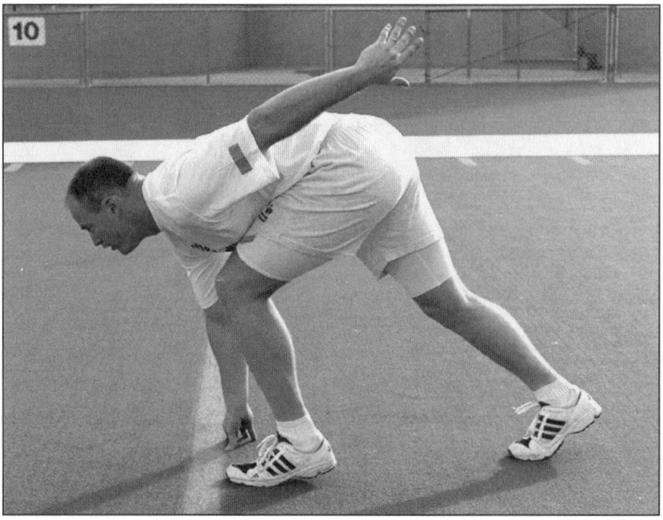

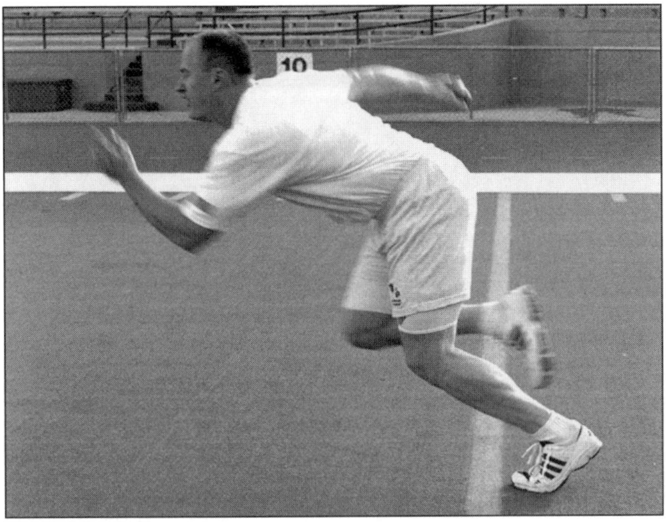


**Rest:** 20 seconds between each repetition

**Key Points:**

1. Do not stand straight up coming out of start.
2. Do not twist feet to side when driving out.
3. Do not take first step with front leg.

## POSITION STARTS

**Purpose:** To develop good acceleration from the player's starting stance

**Procedure:**

1. Get in your on-the-field starting position stance (see Form Starts exercise).
2. On coach's command, explode out of your starting stance for 10 to 15 yards.

**Rest:** 30 seconds between each repetition

# ACCELERATION DRILLS

## BUILDUPS

**Purpose:** To improve acceleration

**Procedure:**

1. Set up a 60-yard course with the 40-yard point marked (figure 6.4).

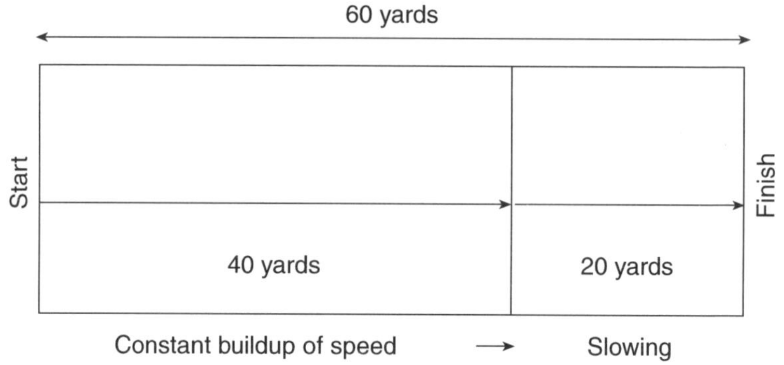


Figure 6.4

2. Start from a standing start into a slow run, concentrating on good running form.
3. Gradually build up speed until you are at full speed at 40 yards.
4. Once full speed is achieved at 40 yards, gradually slow down over the final 20 yards.

**Rest:** 60 seconds between each repetition

**Key Points:**

1. Do not accelerate too fast or too slow.
2. Gradually build your speed for the entire 40 yards. Doing buildups is like driving a car with a stick shift. Run the first 10 yards at a slow run, at 10 yards shift gears into a higher speed, at 20 yards go into a stride, at 30 into a fast stride. You should be reaching full speed at 40 yards. Avoid running at full speed after 40 yards is reached.

## FLYING 10S

**Purpose:** To improve acceleration and stride frequency

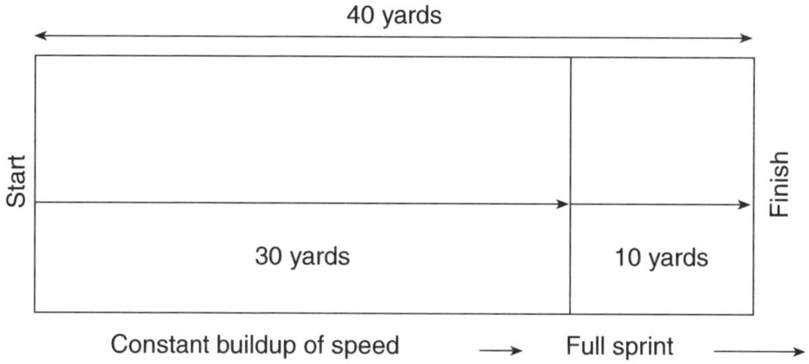


Figure 6.5

**Procedure:**

1. Set up a 40-yard course with the 30-yard point marked (figure 6.5).
2. Start running at half speed, building speed at each stride for 30 yards. By the time you reach the 30-yard mark, you should be running at full speed (flying).
3. Continue this full-speed sprinting for 10 more yards.

**Rest:** 60 to 90 seconds between each repetition

**Key Point:** Do not accelerate too fast or too slow; it is like doing a buildup except you should be running full speed at 30 yards. After sprinting full-speed for 10 yards slow down gradually.

## FLYING 20S

**Purpose:** To improve acceleration and stride frequency

**Procedure:**

1. Set up a 50-yard course with the 30-yard point marked (figure 6.6).

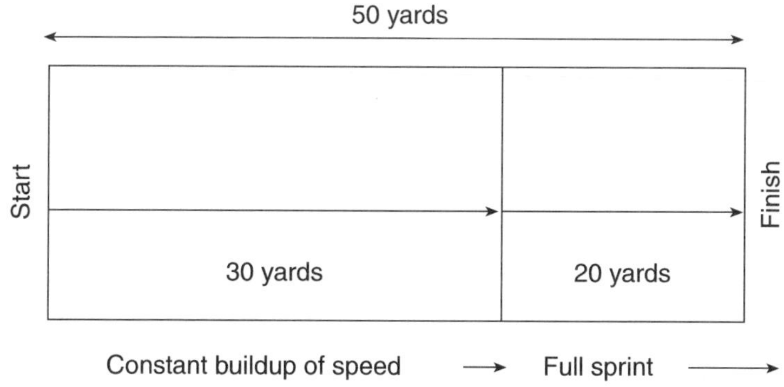


Figure 6.6

2. Start running at half speed, building speed at each stride so that acceleration is continuous for the first 20 yards.
3. By the time you reach the 30-yard mark, you should be running at full speed (flying). Continue this sprint for 20 more yards.

**Rest:** 60 to 90 seconds between each repetition

## FLYING 30S

**Purpose:** To improve acceleration and stride frequency

**Procedure:**

1. Set up a 60-yard course with 30-yard point marked (figure 6.7).
2. Start running at half speed, building speed at each stride so that acceleration is continuous for the first 30 yards.
3. By the time you reach the 30-yard mark, you should be running at full speed (flying) and should continue this sprint for the remaining 30 yards.

**Rest:** 60 to 90 seconds between each repetition

**Key Point:** Do not accelerate too fast or too slow; keep the buildup constant for 30 yards.

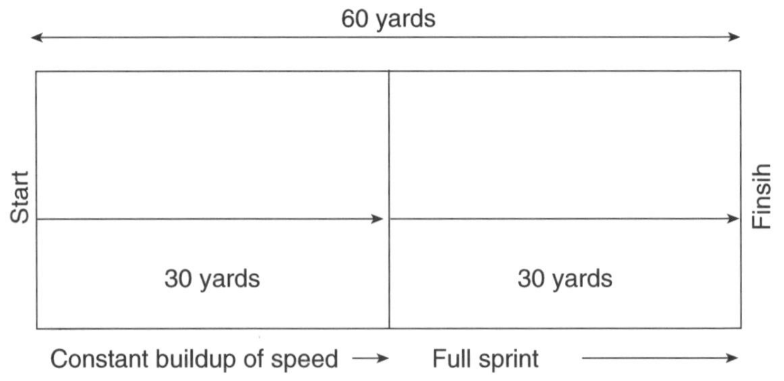


Figure 6.7

## HOLLOW SPRINTS

**Purpose:** To improve acceleration

**Procedure:**

1. Set up a 100-yard course with every 20-yard point marked (figure 6.8).
2. Start running at half speed for first 20 yards.
3. At the 20-yard point accelerate and sprint at full speed for 20 yards.
4. Slow back to the original half-speed run for 20 yards.
5. Repeat this half-speed and sprint pattern until course is complete.

**Rest:** 60 to 90 seconds between each repetition

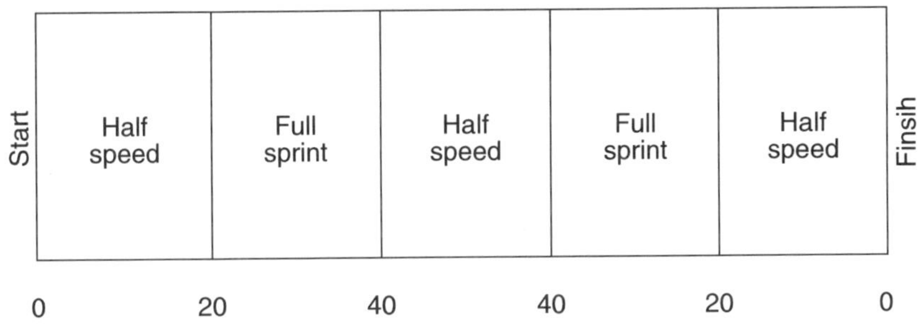


Figure 6.8

## 40-YARD SPRINTS

**Purpose:** To develop acceleration and speed

**Procedure:** Sprint at full speed past the 40-yard marker, using good sprinting form.

**Rest:** 60 to 90 seconds between each repetition

# PLYOMETRICS

The main purpose of plyometric drills is to develop the stretch-shortening cycle—an eccentric contraction followed by a concentric contraction. When the muscle is stretched, it builds elastic energy. The muscle then fights to return to its normal resting length (similar to the stretching of a rubber band). If the muscle shortens immediately after the stretch, greater force and power can be generated.

Special attention must be given to two phases of the plyometric drills: the landing and the countermovement. Land with feet nearly flat (balls of feet touch first, then to heel). Bend at the knees and hips (try to stop the flexion of knees as quickly as possible). Reverse directions and push off the ground with balls of feet as quickly as possible after landing. Avoid doing the countermovement slowly. Be sure to use a surface that is firm, yet has some resiliency for landing, such as a grass field. Do not jump on concrete or wood floors.

## BOUNDING

**Purpose:** To increase explosion and stride length

**Procedure:**

1. Push off forcefully with the front leg.
2. Simultaneously drive the back leg's knee up and out to develop maximal hang time.
3. When leg contacts the ground, immediately push off forcefully and drive through with other leg, repeating the process for 30 to 40 yards.

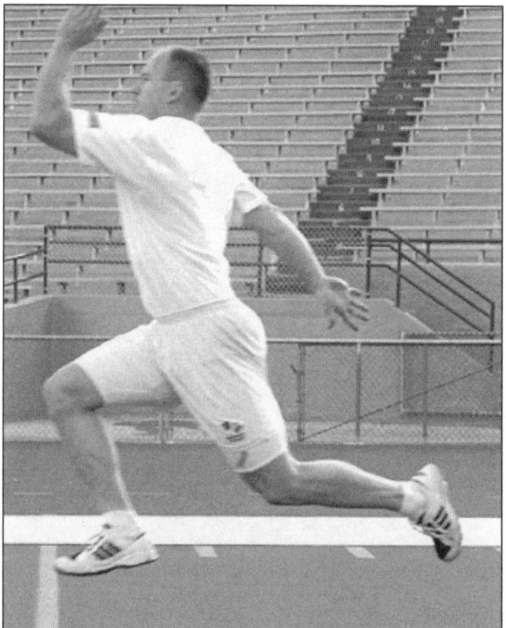

**Rest:** 60 to 90 seconds between each repetition

**Key Points:**

1. Drive knees high so that the thighs are parallel with the ground.
2. Make sure your strides are as long as possible, and keep your time spent on the ground at a minimum.

## POWER SKIPS FOR HEIGHT

**Purpose:** To increase explosive action in the leg and hips

**Procedure:**

1. Begin skipping, pushing off explosively with the back leg.
2. Opposite leg drives knee up as high as possible, trying to achieve maximal height.
3. Prepare for contact with the ground and repeat with opposite leg immediately upon landing. Repeat this pattern for 30 to 40 yards.

**Rest:** 60 seconds between each repetition

**Key Points:**

1. Skip as high as possible with triple extension of the back leg.
2. Drive knee to your chest and use sprinting arm action.

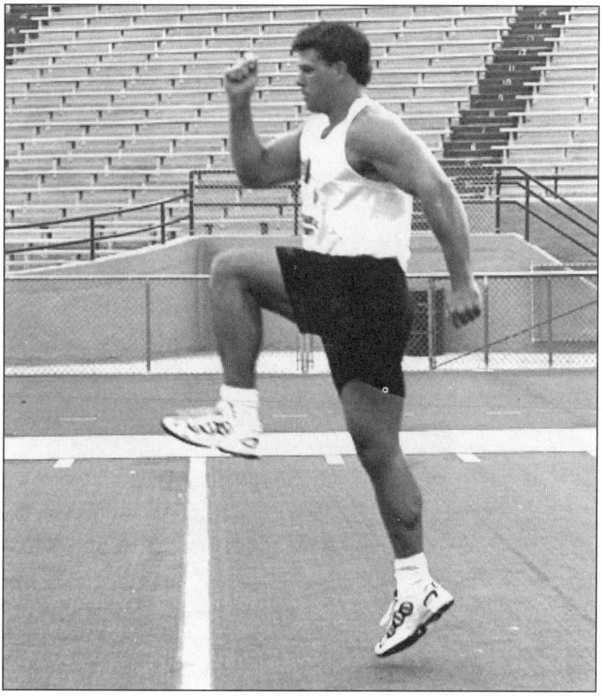

# POWER SKIPS FOR DISTANCE

**Purpose:** To increase explosive action in your legs and hips

**Procedure:**

1. Begin skipping by pushing off explosively with your back leg.
2. Drive your opposite knee up and out as high as possible, trying to achieve maximal distance.
3. Prepare for contact with the ground and repeat with opposite leg immediately upon landing. Repeat this pattern for 30 to 40 yards.

**Rest:** 60 seconds between each repetition

**Key Points:**

1. Skip as far as possible with triple extension of the back leg.
2. Drive your knee up and out.
3. Use proper arm action.

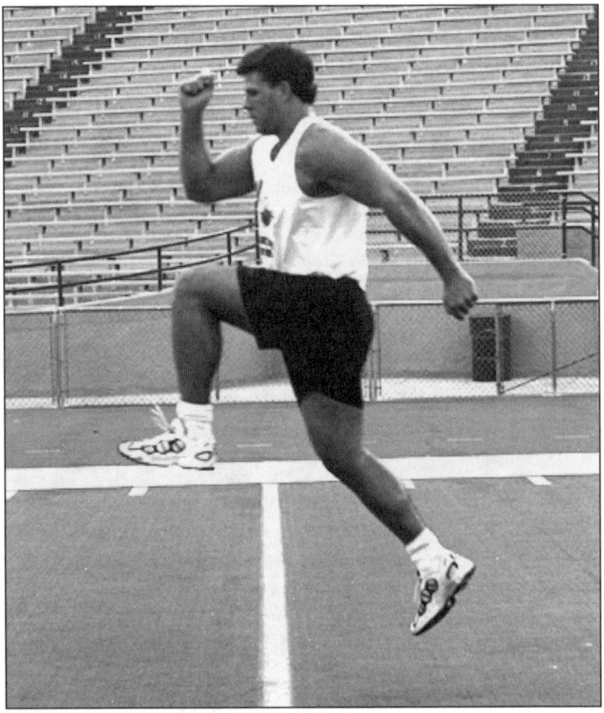

# SPEED SKIPS

**Purpose:** To develop stride frequency

**Procedure:**

1. Begin skipping, pushing off forcefully with your back leg.
2. Quickly bring opposite foot back to the ground and push off forcefully with this leg, repeating this process for 10 to 15 yards.

**Rest:** 60 seconds between each repetition

**Key Point:** Use good arm action and rapid foot contacts.

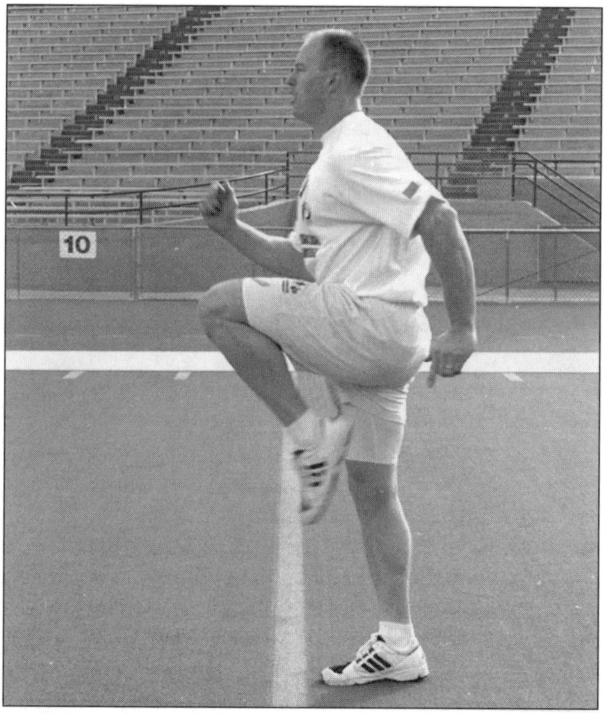

# LATERAL BAG JUMPS

**Purpose:** To develop explosive lateral power

**Procedure:**

1. Stand laterally beside a blocking bag and jump over the bag using both feet. Bring your knees to the chest, not just raising the heels over the bag.
2. Once you make contact with the other side of the bag, jump in the opposite direction to the original starting position, and continue this pattern for 10 repetitions.

**Rest:** 60 to 90 seconds between each repetition

**Key Points:**

1. Do not spend a lot of time on the ground, have quick feet, and do not use stutter steps.
2. Use your arms to explode over the bag.

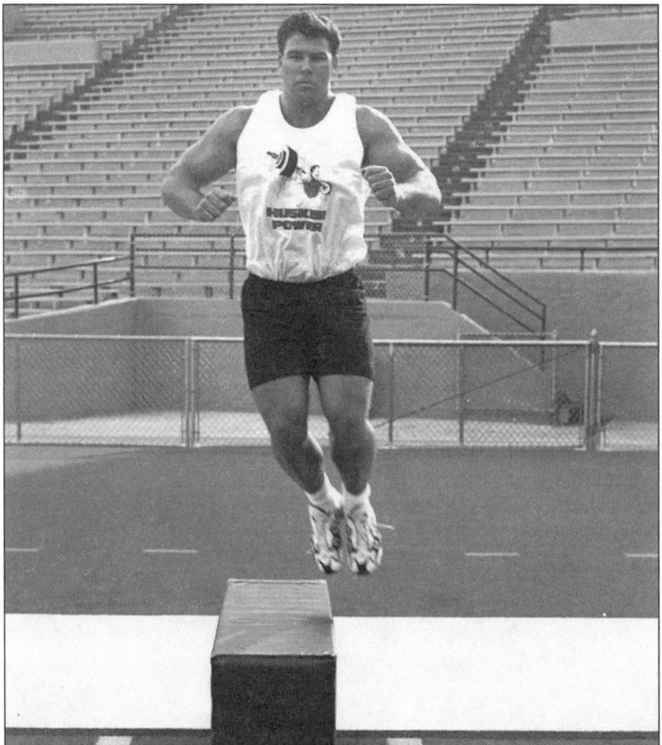

# BAG JUMPS

**Purpose:** To develop explosiveness and acceleration

**Procedure:**

1. Stand facing a series of four to five bags stacked two bags high. Begin by jumping forward over the first set of bags.
2. Assist your jump by moving your arms explosively and bringing your knees to your chest.
3. After contact with ground, quickly jump over second set of bags and continue through all sets of bags.

**Rest:** 60 to 90 seconds between each repetition

**Key Points:**

1. Do not spend a lot of time on the ground and do not stutter step between the bags.
2. Use your arms to help jump over the bags.
3. Make sure your feet come over, not out around the sides, of the bags.

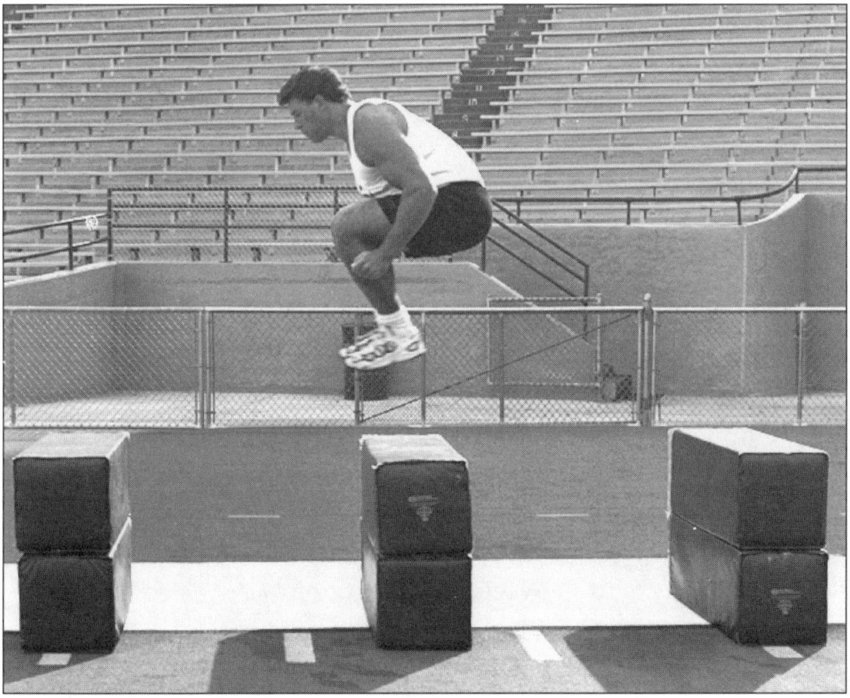

# 10/10 HOPPING

**Purpose:** To develop explosive power

**Procedure:**

1. Set up a 40-yard straight with every 10 yards marked (figure 6.9).
2. Hop for 10 yards on one leg, then switch legs and hop on the other for 10 yards. Concentrate on not spending much time on the ground between hops.
3. Continue alternating legs every 10 yards.

**Rest:** 60 seconds between each repetition

**Key Point:** Use good arm action.

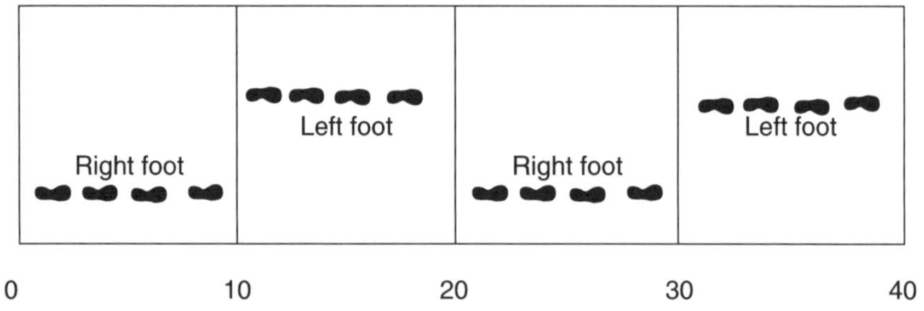


**Figure 6.9**

# SINGLE LEG HOPS

**Purpose:** To develop starting power and acceleration

**Procedure:**

1. Begin by hopping forward and up on one leg.
2. Completely extend the leg as you drive off of it, and bring your heel to your buttocks and quickly swing your knee forward as you land.
3. Repeat for required amount of jumps, then switch legs and repeat the drill.

**Rest:** 60 to 90 seconds between each repetition

**Key Point:** Do not hesitate between hops; keep the motion continuous.

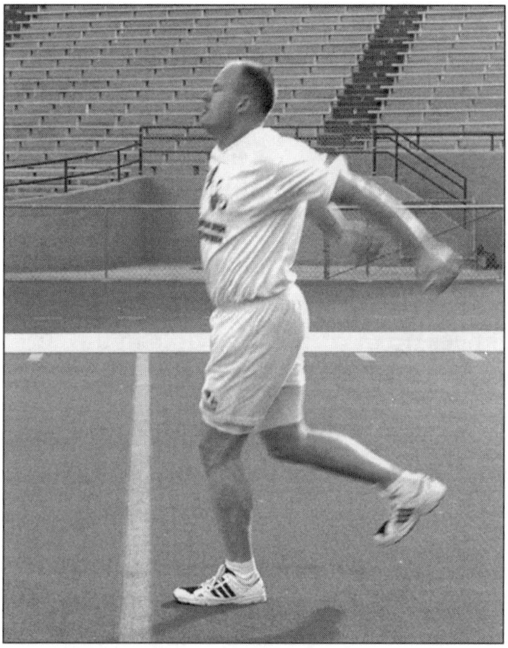

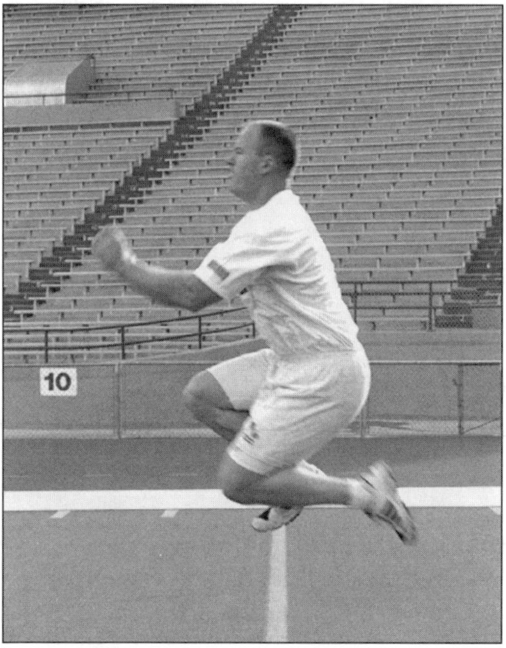
10

# RIGHT, LEFT, JUMP

**Purpose:** To develop explosive power

**Procedure:**

1. Stand with your feet parallel, hip-width apart, and toes pointed straight ahead.
2. Swing arms backward, bend your knees and hips, and explosively jump forward and up, simultaneously swinging the arms forward.
3. Pull your knees up to your body while in the air.
4. Land on your right foot, bending at the knee to absorb the shock.
5. Explosively jump by extending the right leg.
6. Land on your left foot, bending at the knee to absorb the shock.
7. Explosively jump, extending with the left leg.
8. Finally land on both feet (figure 6.10).

**Rest:** 60 seconds between each repetition

**Key Points:**

1. Achieve as much distance as possible on each jump, and work to keep the movement continuous.
2. Many variations can be used with this drill. Some examples are: right, left, jump; right, left, right, jump; right, right, left, jump, etc. (see figure 6.10).

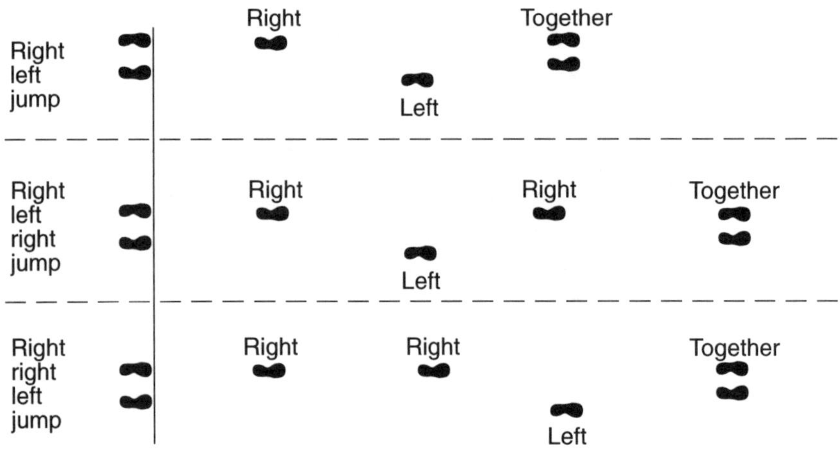


**Figure 6.10**

# RESISTED SPEED

Resisted speed drills make the sprinting action harder than normal by adding resistance. The resistance can be a harness held by a partner or running uphill (stadium steps or hills). Other forms of resistance running, such as attaching bungee cords and parachutes to the runner, are not covered in this book; it is difficult to use these devices when working with large groups.

When doing resisted speed drills it is important to use the proper resistance. When doing the harness drill, for example, don't pull so hard on the player running that he is unable to run with proper form. Pull just hard enough to make him work, but allow smooth running form. The same holds true with running uphill; don't run hills so steep they take away from good running mechanics.

## HARNESS STARTS

**Purpose:** To provide added resistance coming out of the start

**Procedure:**

1. After putting on harness, assume a three-point start stance.
2. Against proper resistance, explode out of the start.
3. Continue to accelerate for the required distance.

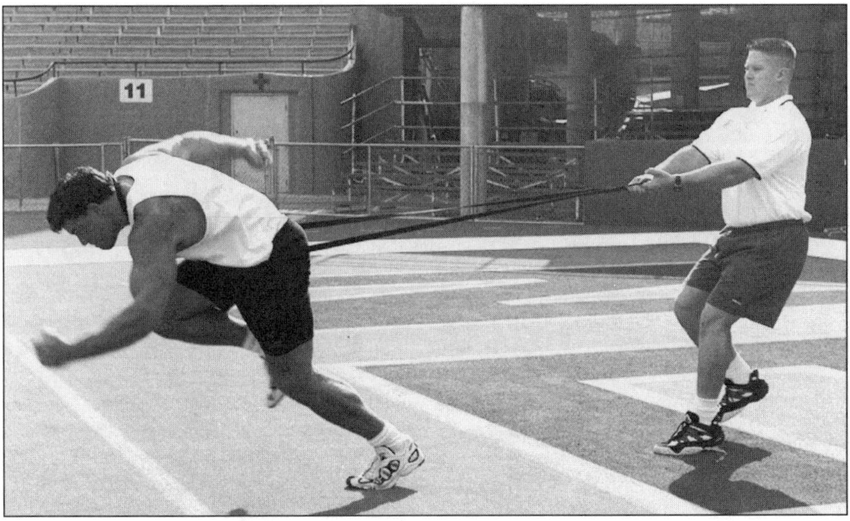

**Rest:** 60 seconds between each repetition

**Key Points:**

1. Make sure to use good form and quickly pump your arms.
2. Apply the proper resistance.
3. You need to have a forward body lean—feet behind the waist and when striking ground, and shoulders in front of the waist—and good running form.

## HARNESS DRILL

**Purpose:** To develop acceleration and reach top speed quickly

**Procedure:**

1. Find a flat, 50- to 60-yard course.
2. Run forward with a harness, focusing eyes 20 to 30 feet ahead, driving off back leg, and extending completely at ankles, knees, and hips.
3. Carry leg to high knee and maintain a good forward lean.
4. Hold arms at a 90-degree angle. Drive elbows back and up on backswing and bring hands level with shoulders on forward swing.

**Rest:** 60 seconds between each repetition

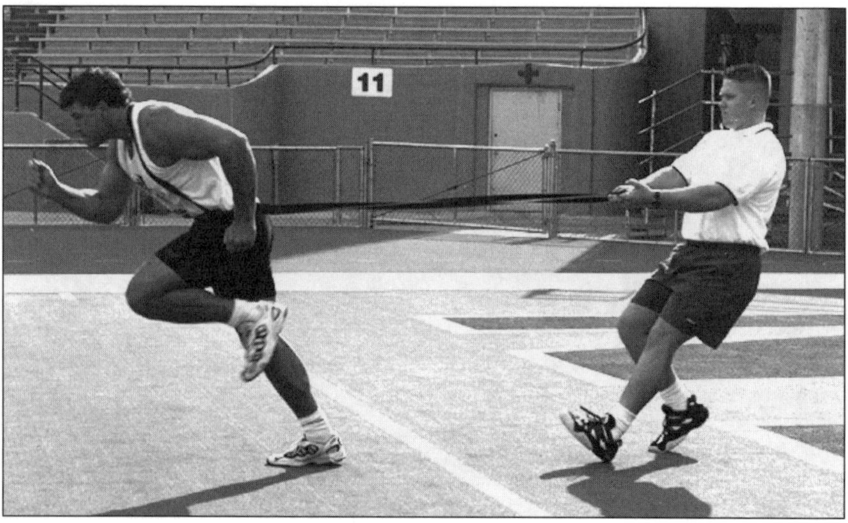

**Key Points:**

1. Pump arms quickly and use good form, running upright with the feet striking the ground directly below the waist.
2. Apply the proper resistance.
3. Drive knees and heels up.

## HILL SPRINTS

**Purpose:** To develop explosiveness and stride length

**Procedure:**

1. This drill can be used in place of stadium steps. Find a hill that is 50 to 100 yards long with a 10- to 15-degree angle.
2. Start at the bottom of the hill.
3. Concentrate on driving off hind leg, extending completely at ankles, knees, and hips.
4. Drive knees and heels up as your leg carries forward.
5. Hold your arms at 90-degree angles with a straight swinging motion, driving elbows back and up on backswing and bringing hands to shoulder level on forward swing.
6. Jog down the hill and run back up as soon as you reach the bottom.

**Rest:** 60 to 90 seconds between each set

**Key Points:**

1. Make sure the hill is not too steep.
2. Get triple extension at the ankles, knees, and hips, and drive with your legs.
3. Use good arm action.

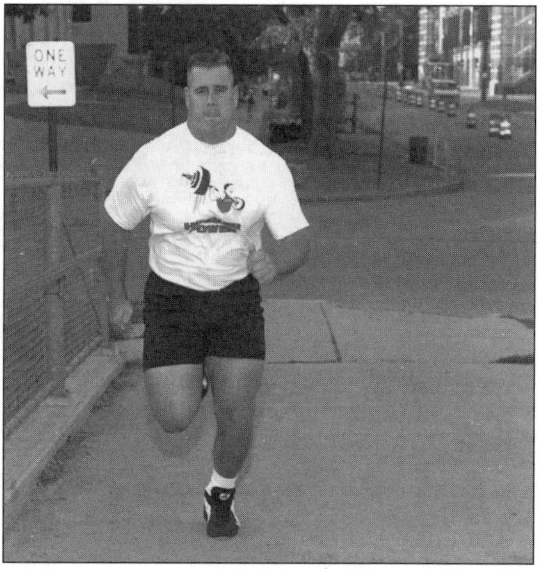

# STADIUM STEPS

**Purpose:** To develop explosiveness and stride length

**Procedure:**

1. Find a set of 30 stadium steps.
2. Run repetitions of the steps, concentrating on driving off the hind leg and extending completely at ankles, knees, and hips.
3. Drive knees and heels up as you carry your leg forward.
4. Hold your arms at 90-degree angles, with a straight swinging motion; drive elbows back and up on backswing and bring hands level with shoulders on forward swing.
5. Once you reach the top, walk back to the bottom of the steps and run the next set as soon as you reach the bottom. Continue until all sets are completed.

**Rest:** 60 seconds between each set

**Key Points:**

1. Get triple extension at the ankles, knees, and hips, and drive with the legs.
2. Use good arm action.
3. Once you reach bottom of steps, repeat drill.

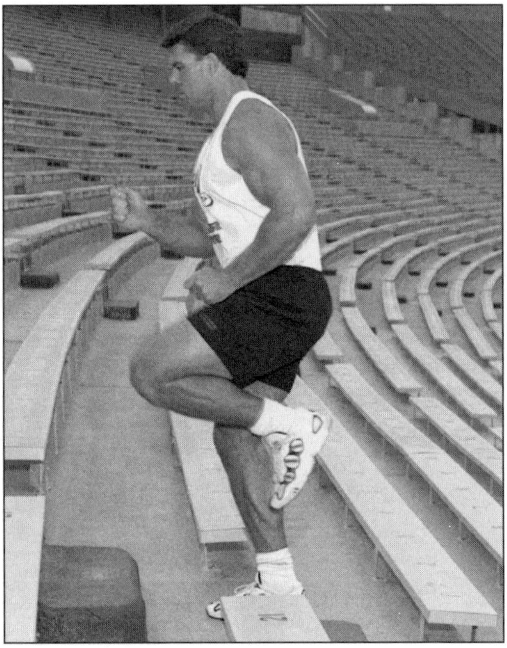

**Variations:** The following are three variations of the stadium step drill to try. Use your imagination and come up with some of your own variations.

1. Running every step
2. Running every other step
3. 10/10 hopping—hop 10 steps on right foot, then 10 steps on left foot, alternating to top

# CHAPTER 7

# AGILITY DRILLS

Agility is the ability to accelerate, decelerate, and change direction quickly while maintaining good body control. In chapter 1 we said football is not played straight ahead, but requires changes of direction in which cutting maneuvers (side steps or crossover steps) are used in the several planes of movement simultaneously. Football is played in short bursts of 5 to 10 yards or less before a change of direction is required. So, acceleration is an important aspect of agility during a football game.

Whether you're a defensive back breaking toward a pass or a guard pulling to make a block, agility is a key and sometimes overlooked component of football. A good agility program should be incorporated into a total conditioning program. The agility drills in this chapter require the skill to stop quickly and accelerate in a different direction.

Seriously consider the concept of specificity when designing your agility program. The footwork encountered by a lineman is different from that of a linebacker, which is also different from that of a running back. The drills on the following pages have proven to be successful in developing agility. You should not, however, limit yourself only to these drills. In any agility program you should create a variety of drills specific to the movements encountered on the field. Changing the order, or making small changes in the drills themselves (such as reversing directions), helps keep players mentally fresh.

Before describing the various agility and position-specific drills, it is necessary to have a clear understanding of some of the terms used to describe the drills.

**Shuffle step.** Lateral movement, stepping first with the right foot and then sliding the left foot to the right foot. Keep knees bent, body squared, and don't cross your legs. Repeat, leading with left foot.

**Lateral step.** Moving your feet by stepping sideways and lifting your knees over a series of bags or through the open spaces of ropes or tires. Keep your body squared as you move laterally.

**Double chop step.** Moving your feet by taking two quick steps (double step) or a stutter step. The double chop can be used during forward or lateral movements.

**Carioca.** Lateral movement, crossing right foot over in front of the left, stepping laterally with the left, and then bringing the right foot behind the left foot on the next step. While moving, keep knees flexed and shoulders squared with a good hip rotation.

**Backpedal.** Run backward, keeping the shoulders and body weight forward. Step, keeping feet low to ground and eyes focused upfield.

**Drop action.** Running diagonally looking back over the shoulder.

**Drop step.** If moving to the right, move the right foot backward diagonally and slide the left foot to the right foot. If moving to the left, move the left foot backward diagonally and slide the right foot to the left foot. Keep the head up and knees flexed, and keep the hips pointing upfield.

**Side step.** Plant outside foot and cut in the opposite direction. (If you plant on right foot, cut to the left.) This is also known as a straight cut.

**Crossover step.** Plant foot and cut in direction of planted foot by crossing in front with other foot.

**Reverse pivot.** If cutting to the right, plant right foot and throw left shoulder counterclockwise, pivoting on the right foot. If cutting to the left, plant left foot and throw right shoulder clockwise, pivoting on the left foot.

The agility drills are divided into the following six categories:

1. Rope drills
2. Bag drills
3. Backpedal drills
4. Cone drills
5. Line drills
6. Jump rope drills

## ROPE DRILLS

In rope drills for football offensive linemen keep the ropes low to the ground, adjusted no higher than 3 to 4 inches. All other football position players should do the drills with ropes adjusted to 12 to 18 inches. When doing these drills keep your head up and eyes focused straight ahead, and concentrate on getting your feet off the ground and back down as quickly as possible.

### EVERY OTHER HOLE

**Purpose:** To develop high knee action, peripheral vision, flexibility, and footwork

**Procedure:**

1. Run forward through ropes using high knee action with a slight forward lean.
2. Hit every other hole on right side with right foot; hit every other hole on left side with left foot (figure 7.1).
3. Use good pumping arm action.

**Rest:** 30 seconds between each repetition

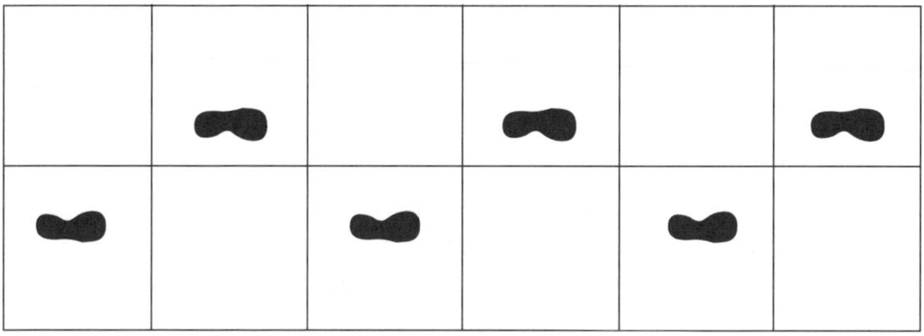

**Figure 7.1**

## EVERY HOLE

**Purpose:** To develop high knee action, peripheral vision, and footwork

**Procedure:**

1. Run forward, using high knee action and good arm action.
2. Right foot hits every hole on right side, left hits every hole on left side (figure 7.2).

**Rest:** 30 seconds between each repetition

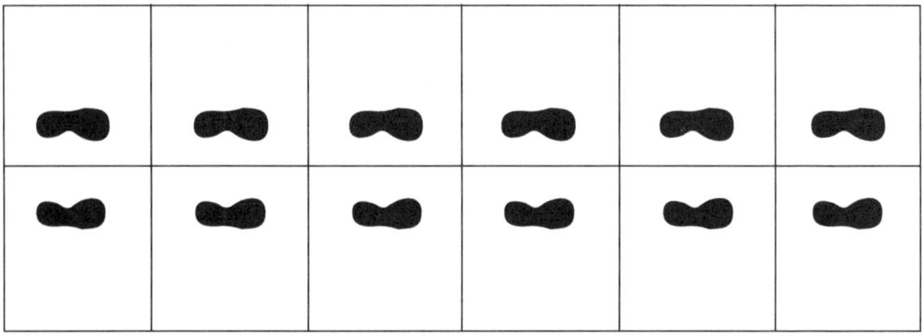

**Figure 7.2**

## DOUBLE CHOP

**Purpose:** To improve foot quickness

**Procedure:**

1. Step forward on either right or left side of the ropes, using good arm action.
2. Chop the feet twice in each hole (figure 7.3).

**Rest:** 45 seconds between each repetition

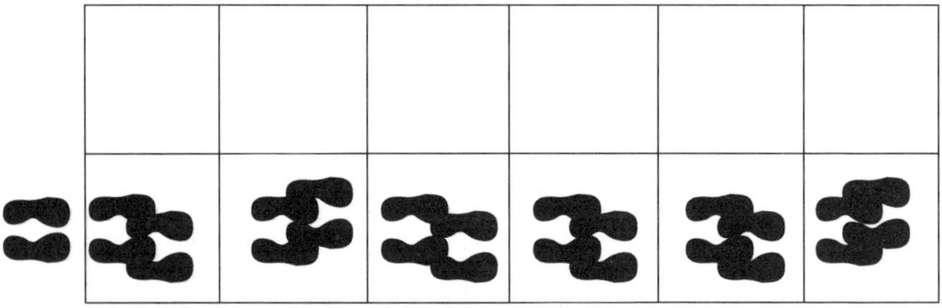

**Figure 7.3**

## LATERAL STEP

**Purpose:** To develop foot quickness, flexibility, and peripheral vision

**Procedure:**

1. Run laterally through one side of rope holes, using high knee action and hitting every hole (figure 7.4).
2. Go one direction leading with left foot and come back other direction leading with right foot.

**Rest:** 30 seconds between each repetition

**Key Point:** Keep shoulders and hips squared.

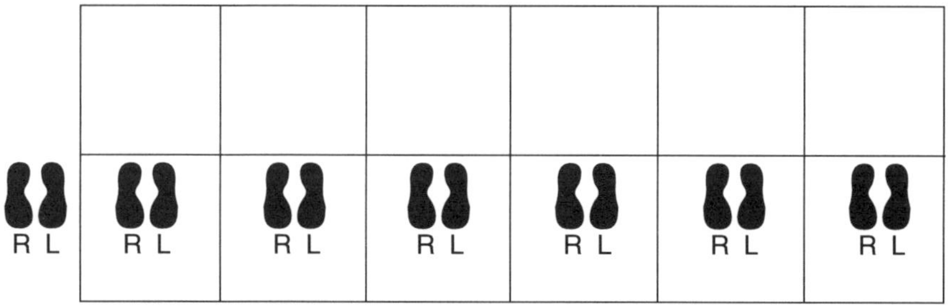


**Figure 7.4**

## LATERAL STEP WITH DOUBLE CHOP

**Purpose:** To develop foot quickness, flexibility, and peripheral vision

**Procedure:**

1. Run laterally, using only one row of holes. Use high knee action to chop the feet twice in each hole (figure 7.5).

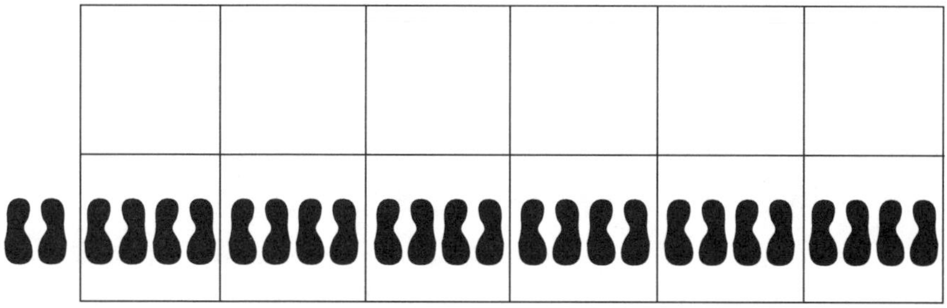

**Figure 7.5**

2. Go one direction leading with right foot, go other direction leading with left foot.

**Rest:** 45 seconds between each repetition

**Key Point:** Keep shoulders and hips squared.

## BUNNY HOP

**Purpose:** To improve foot quickness and provide plyometric benefits

**Procedure:**

1. With feet together, hop diagonally through ropes, hitting every other hole; spend a minimum amount of time on the ground (figure 7.6).
2. Pump both arms at same time during each hop.

**Rest:** 45 seconds between each repetition

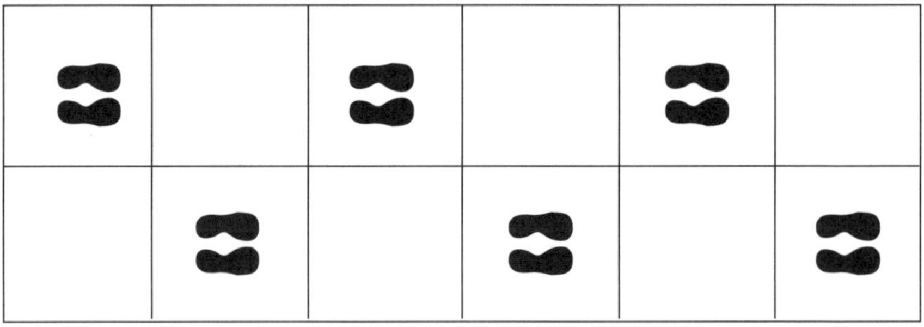

**Figure 7.6**

## CROSSOVER STEP

**Purpose:** To improve footwork and hip flexibility

**Procedure:** Run forward, placing right foot in every other left-side hole and left foot in every other right-side hole (figure 7.7).

**Rest:** 30 seconds between each repetition

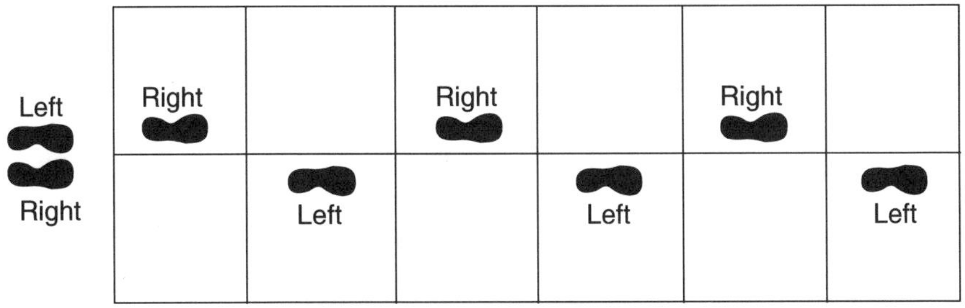


Figure 7.7

## ROPE WEAVE

**Purpose:** To improve change of direction

**Procedure:**

1. Starting by the outside corner of the right-side hole, place your left foot in the right-side hole.
2. Continue, using quick foot action and moving diagonally with the right foot in the left-side hole and taking the next step with the left foot outside the rope (figure 7.8).
3. Change direction with a slight pivot and move the right foot into the left-side hole.
4. Continue weaving in and out through the ropes.

**Rest:** 30 seconds between each repetition

**Key Points:**

1. Make sure your foot movement and pivots are quick.
2. Take the initial step with the correct foot.

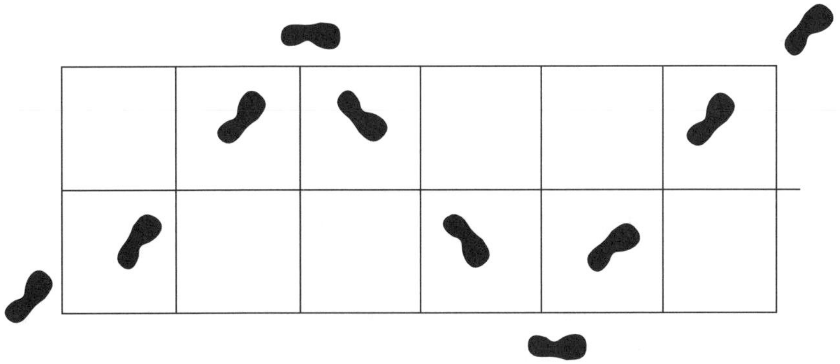

Figure 7.8

# BAG DRILLS

The best kind of bags to use are the square blocking bags used for football practices, since they can lay flat without being rolled. If someone kicks a bag out of place, stop the drill and replace it in its correct position. This will keep the players from tripping on them and running into each other. Space the bags about two and one-half feet apart. Players should keep their heads up and eyes focused straight ahead for all of these drills.

## STRAIGHT RUN

**Purpose:** To develop quick foot action, flexibility, and high knee action

**Procedure:** Run forward over bags using high knee action with a slight forward lean (figure 7.9).

**Rest:** 30 seconds between each repetition

**Key Points:**

1. Do not lean backward.
2. Pick up knees; do not throw feet around ends or sides of bags.

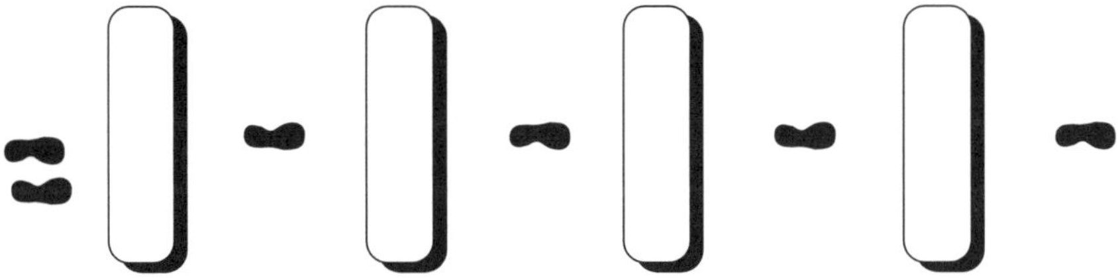

Figure 7.9

## FORWARD WITH DOUBLE CHOP

**Purpose:** To develop quick foot action, flexibility, and high knee action

**Procedure:**

1. Run forward over bags using high knee action with a slight forward lean.
2. Chop feet twice between each bag (figure 7.10).

**Rest:** 45 seconds between each repetition

**Key Point:** Do not lean backward.

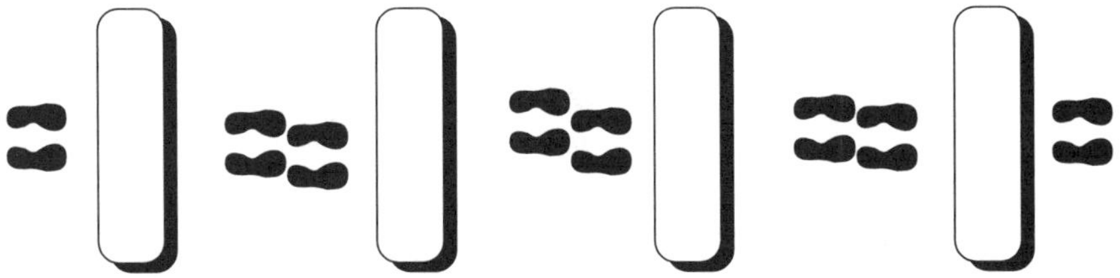

**Figure 7.10**

## LATERAL STEP (BAG)

**Purpose:** To develop quick foot action, flexibility, and high knee action.

**Procedure:**

1. Run laterally over bags using high knee action. Start with leg closest to bag (figure 7.11).
2. Go one direction leading with right foot, go the other direction leading with left foot.

**Rest:** 30 seconds between each repetition

**Key Point:** Keep shoulders and hips squared.

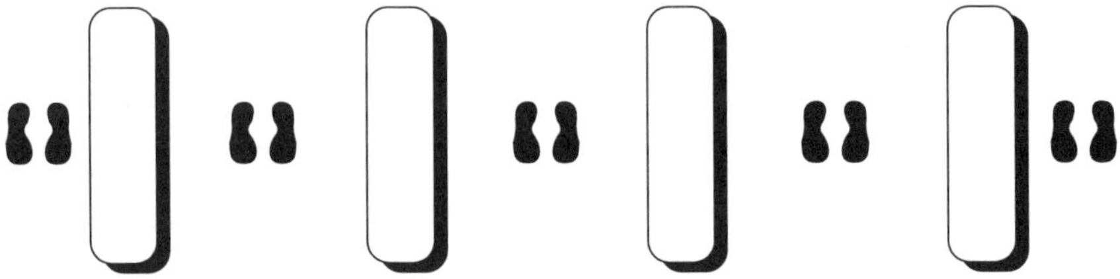

**Figure 7.11**

## LATERAL STEP WITH DOUBLE CHOP (BAG)

**Purpose:** To develop quick foot action, flexibility, and high knee action

**Procedure:**

1. Run laterally using high knee action.
2. Chop feet twice between each bag (figure 7.12).

**Rest:** 45 seconds between each repetition

**Key Point:** Keep shoulders and hips squared.

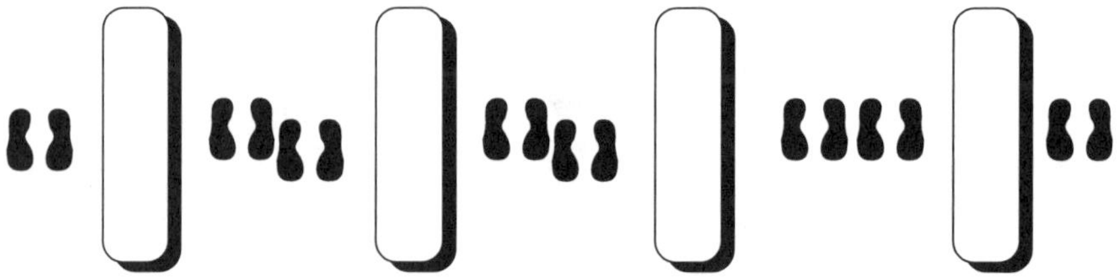

Figure 7.12

## TAP

**Purpose:** To develop quick foot action and ability to stay low

**Procedure:**

1. Start from a two-point stance with knees slightly bent, torso upright, head up, and hands and arms away from body.
2. On command, laterally step over the bags, tapping each bag with both hands (figure 7.13).
3. Upon completion of last bag, sprint forward for five yards.

**Rest:** 45 seconds between each repetition.

**Key Point:** Keep your rear end down and head up as you move through the bags.

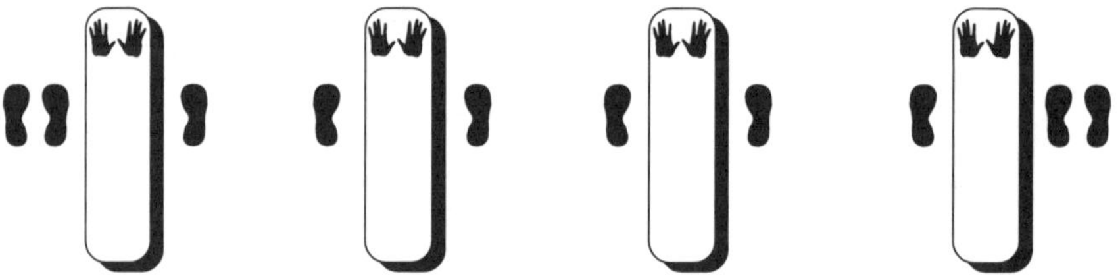

Figure 7.13

## CHANGE OF DIRECTION

**Purpose:** To develop quick foot action and change of direction

**Procedure:**

1. Start at one end of the bags on right or left side and run forward toward other side of bag.

2. Planting outside foot at the end of bag, use a side step to explode forward toward the other end of the next bag.
3. Continue through bags (figure 7.14).

**Rest:** 45 seconds between each repetition

**Key Point:** Push off with your outside foot and accelerate through the bags.

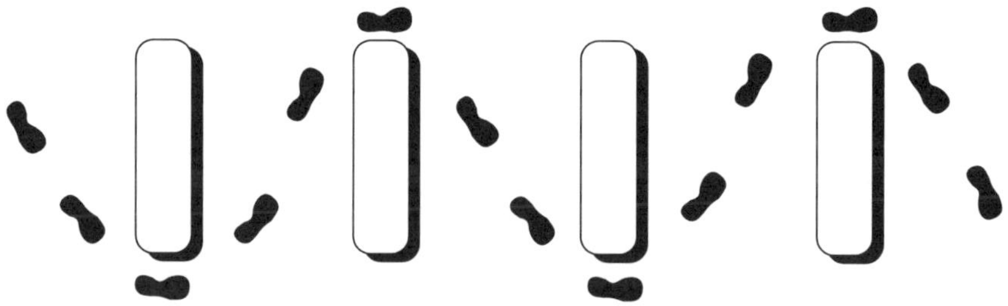

**Figure 7.14**

## FORWARD-BACK

**Purpose:** To develop quick foot action, flexibility, and high knee action

**Procedure:**

1. Start from a two-point stance with knees slightly bent, torso upright, head up, and hands and arms away from body.
2. On command, run forward to end of bag.
3. Backpedal through bags to other end, then move forward again (figure 7.15).
4. Repeat through all bags, ending with five-yard sprint.

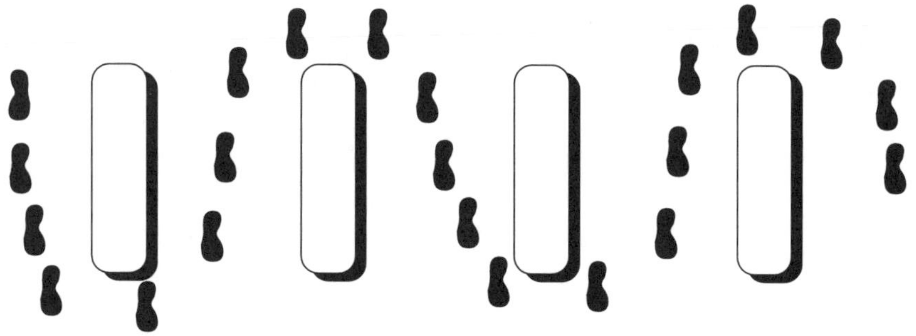

**Figure 7.15**

**Rest:** 30 seconds between each repetition

**Key Points:**

1. Stay low throughout drill.
2. Keep weight forward during backpedal segment.
3. Eliminate false steps when changing directions.

## ZIGZAG OR SHUFFLE

**Purpose:** To develop foot coordination, quickness, strength, and flexibility in abductors and adductors

**Procedure:**

1. Start at one end of the bags on either right or left side, facing the row of bags.
2. Shuffle diagonally beyond first bag.
3. Change directions and shuffle diagonally to end of second bag and continue shuffling through bags (figure 7.16).

**Rest:** 30 seconds between each repetition

**Key Points:**

1. Stay low throughout the drill.
2. Do not cross feet.
3. Push off with trailing foot; push off with outside foot when changing direction.

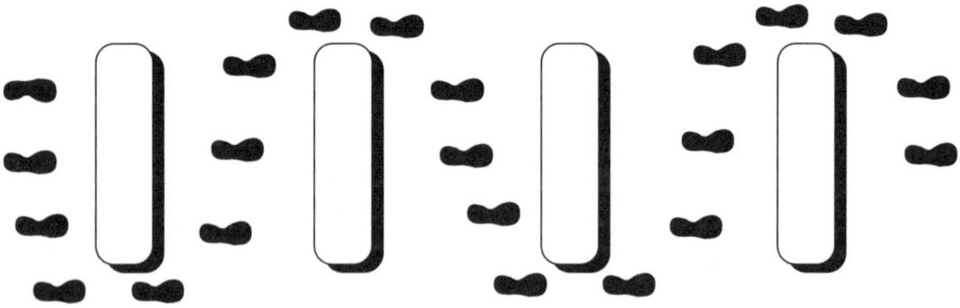

Figure 7.16

## COMBO LATERAL/FORWARD-BACK

**Purpose:** To develop quick foot action, flexibility, change of direction, and high knee action

**Procedure:**

1. Start from a two-point stance with knees slightly bent, torso upright, head up, and hands and arms away from body.
2. Run laterally over the first two bags.
3. Sprint five yards to the front of the third bag and shuffle step.
4. Backpedal five yards and laterally step over bags four and five.
5. Continue through the bags in this pattern (figure 7.17).

**Rest:** 45 seconds between each repetition

**Key Points:**

1. Accelerate.
2. Stay low during backpedal.
3. Keep hips and shoulders squared during lateral steps.

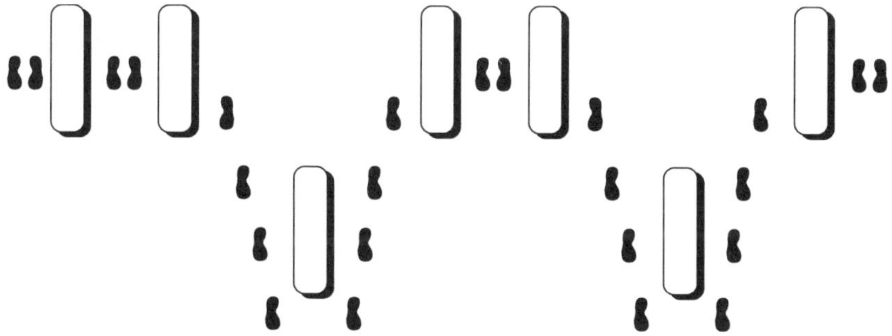

Figure 7.17

## WAVE

**Purpose:** To develop quick foot action and reactions

**Procedure:**

1. Start from a two-point stance with knees slightly bent, torso upright, head up, and hands and arms away from body.
2. Watch the coach's hand signals and respond to the direction he points by laterally stepping over the bags using quick high knee action (figure 7.18).
3. Finish the drill by sprinting 10 yards forward.

**Rest:** 45 seconds between each repetition

**Key Points:**

1. Always move at right angles when changing directions; don't anticipate the change of direction.
2. Run hard.

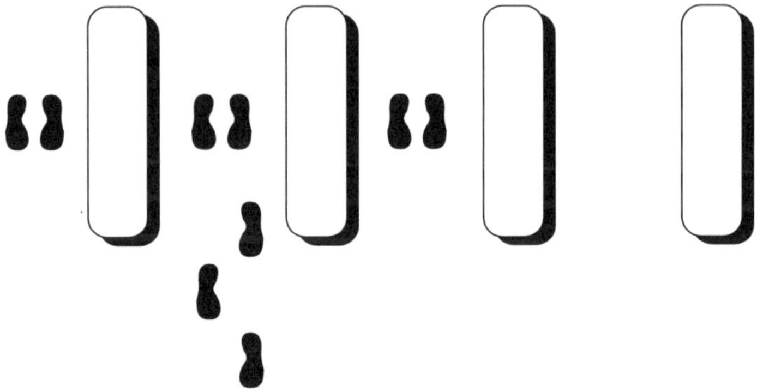

Figure 7.18

## ROTATION

**Purpose:** To improve hip flexibility and foot quickness

**Procedure:**

1. Using quick feet, laterally step over first two bags.
2. Pivot 180 degrees by turning the hips, and laterally step over third bag.
3. Laterally step over next two bags.
4. Continue this pattern through the bags (figure 7.19).

**Rest:** 45 seconds between each repetition

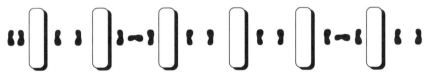

Figure 7.19

## BUNNY HOP ROTATION

**Purpose:** To improve hip flexibility and foot quickness and provide plyometric benefits

**Procedure:**

1. Laterally hop over the first bag, rotating 180 degrees while in the air.
2. After contact quickly hop over second bag, rotating 180 degrees in the opposite direction.
3. Continue hopping and rotating over the bags (figure 7.20).

**Rest:** 45 seconds between each repetition

**Key Points:**

1. Use quick feet; do not spend a lot of time on the ground.
2. Twist with the hips when rotating.

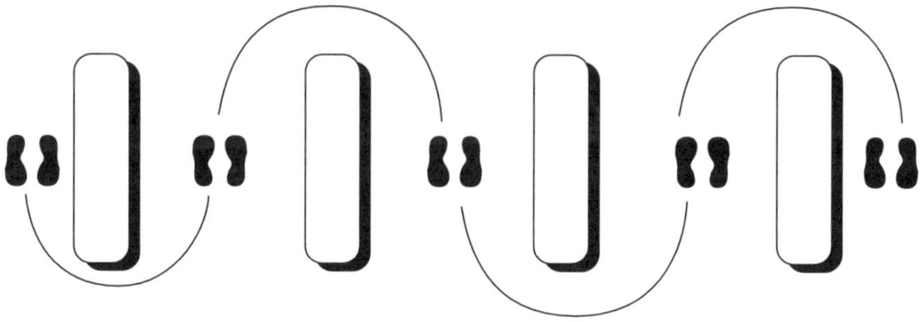

Figure 7.20

## WHEEL

**Purpose:** To develop quick foot action and balance

**Procedure:**

1. Arrange bags as in figure 7.21; start at point A with both hands in the middle on the X formed by the bags.
2. On the coach's command, chop feet over each bag while pivoting around all four bags on your hands until you are back at the original starting position.
3. Quickly change directions and rotate back, chopping feet over all four bags.
4. Finish the drill by quickly sprinting out of bags over the fifth bag.

**Rest:** 45 seconds between each repetition

**Key Points:**

1. Take one foot over the bag at a time, moving quickly.
2. Keep on fingertips.

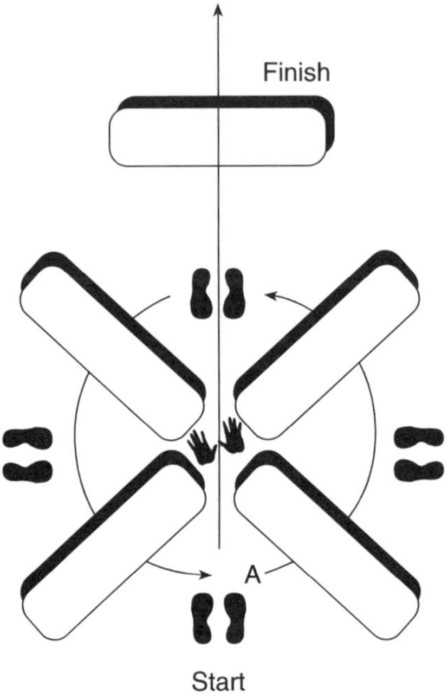


**Figure 7.21**

## LATERAL SPEED

**Purpose:** To develop change of direction, acceleration, and reaction

**Procedure:**

1. Sprint to side of first bag and take a lateral step over bag by pushing off with outside foot.
2. Once over the bag, push off with outside foot and sprint to next bag and repeat steps.
3. At end of row of bags, sprint either right or left in direction of coach's signal (figure 7.22).

**Rest:** 45 seconds between each repetition

**Key Point:** Push off with outside foot and accelerate from bag to bag, using quick feet over the bag.

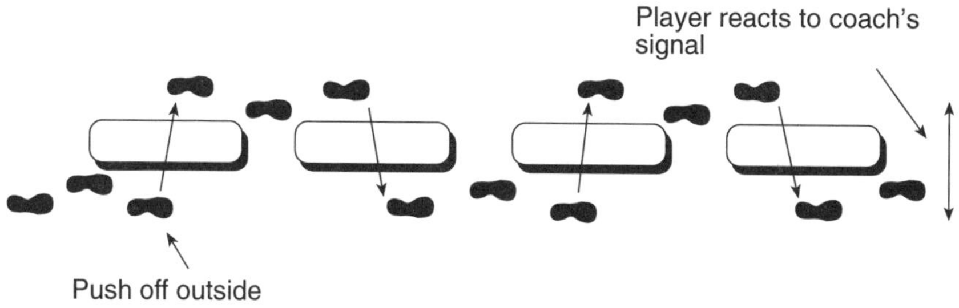


Figure 7.22

## COMBO LATERAL STEP/HIGH KNEE

**Purpose:** To develop lateral movement and high knee action

**Procedure:**

1. Set up bags as illustrated in figure 7.23.
2. From a two-point stance with knees slightly bent, torso upright, head up, and hands and arms away from body, use a lateral step and begin running diagonally through bags.
3. At completion of angled bags, burst for three to five yards.
4. Turn and run straight through next series of bags, using high knee action.

**Rest:** 45 seconds between each repetition

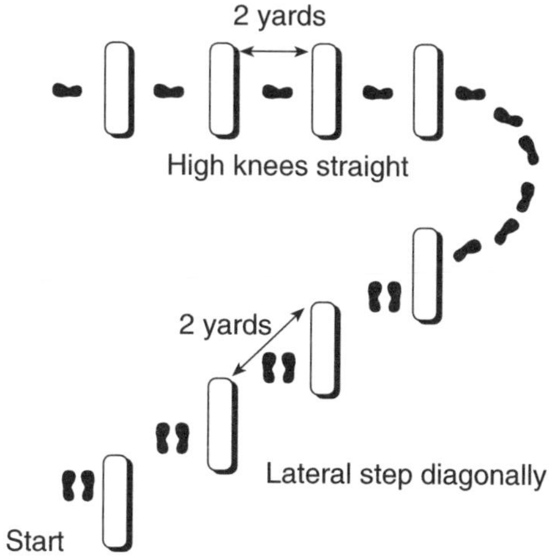


Figure 7.23

**Key Points:**

1. Do not cross legs on side step.
2. Keep eyes up (not looking at bags), and maintain a low position throughout drill.
3. Have hands out in front where you can use them.
4. Change direction of angled bags to get footwork in both directions.

## BACKPEDAL DRILLS

Defensive backs are the only players who do all of the backpedal drills (though linebackers do many of these drills). Because defensive backs cover receivers, they start most plays by backpedaling—running backward, keeping their shoulders and body weight forward. They step keeping their feet low to the ground and their eyes focused upfield. After a receiver makes his cut, the defensive back must be able to react by switching to a different movement pattern. Almost every backpedal drill requires a change of direction by switching from one movement pattern to another. All backpedal drills start from a two-point stance.

### COMEBACK

**Purpose:** To develop change of direction and reaction

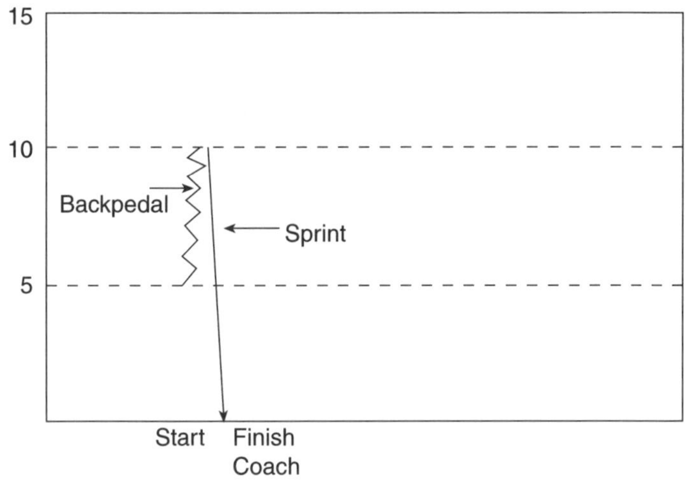


Figure 7.24

**Procedure:**

1. Backpedal on the coach's command.
2. Sprint forward, concentrating on accelerating, on coach's hand signal (figure 7.24).

**Rest**: 45 seconds between each repetition

**Key Points:**

1. Keep shoulders and body weight forward and low.
2. Keep feet moving during change of direction; do not be caught "flatfooted."

## 90-DEGREE

**Purpose:** To develop change of direction and reaction

**Procedure:**

1. Backpedal on the coach's command.
2. Watch the coach's hand signals, responding to the direction he points (right or left).
3. Push at a 90-degree angle in the direction coach points and sprint 10 yards (figure 7.25).

**Rest:** 45 seconds between each repetition

**Key Points:**

1. If cut is to the left, plant and pivot off right foot and vice versa.

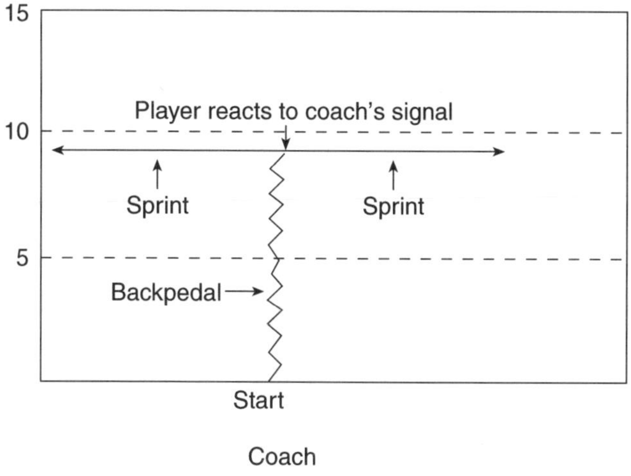


**Figure 7.25**

2. Make cuts at full speed.
3. Keep shoulders and body weight forward and low.

## 45-DEGREE

**Purpose:** To develop change of direction and reaction

**Procedure:**

1. Backpedal on the coach's command.
2. Watch the coach's hand signals, responding to the direction he points (right or left).
3. Reverse your direction and sprint at 45-degree angle to the direction to which coach points (figure 7.26).

**Rest:** 45 seconds between each repetition

**Key Points:**

1. Keep shoulders and body weight forward and low.
2. Show good acceleration during the forward cut.

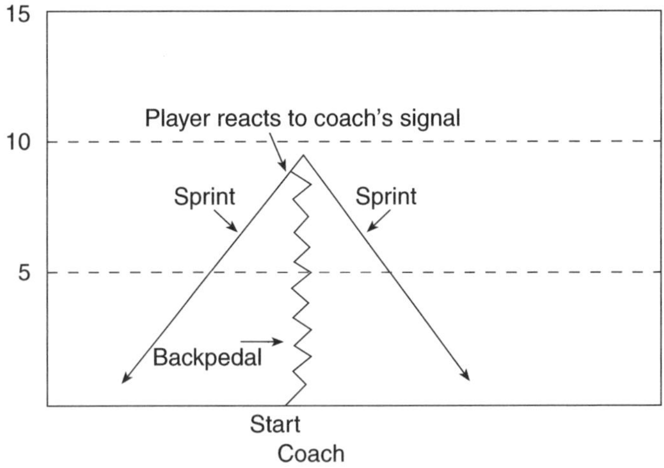


Figure 7.26

## POST/CORNER

**Purpose:** To develop change of direction and acceleration after a turn

**Procedure:**

1. Backpedal on the coach's command.
2. Watch the coach's hand signals, responding to the direction he points (right or left).
3. Turn, accelerate, and break deep at a 45-degree angle for 20 yards (figure 7.27).

**Rest:** 45 seconds between each repetition

**Key Point:** Keep shoulders and body weight forward and low during backpedal.

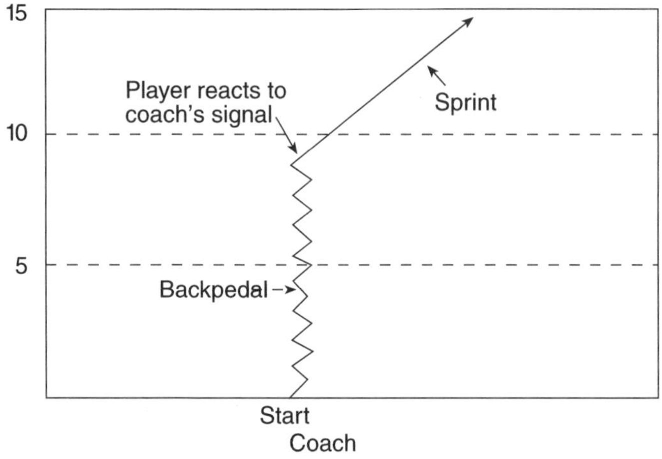


**Figure 7.27**

# CENTERFIELD

**Purpose:** To develop change of direction, reaction, and acceleration after a turn

**Procedure:**

1. Backpedal on the coach's command.
2. Watch the coach's hand signals, responding to the direction he points.
3. Push right or left at a 45-degree angle for a couple of steps and then turn the opposite direction, accelerate, and break deep at a 45-degree angle in the opposite direction (figure 7.28).

**Rest:** 45 seconds between each repetition

**Key Points:**

1. Keep shoulders and body weight forward and low during back-pedal.
2. Quickly turn body and head.

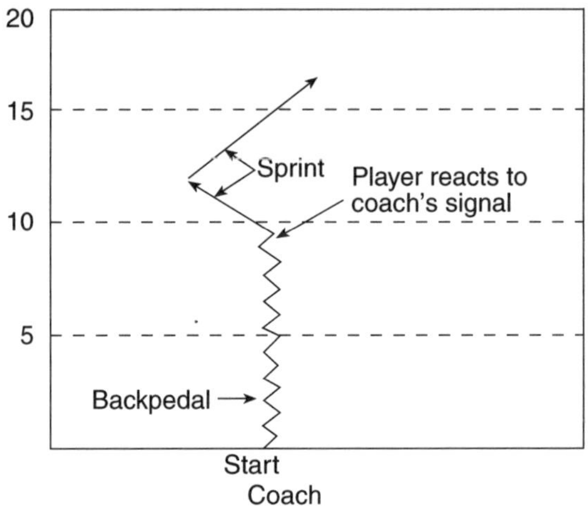


**Figure 7.28**

## HIP FLIP ON LINE

**Purpose:** To develop hip flexibility

**Procedure:**

1. Start in two-point ready position; on command begin backpedaling on the line.
2. With coach's direction, pivot hips and run, staying on the line with eyes on coach.
3. Coach will direct you in opposite direction; pivot to opposite direction, keeping eyes on coach.
4. Repeat steps 2 and 3. After four pivots, turn and sprint for 10 yards (figure 7.29).

**Rest:** 45 seconds between each repetition

**Key Points:**

1. Stay low with weight over balls of feet.
2. When pivoting it is helpful to throw elbow to help get around.
3. Stay on the line.

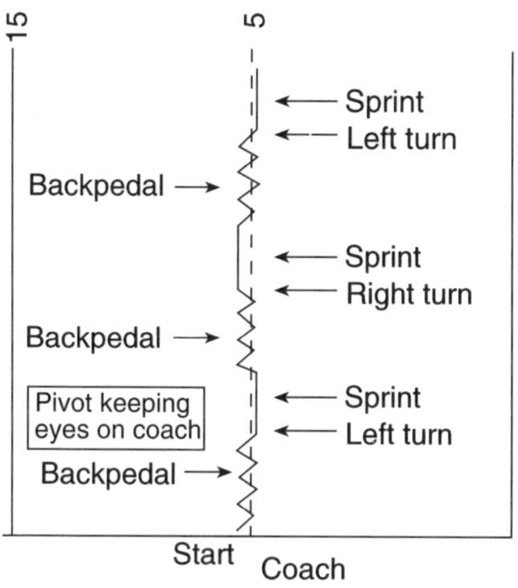


Figure 7.29

## W BACKPEDAL-BREAK

**Purpose:** To hone your ability to quickly change direction

**Procedure:**

1. Backpedal for five yards at a 45-degree angle.
2. Plant outside foot and sprint forward at 45-degree angle for five yards (figure 7.30).
3. Repeat twice.

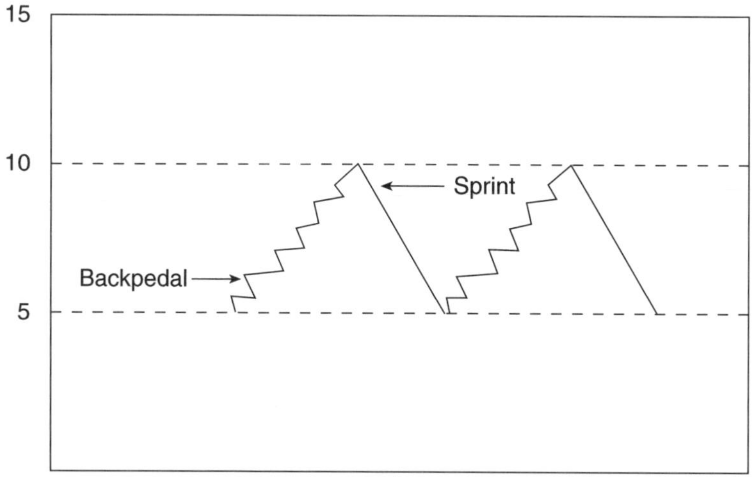


Figure 7.30

**Rest:** 45 seconds between each repetition

**Key Points:**

1. This is not a race; emphasize proper backpedal, then sprint.
2. Do drill in both directions.

## WET FIELD

**Purpose:** To warm up and develop change of direction and quick feet

**Procedure:**

1. Backpedal 10 yards as fast as possible.
2. When hitting the 10-yard strip (if on football field), plant foot and take quick steps with high knees as you sprint forward to starting line (figure 7.31).
3. Repeat four times.

**Rest:** 45 seconds between each repetition

**Key Point:** Make sure feet are pointing straight ahead when planting them to change directions; if you try to turn foot sideways to change direction it will slip.

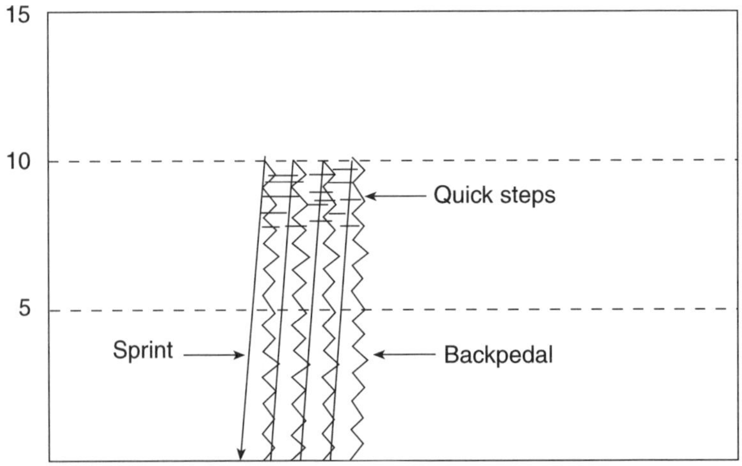


**Figure 7.31**

# BACKPEDAL WEAVE

**Purpose:** To warm up and work on backpedal technique

**Procedure:**

1. Backpedal in a weaving motion, changing direction every three or four steps.

**Rest:** 45 seconds between each repetition

**Key Point:** Stay low on the backpedal.

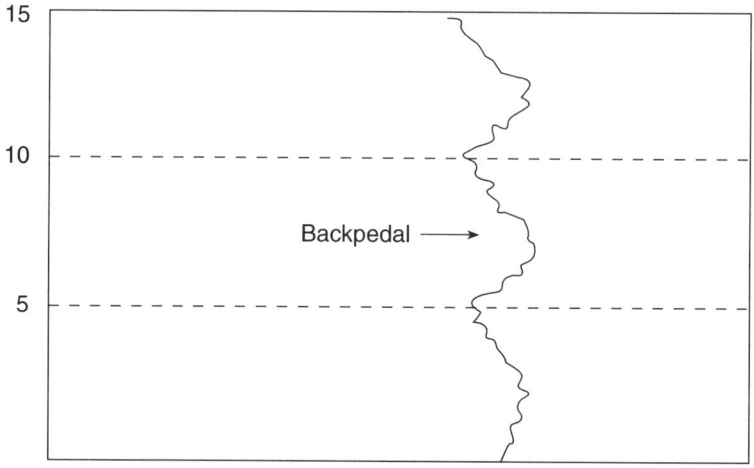


Figure 7.32

# MIRROR

**Purpose:** To warm up and develop footwork

**Procedure:**

1. Two players are needed to run drill: a receiver and a defender.
2. Receiver runs a weaving pattern (figure 7.33).
3. Having been lined up over the receiver's shoulder, defender backpedals keeping proper procedure on receiver.
4. This can progress with weave to outs, posts, etc.

**Rest:** 45 seconds between each repetition

**Key Point:** The receiver should not line up directly in front of the defender. He should line up one or two yards to the side of defender.

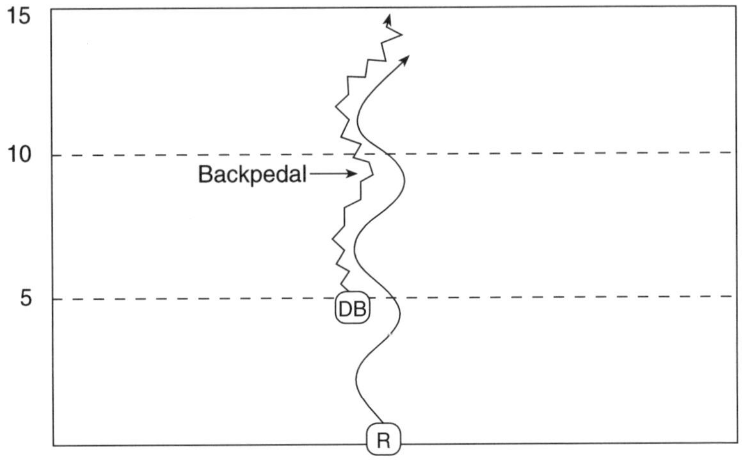


Figure 7.33

## CONFIDENCE

**Purpose:** To develop defensive backs' confidence to stay in backpedal for greater distance before having to turn and run with receiver

**Procedure:**

1. Using a defender and receiver, defender lines up three yards from receiver (figure 7.34).
2. Receiver runs straight forward as fast as possible until he passes defender.

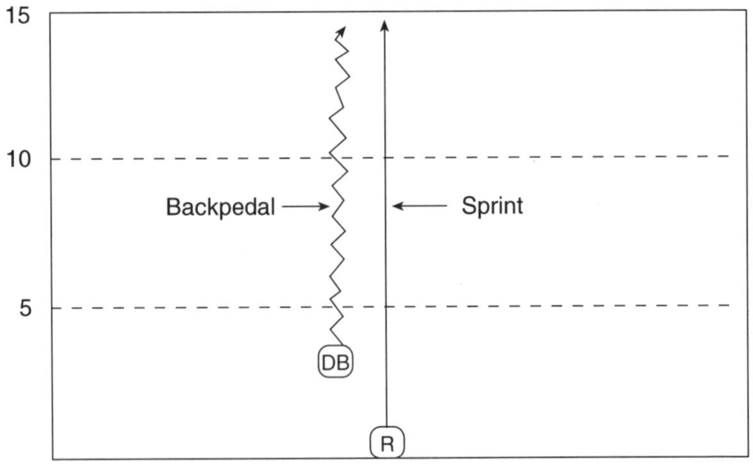


Figure 7.34

3. Defender backpedals as fast as possible, for greatest distance possible.

**Rest:** 45 seconds between each repetition

## CONE DRILLS

Perform cone drills on artificial turf or natural grass, using 5 to 10 cones. For the safety of the athlete, coaches should choose cones that are 8 to 12 inches high and made of a flexible orange rubber. Perform the drills at full speed with correct running form. Emphasize good acceleration and deceleration between cones. Cones should not be knocked over while performing the drills.

The following five exercises are variations of the four-corner drill. Use your imagination to vary the drill depending on your purpose. For example, you can do each of these drills on the opposite side. Each drill uses four cones at 5 yards or 10 yards apart, whichever you prefer.

### FOUR-CORNER CARIOCA

**Purpose:** To improve change of direction, footwork, and flexibility in hips

**Procedure:**

1. Start on the right side of the square and accelerate forward.
2. At the first cone make a reverse pivot.
3. Carioca to the next cone.
4. Reverse pivot and backpedal to the next cone.
5. Reverse pivot and carioca to the finish (figure 7.35).

**Rest:** 60 seconds between each repetition

**Key Points:**

1. Make sure you are facing the proper direction when doing the carioca.
2. To make it easy to remember which way to make a reverse pivot, always turn to the inside toward the cones.

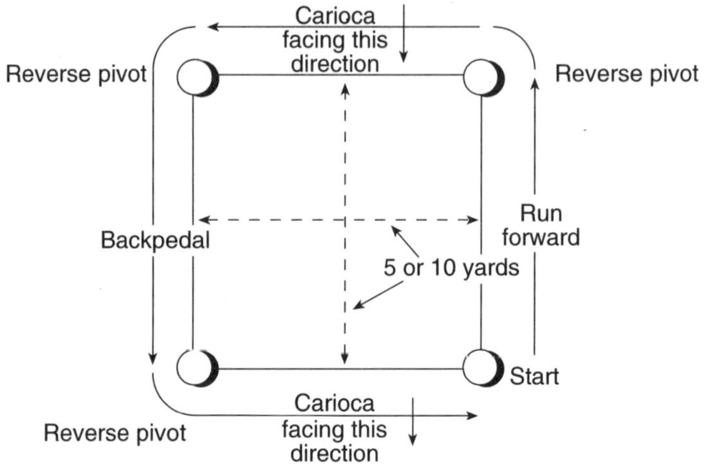


**Figure 7.35**

## FOUR-CORNER SHUFFLE

**Purpose:** To improve footwork and flexibility, and strength in groin area

**Procedure:**

1. Start on the right side of the square and accelerate forward.
2. At the first cone make a reverse pivot by throwing your right shoulder clockwise.
3. Shuffle to the next cone.

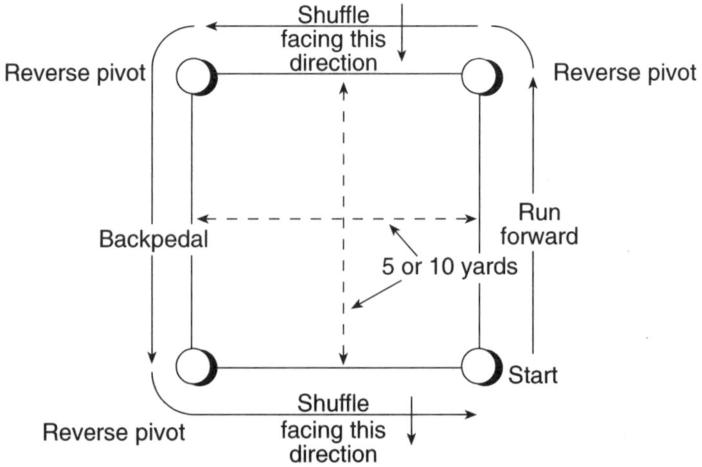


**Figure 7.36**

4. Reverse pivot and backpedal to the next cone.
5. Reverse pivot and shuffle to the finish.

**Rest:** 60 seconds between each repetition

**Key Points:**

1. Make sure you are facing the proper direction when doing the shuffle and that you back pivot.
2. Do not cross feet during the shuffle.

## FOUR-CORNER COMEBACK

**Purpose:** To improve footwork, backpedal, and change of direction

**Procedure:**

1. Start on the right side of the square and backpedal to first cone.
2. At the first cone sprint diagonally to the second cone.
3. Backpedal to the third cone.
4. At the third cone sprint diagonally to the fourth cone (figure 7.37).

**Rest:** 60 seconds between each repetition

**Key Points:**

1. Stay low during the backpedal.
2. Make sure each quick change of direction is followed by good acceleration.

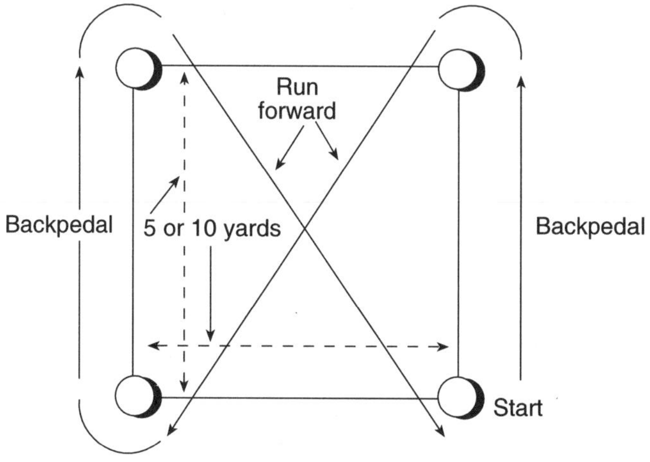


**Figure 7.37**

# FOUR-CORNER DROP

**Purpose:** To improve footwork and change of direction

**Procedure:**

1. Start on the right side of the square and sprint to the first cone.
2. At the first cone run to the second cone using a drop angle.
3. Sprint to the third cone.
4. At the third cone run to the fourth cone using a drop angle (figure 7.38).

**Rest:** 60 seconds between each repetition

**Key Point:** Maintain good acceleration and deceleration while sprinting to the cones.

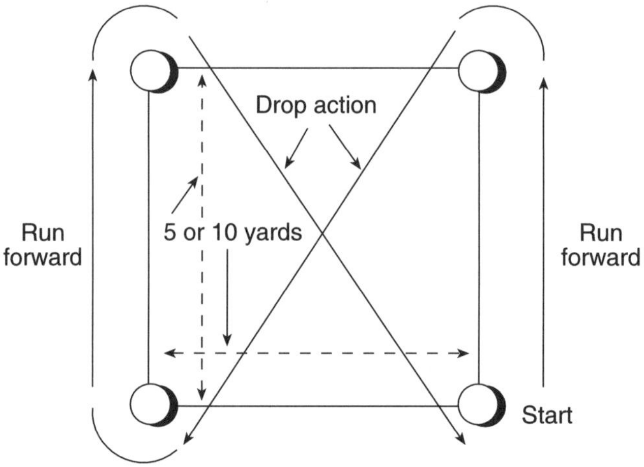


**Figure 7.38**

# FOUR-CORNER SQUARE-IN

**Purpose:** To improve change of direction and acceleration

**Procedure:**

1. Backpedal to first cone.
2. Turn at first cone and sprint forward to second cone.
3. At second cone backpedal to third cone.
4. At third cone sprint to fourth cone (figure 7.39).

**Rest:** 60 seconds between each repetition

**Key Points:**

1. Stay low on the backpedal.
2. Have good acceleration and deceleration while sprinting to the cones.

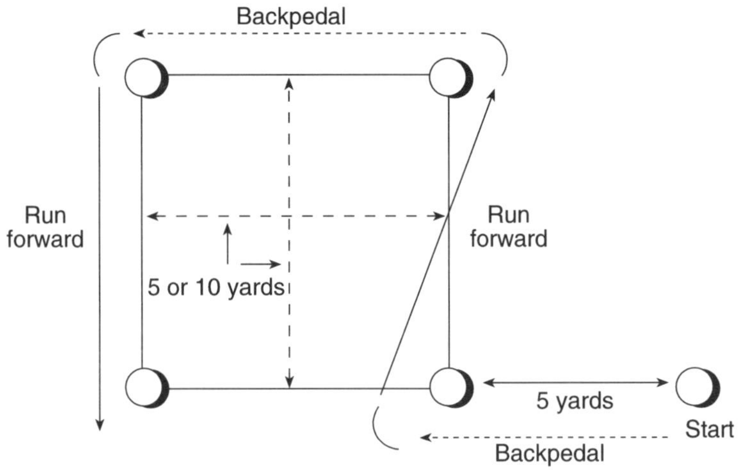


**Figure 7.39**

## RAG

**Purpose:** To improve footwork, flexibility in legs and hips, foot speed, and quickness

**Procedure:**

1. Put four rags or towels approximately 10 yards apart in a square (figure 7.40).
2. Start at one corner and run to the first rag and rotate 360 degrees on the right hand.
3. Go to the second rag and rotate 360 degrees on the left hand.
4. Go to the third rag and rotate 360 degrees on the right hand.
5. Go to the fourth rag and rotate 360 degrees on the left hand.

**Rest:** 60 seconds between each repetition

**Key Point:** Emphasize foot movement, quick feet, head up, hips parallel to the ground, and full extension of legs and feet.

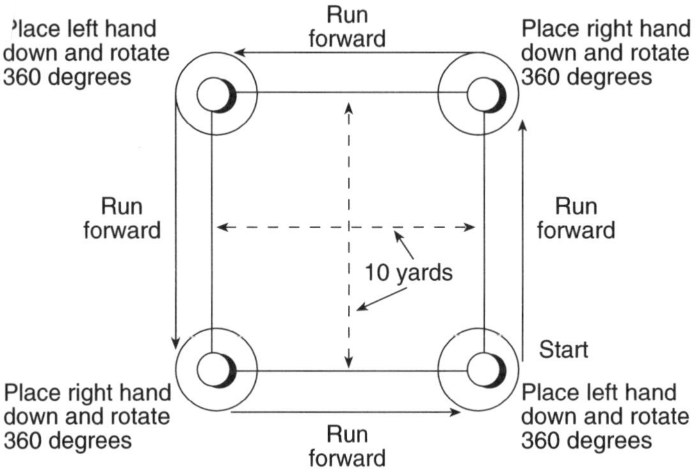


**Figure 7.40**

## THREE-CORNER

**Purpose:** To improve footwork, change of direction, acceleration, and deceleration

**Procedure:**

1. Start in a three-point stance on first line (figure 7.41).
2. Sprint to the first cone; drive off your left foot using a side step, and shuffle right to second cone.
3. At second cone backpedal to third cone.

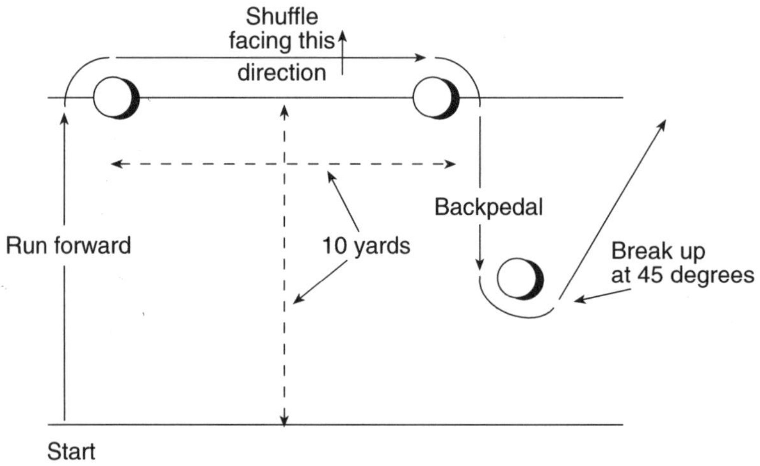


**Figure 7.41**

4. At third cone, plant left foot and break at a 45-degree angle to the right as you would breaking for the ball.

**Rest:** 60 seconds between each repetition

**Key Points:**

1. Maintain good acceleration while sprinting to the first cone and after third cone.
2. Don't cross legs on shuffle step.
3. Stay low on backpedal.

## DODGING RUN

**Purpose:** To improve foot quickness

**Procedure:**

1. Starting in a three-point stance, sprint to the first cone, plant the outside foot, use a side step, and cut around it (figure 7.42).
2. Continue to sprint to each cone, planting outside foot and using a side step to cut hard.

**Rest:** 45 seconds between each repetition

**Key Point:** Maintain good acceleration from cone to cone.

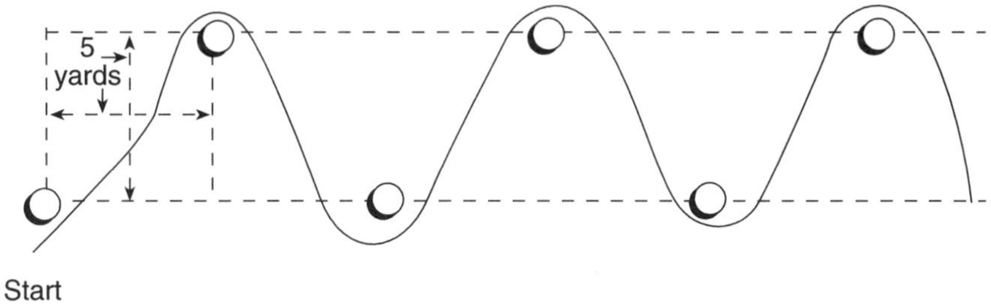


**Figure 7.42**

## ZIGZAG

**Purpose:** To improve footwork and quickness

**Procedure:**

1. Stand facing a row of 10 cones, each cone one yard apart (figure 7.43).
2. Step forward diagonally with the right foot to the right of the first cone and then slide left foot to the right foot.

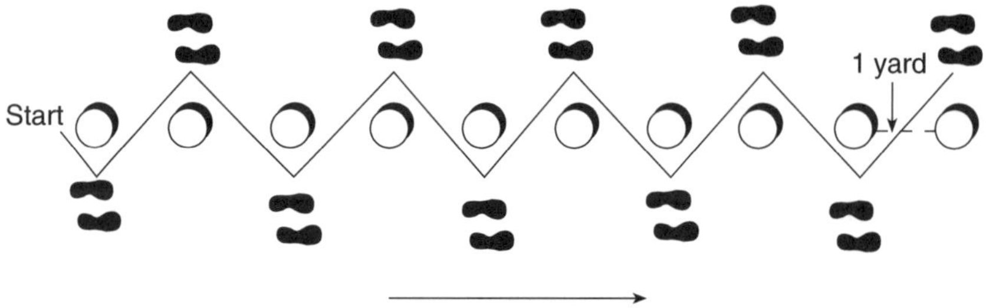


Figure 7.43

3. Lead with the left foot to the left side of the next cone and then slide the right foot to the left foot.
4. Zigzag through all the cones quickly and explosively.

**Rest:** 45 seconds between each repetition

**Key Points:**

1. Keep hips and shoulders squared.
2. Plant both feet as you move to each side of the cone.
3. Push off with your outside foot.

## BACKWARD ZIGZAG

**Purpose:** To improve foot quickness and coordination

**Procedure:**

1. Stand with your back to a row of 10 cones, each cone one yard apart (figure 7.44).
2. Step diagonally backward, leading with the left foot to the left of the first cone and sliding the right foot to the left foot.

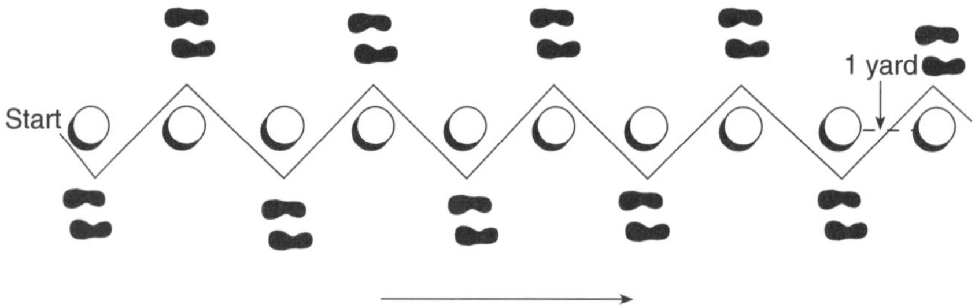


Figure 7.44

3. Step diagonally backward with the right foot to right of the next cone, sliding the left foot to the right foot.
4. Repeat the action through all the cones.

**Rest:** 45 seconds between each repetition

**Key Points:**

1. Keep your hips and shoulders squared as you move backward.
2. Keep low with your knees bent, head up, and back straight.

## COMBO ZIGZAG

**Purpose:** To improve foot quickness, coordination, and change of direction

**Procedure:**

1. Stand with your back to the first cone in a row of 10 cones, each one yard apart (figure 7.45).
2. Step diagonally backward leading with your left foot facing the second cone and slide your right foot toward your left foot.
3. Then step diagonally forward with your left foot back to the third cone and slide your right foot toward your left foot.
4. Repeat going in opposite direction.

**Rest:** 60 seconds between each repetition

**Key Point:** Keep your hips squared, eyes forward, and feet quick.

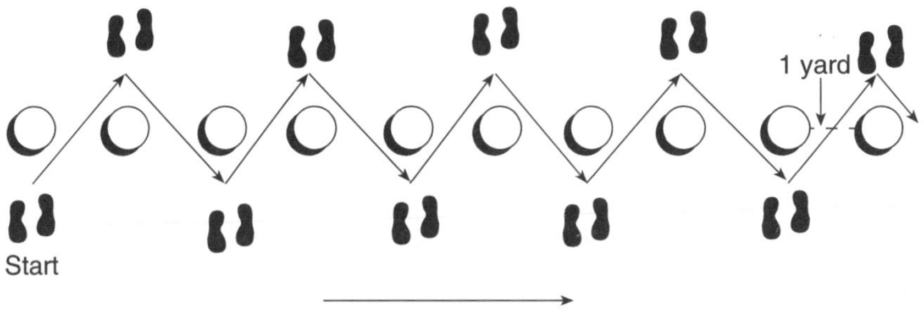


**Figure 7.45**

## NEBRASKA AGILITY

**Purpose:** To improve foot quickness and change of direction

**Procedure:**

1. Set up cones five yards apart as illustrated in figure 7.46.
2. Start in a three-point stance on the first line; sprint to the first cone and make a right-hand turn.
3. Return to the starting line. Go around the second cone with a left-hand turn.
4. Run to the five-yard line and touch it with your fingers, then backpedal across the starting line to the finish.

**Rest:** 45 seconds between each repetition

**Key Points:**

1. Do not knock the cones over.
2. Stay low on the backpedal.
3. Keep feet moving around the cones as quickly as possible while staying low.

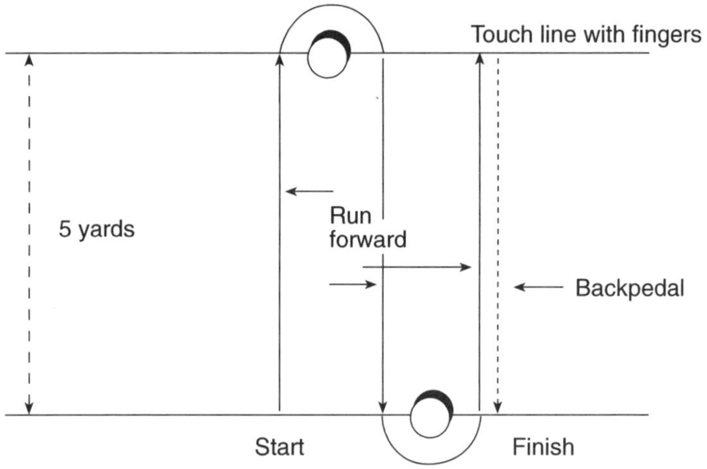


**Figure 7.46**

## LINE DRILLS

Perform line drills on artificial turf or natural grass. Line the field as a standard football field for 15 yards. Be sure to touch lines with alternating feet; push off with both feet so you aren't running in circles. Perform the drills at full speed with correct running form. Emphasize good acceleration out of your turns.

# PRO AGILITY

**Purpose:** To improve footwork, change of direction, and reaction time

**Procedure:**

1. From a two-point stance straddle the middle line.
2. Sprint to the right line and touch it with your right hand.
3. Push off forcefully and sprint back across the middle line to the left line and touch it with your left hand.
4. Sprint back to the right, finishing at the middle line (figure 7.47).

**Rest:** 60 seconds between each repetition

**Key Points:**

1. When running to the right always touch the line with your right hand, and touch it with your left hand when running to the left. This ensures that you will push off with opposite feet.
2. Up to five players can do this drill at the same time and race each other.
3. A player or coach can stand in front and point to the right or left to start the players.
4. Stay low when changing directions.

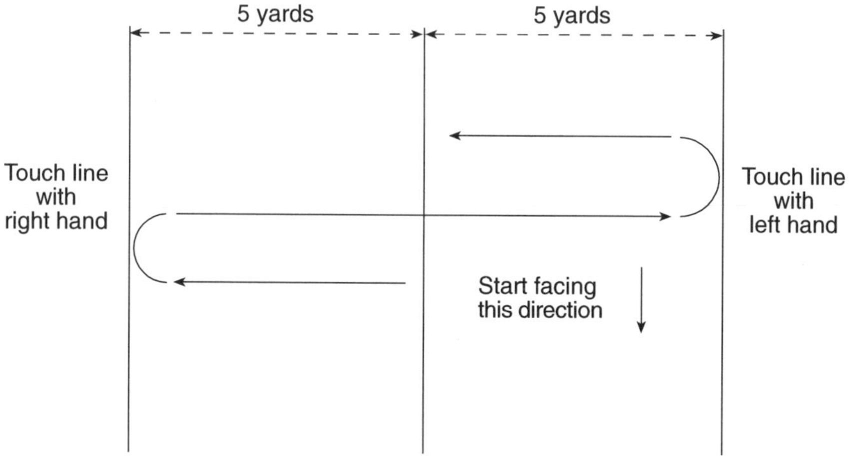


**Figure 7.47**

# SQUIRM

**Purpose:** To improve footwork and reaction time

**Procedure:**

1. Start in a three-point stance and on the coach's command, sprint five yards.
2. On the coach's command (right or left) the players put the designated hand down, rotate 360 degrees, and sprint another five yards.
3. After the players have rotated twice the coach points either right or left. The players then react and run in that direction (figure 7.48).

**Rest:** 60 seconds between each repetition

**Key Points:**

1. Keep full weight on your hand.
2. Emphasize quick foot movement, head up, hips parallel to the shoulders, and full extension of legs and feet.

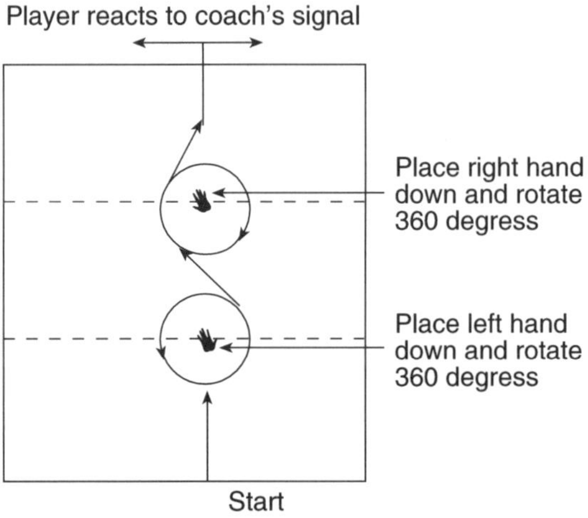


Figure 7.48

# LADDER DRILLS

The following are variations of the ladder drill. Use your imagination to vary these drills, depending on your purpose. Run any combination of distances. Running 5/10/5 yards is the basic combination. Be sure all runs are done at full speed.

## LADDER—5/10/5 SPRINT

**Purpose:** To develop agility and conditioning

**Procedure:**

1. Begin in a three-point stance on the starting line.
2. Sprint to the first line (5 yards), touch the line with your right foot, and return to the starting line and touch it with your left foot.
3. Sprint to the second line (10 yards), touch the line with your right foot, and return to the starting line and touch it with your left foot.
4. Sprint to the first line (5 yards), touch the line with your right foot, and return to the starting line (figure 7.49).

**Rest:** 60 seconds between each repetition

**Key Point:**

Always touch the line at the five-yard intervals with the right foot and the starting line with the left foot. This is so you push off each leg and don't run in circles by pushing off the same leg all the time.

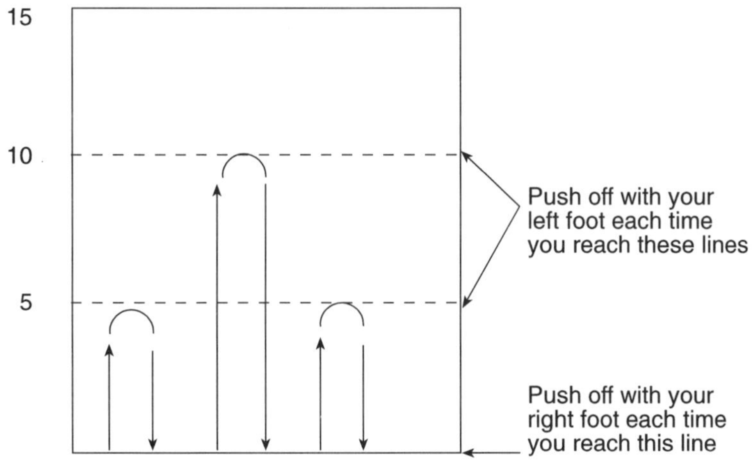


**Figure 7.49**

## LADDER—5/10/5 SHUFFLE

**Purpose:** To develop agility, conditioning, strength, and flexibility in abductors and adductors

**Procedure:**

1. Begin in a two-point stance, standing perpendicular to the start line.

2. Shuffle to the first line, touch the line with your right foot, and shuffle to the starting line and touch with the left foot.
3. Shuffle to the second line, touch the line with your right foot, and shuffle to the starting line and touch with the left foot.
4. Shuffle to the first line, touch the line with your right foot, and shuffle to the starting line (figure 7.50).

**Rest:** 60 seconds between each repetition

**Key Points:**

1. Always touch thc interval lines with your right foot and the starting line with your left foot so that you push off each leg and don't run in circles by pushing off the same leg all the time.
2. Coach positions himself so athletes are always facing him.
3. Do not cross feet.
4. Keep back straight while staying low.

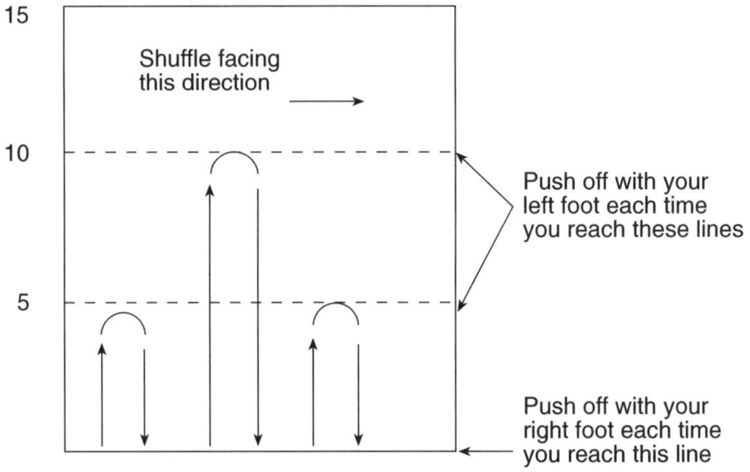


Figure 7.50

## LADDER—5/10/5 BACKPEDAL-FORWARD

**Purpose:** To develop agility, conditioning, and change of direction

**Procedure:**

1. Begin in a two-point stance, standing with your back to the starting line.

2. Backpedal to the first line, touch the line with either foot, and sprint to the starting line and touch it with either foot.
3. Backpedal to the second line, touch the line with either foot, and sprint to the starting line and touch it with either foot.
4. Backpedal to the first line, touch the line with either foot, and sprint to the starting line (figure 7.51).

**Rest:** 60 seconds between each repetition

**Key Point:** Keep low on the backpedal and show good acceleration coming out of the backpedal.

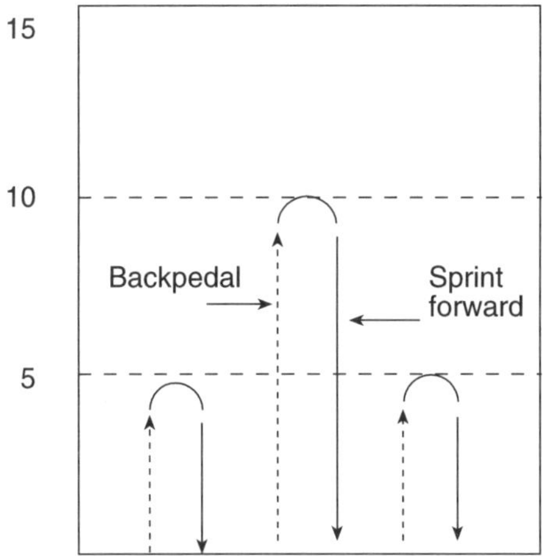


**Figure 7.51**

## LADDER—BACKPEDAL-SPRINT

**Purpose:** To develop agility, conditioning, and acceleration after a change of direction

**Procedure:**

1. Begin in a two-point stance, standing with your back to the starting line.
2. Backpedal 10 yards, pivot to the right 180 degrees, and sprint 10 more yards and touch the line with either foot.
3. Backpedal 10 yards, pivot to the left 180 degrees, and sprint 10 yards to the starting line (figure 7.52).

**Rest:** 60 seconds between each repetition

**Key Points:**

1. Keep shoulders and body weight forward during the backpedal.
2. Accelerate after the turn.

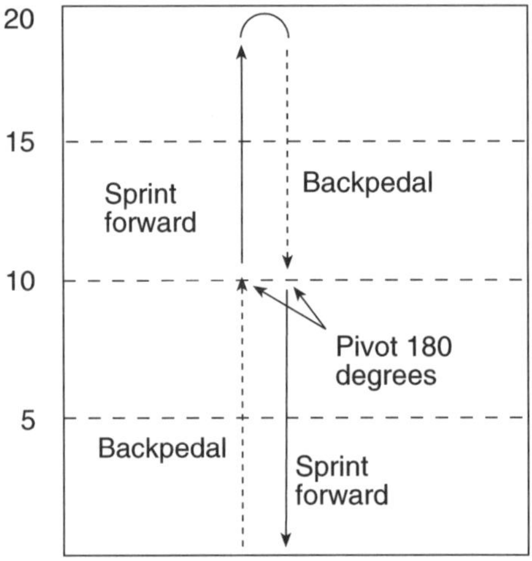


**Figure 7.52**

## JUMP ROPE DRILLS

Test the length of the jump rope by stepping on the middle of the rope and extending the handles to each armpit. To start, hold the handles loosely in your hands and use your wrists to turn the rope. The drills are listed in order of difficulty; learn the easy drills first, then advance to the tougher drills. Do the drills in place until you get the rhythm of the movement. Next, work on smooth movements. Do all the drills starting from the sideline of an artificial turf field (grass fields won't work) and going to the hash marks already on the playing field. Use the yard lines as reference as you do the drills. Remember to keep your head up and eyes focused forward. As your movements become smooth, work on quickness. It is important to use a surface that allows you to jump freely and has a line 15 to 20 yards long.

## DOUBLE BUNNY HOP

**Purpose:** To develop timing, agility, and balance

**Procedure:**

1. Stand with both feet together at the sideline and to one side of a yard line.
2. Jump back and forth over the line, emphasizing quickness as you move forward (figure 7.53).
3. Go to the hash marks that are already on the field, or 15 yards.

**Rest:** 60 seconds between each repetition

**Key Points:**

1. Stay as close to the line as possible.
2. This drill can also be done going backward.

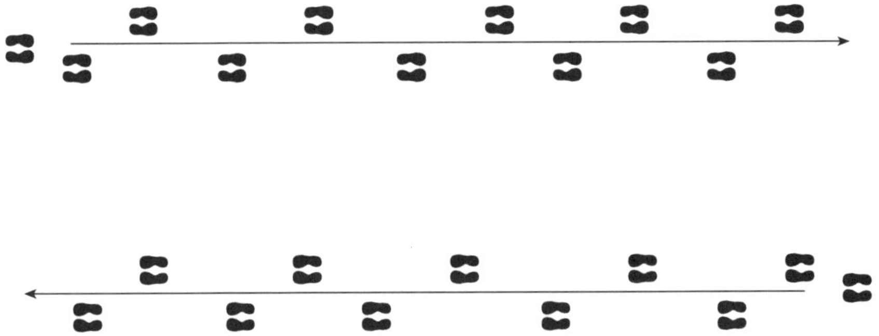

Figure 7.53

## SINGLE BUNNY HOP

**Purpose:** To develop timing, agility, balance, and leg strength

**Procedure:**

1. Stand at the sideline with one foot to one side of a yard line.
2. Jump back and forth over the line with one foot as you move forward.
3. Switch feet at the halfway point without stopping.

**Rest:** 60 seconds between each repetition

**Key Points:**

1. Stay as close to the line as possible.
2. This drill can also be done going backward.

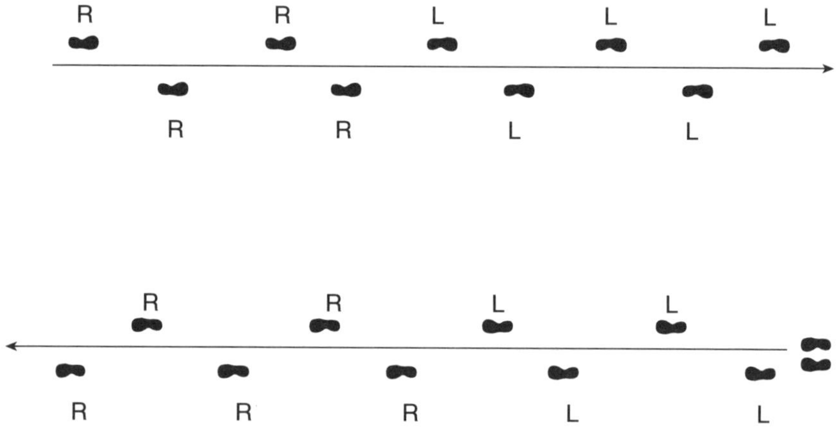


Figure 7.54

## SHUFFLE STEP

**Purpose:** To develop timing, agility, balance, and lateral movement

**Procedure:**

1. Stand sideways at the sideline with both feet on the yard line.
2. Shuffle step down the line (figure 7.55).

**Rest:** 60 seconds between each repetition

**Key Points:**

1. Stay on the line as you shuffle step.
2. Go to the right and left.

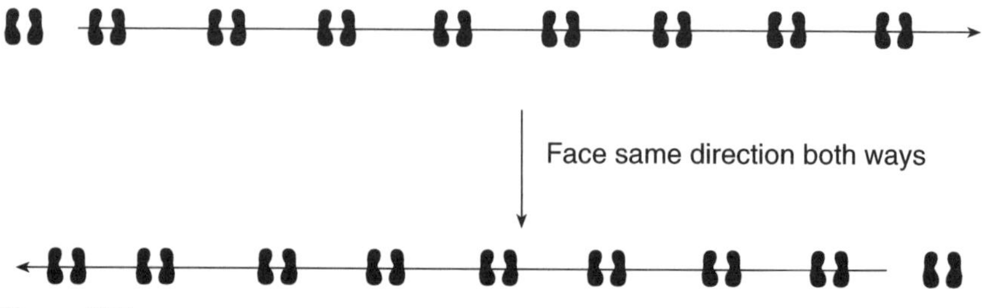


Figure 7.55

## ALI SHUFFLE

**Purpose:** To develop timing, agility, balance, and coordination

**Procedure:**

1. Stand sideways at the sideline with both feet to one side of the yard line.
2. Do the Ali shuffle as you move laterally down the line—one foot goes forward of the line as one foot stays behind the line. Switch feet as you jump in the air to the front and back of line (figure 7.56).

**Rest:** 60 seconds between each repetition

**Key Points:**

1. Go to front and back of line as you switch feet.
2. Go to the right and left.

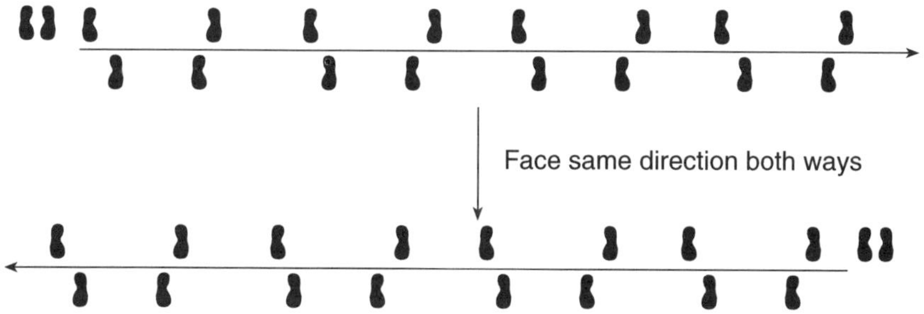


**Figure 7.56**

## SCISSORS STEP

**Purpose:** To develop timing, agility, balance, and coordination

**Procedure:**

1. Stand at the sideline with feet straddling the yard line.
2. Do scissors step as you move forward down the line—the feet cross over each other to the front and back. The feet should be crossed on both sides of the line. Switch feet as you jump in the air (figure 7.57).
3. Go to the hash marks that are already on the field, or 15 yards.

**Rest:** 60 seconds between each repetition

**Key Point:** Feet go on both sides of line as you switch.

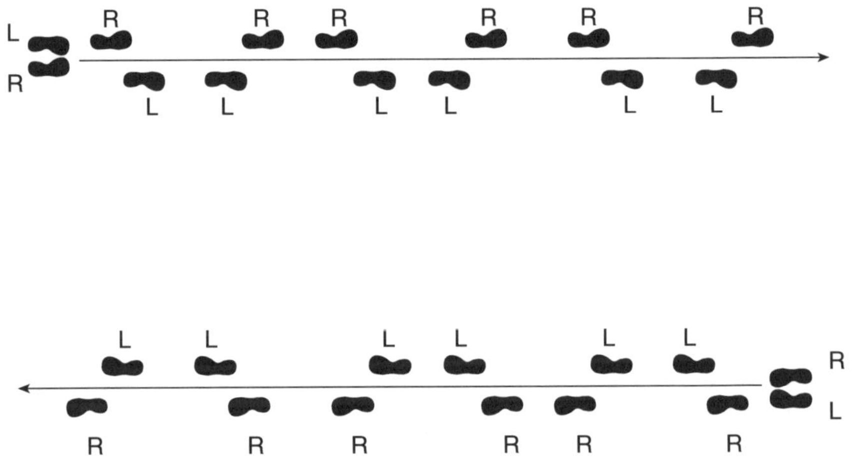


Figure 7.57

## THREE TO NINE

**Purpose:** To develop timing, agility, balance, and hip flexibility

**Procedure:**

1. Stand at the sideline with both feet to one side of the yard line in six o'clock position.
2. With both feet jump a quarter turn to nine o'clock position (to the left) as you move forward.
3. Next, with both feet jump a half turn to three o'clock position (to the right) as you move forward.
4. Repeat the half turns, going from a nine o'clock position to a three o'clock position (figure 7.58).
5. Go to the hash marks that are already on the field, or 15 yards.

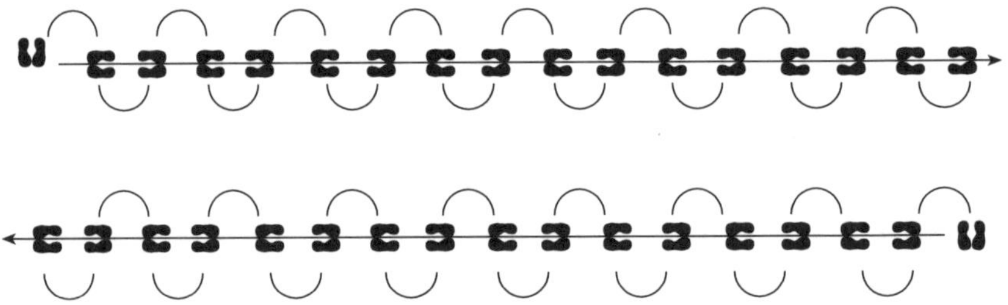

Figure 7.58

**Rest:** 60 seconds between each repetition

**Key Points:**

1. As you turn your feet, they should be parallel to the sideline (rotate your hips).
2. Lead the action with the feet and let the hips follow.
3. Keep your shoulders squared and facing up the field.

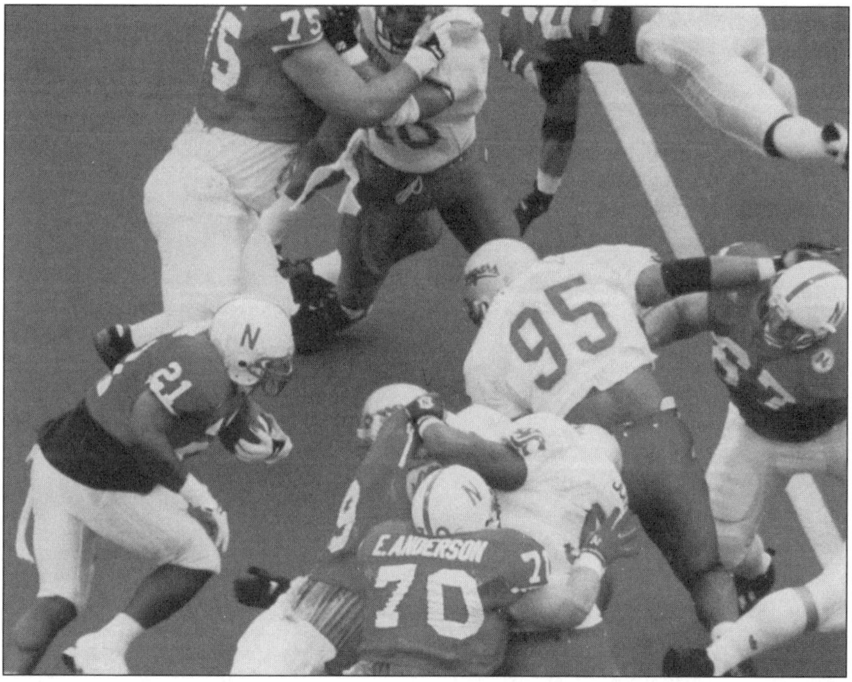

CHAPTER 8

# NUTRITION AND REST

Chiseled into one corner of Memorial Stadium at the University of Nebraska are the words, "Not the victory, but the action. Not the goal, but the game. In the deed, the glory." This quotation reminds us that goals and victories are important, but without resolve, discipline, courage, and perseverance they can't be attained. Goals are achieved and victories happen only when you take action by lifting, running, and stretching according to your workout plan, and eating properly and getting plenty of rest on a daily basis.

Conditioning has to do not only with physical training but also with the ability to recover through nutrition and rest. Typically about 6 to 8 percent of an athlete's time is spent training. Yet, an athlete's character during the rest of the time is what determines the outcome of the training. As we discussed in chapter 1, character is the basis for being the best player you can be. Character is based on a person's attitudes and is reflected in a person's behavior. The best training efforts can be destroyed with just one bad behavior or can be helped by a good behavior. Our behaviors can take us down one of two roads. One road leads to peak performance, the other leads to overtraining and self-destruction.

Overtraining is one road that can lead to defeat. Overtraining occurs when the energy output of training exceeds the energy input of recovery to the point where performance is decreased. After several weeks of training you may notice a leveling off or a decrease in performance associated with a loss of muscular strength, muscle soreness, decreased appetite, weight loss, sleep disturbances, increased irritability, excessive anxiety, injury, and illness. These are the symptoms of overtraining. To prevent overtraining it is important to combine a properly designed strength and conditioning program with good daily lifestyle habits that aid recovery. A basic understanding of metabolism can give greater insight to the processes of recovery and avoiding overtraining.

## TRAINING YOUR METABOLISM FOR RECOVERY

Metabolism is the sum of the catabolic and anabolic cellular reactions that contribute to all the energy needs of every cell of the body. The catabolic reaction, or *catabolism,* releases energy to contribute to the digestion of the food we eat, the breakdown of muscle tissue during exercise, and the subsequent production of waste matter. Anabolic reactions, or *anabolism*, on the other hand, utilize energy to excrete waste matter, build muscle tissue, and store energy from the digested food we eat. For conditioning purposes catabolism refers to the tearing down of muscle and the release of energy during workouts. Anabolism refers to the building up of muscle tissue and the increase of energy capacity during recovery. This process of metabolism is what conditioning is all about.

Living with healthy habits through proper nutrition, adequate sleep, and controlling our stress levels and emotions enables the balance to be in favor of anabolism. The body responds by growing stronger and increasing its energy capacity. Decay or overtraining favors catabolism. A consistent lack of sleep caused by lack of discipline, excessive emotional stress, or substance abuse can divert energy from anabolic or building-up processes, forcing the body to take longer to recover. Recovery is further compromised if energy stores aren't replenished through a proper diet. If during the next workout the body has not fully recovered, the balance is in favor of the catabolic state, and too many workouts strung together in this manner lead to overtraining and possible injury. However, a proper balance between exercise overload and appropriate recovery will put you on the road to reaching your performance potential. The principles of progressive overload, periodization, split routines, and hard-easy systems (see chapter 2) help prevent overtraining and promote long-term adaptations of the body.

## EATING RIGHT

Proper nutrition can meet the energy needs of metabolic processes. Therefore, proper nutrition becomes even more important for an athlete in training. The body requires six separate types of nutrients in order to function properly: carbohydrates, fats, proteins, vitamins, minerals, and water. Various foods contain assorted proportions of these six nutrients. Therefore, it is important to consume a balance of different types of food to supply the necessary nutrients. An imbalance of these nutrients may cause undesirable adaptations, such as an excessive increase of body fat. The following three steps help ensure a proper balance of nutrients to increase lean muscle mass, limit fat storage, and improve performance. We've also included the three steps on a shopping list to help you properly select food when grocery shopping (table 8.1).

### Step 1: Incorporate Fruits, Vegetables, Seeds, and Nuts Into Your Diet

Fruits, vegetables, seeds, and nuts provide a variety of vitamins and minerals to the diet in addition to calories from carbohydrates and fats. Vitamins and minerals cannot be manufactured by the cells of the body and, when lacking in the diet, can cause metabolic deficits. Every month more and more agents are being identified in vegetables and fruits that enhance anabolic metabolism and health. Many of the natural sources of vitamins and minerals from fruits and vegetables are not available in supplemental form. Thus, natural, fresh produce is especially important for football players to aid recovery during intense training.

There are too many vitamins and minerals, and their contributions to metabolic functioning, to mention here. The following are some of the more important ones.

• *Vitamins* are organic compounds needed for normal growth and repair of muscle tissue. They also act as coenzymes playing a part in a variety of energy reactions. Vitamin C is necessary for growth and maintenance of muscle, cartilage, and bone. Without it, wounds do not heal and bones do not grow. Without vitamin A the body has a higher incidence of infections in the lungs, eyes, and kidneys. Lack of vitamin E in the diet causes the cells of the body, including muscle tissue, to deteriorate.

• *Minerals* are inorganic compounds required as catalysts to start many metabolic reactions. The following are some of the more important ones. Iron is essential for the transport of oxygen to the muscle cells. Zinc is responsible for many cellular reactions, including the digestion of proteins. Without magnesium, carbohydrates cannot break down into ATP. Without phosphorous, the muscle cells cannot utilize ATP for immediate energy production. Without calcium and potassium, nerve transmission for muscle contraction is not possible.

We emphasize fruits and vegetables in step 1 because of the predominant presence of vitamins A and C in these sources. Your best sources of vitamin A are typically found in vegetables with dark green, yellow, orange, and red colors. Your best sources of vitamin C (ascorbic acid) are typically found in citrus fruits such as oranges and in some vegetables such as cauliflower, green peppers, and green beans. When trying to cut calories, fruits and vegetables become even more important and should not be avoided! They are naturally dense in vitamins, minerals, and other nutrients necessary for good health. Every day researchers are discovering compounds in fruits and vegetables not typically found in supplements. Many of these compounds aid the immune system in combating greater stress when daily calorie needs are not being met. Become familiar with the fruits and vegetables on the high priority list in table 8.1 which carry both vitamins A and C.

Nuts and seeds, on the other hand, contain abundant quantities of vitamin E, along with essential fats. Fat is a necessary vehicle for transporting fat-soluble vitamins A, D, E, and K. Certain fatty acids play essential roles in the formation of hormones and immune factors. Athletes who have become "fat a-phobic" need to understand that sources of fat that supply vitamin E are some of the best sources of essential fatty acids like omega-3 fatty acids and other monounsaturated fats that help regulate metabolism. Fat also provides the structure of almost all cell membranes and acts as an insulator for vital organs of the body. But the primary function of fat is to provide energy.

**Table 8.1 Three Winning Steps Shopping List**

| Step #1 | Vitamin E | High priority list—vitamins A and C | | Vitamin A | Vitamin C |
|---|---|---|---|---|---|
| Incorporate fruits, vegetables, and seeds into your meal. | __ Almonds | __ Broccoli | __ Brussels sprouts | __ Apricots | __ Cauliflower |
| | __ Avocados or guacamole | __ Cantaloupes | __ Dark salad greens | __ Carrots | __ Green beans |
| | __ Corn oil | __ Dried papayas | __ Grapefruits (pink or red) | __ Cheese | __ Kiwis |
| | __ Mayonnaise | __ Red peppers | __ Guavas | __ Green peas | __ New potatoes with skin |
| | __ Olive oil | __ Red marinara | __ Mandarin oranges | __ Peaches | __ Oranges |
| | __ Peanut butter | __ Salsa | __ Mangos | __ Pumpkin | __ Pineapples |
| | __ Peanuts | __ Tomato juice | __ Sweet potatoes | __ Skim milk | __ Raisins |
| | __ Salmon | __ Tomato sauce | __ Tangerines | __ Yogurt | __ Strawberries |
| | __ Soybean oil | __ Tomatoes | __ Watermelons | __ Chili powder | __ Pea pods |
| | __ Sunflower seeds or oil | __ V-8 (vegetable drink) | __ Yams | __ Tomato catsup or BBQ | __ Radishes |
| | __ Walnuts | __ Winter squash | | __ Egg yolks | __ Green/yellow peppers |

**Carbohydrates**

| Step #2 | Best choice | Second choice | | Third choice | |
|---|---|---|---|---|---|
| Alter your carbohydrate intake relative to your activity. | __ Acorn squash | __ All-Bran cereal | __ Apples | __ Baked russet potatoes | **Things to remember!** |
| | __ Black beans | __ Baked beans | __ Banana cake | __ Candy | • Fresh produce is best, but to avoid spoilage and to ensure availability buy a combination of fresh, frozen, and canned fruits and vegetables. |
| | __ Butter beans | __ Bran Chex | __ Bananas | __ Cartoon character cereals | • Try to include carbohydrates from all three groups when shopping. |
| | __ Cherries | __ Brown or wild rice | __ Cornmeal | __ Doughnuts | • When not active, reduce your total carbohydrate intake (especially third choice carbohydrates). |
| | __ Cucumbers or pickles | __ Cheerios | __ Grapes | __ French bread | |
| | __ Egg noodles | __ Cream of Wheat | __ Green peas | __ French fries | |
| | __ Eggplant | __ Lima beans | __ Macaroni | __ Golden Grahams | |
| | __ Fettucini | __ Mini or Shredded Wheat | __ Oatmeal cookies | __ Grapenuts | |
| | __ Green beans | __ Multi-grain bread | __ Popcorn | __ Hashbrowns | |
| | __ Kidney beans | __ New boiled potatoes with skin | __ Pound cake | __ Mashed potatoes | |
| | __ Lentils | __ Oat bran | __ Raisins | __ Melba toast | |
| | __ Mushrooms | __ Oatmeal | __ Ravioli | __ Puffed rice | |
| | __ Nectarines | __ Pita bread | __ Spaghetti | __ Refried beans | |
| | __ Onions | __ Rye bread | __ Sweet corn | __ Sweetened drinks | |
| | __ Pears | __ Special K cereal | __ Sweet potatoes | __ Total cereal | |
| | __ Plums | __ Tortillas | __ Water crackers | __ White bread | |
| | __ Split peas | __ Unsweetened fruit juice | __ Wheat crackers | __ White flour | |
| | __ Summer squash | __ Whole grain bread | __ Whole wheat flour | __ White rice | |

*(continued)*

**Table 8.1** *(continued)*

| Step #3 | Best choice | Protein<br>Second choice | | Third choice | |
|---|---|---|---|---|---|
| Select a lean protein source. | __ 95% lean ground beef<br>__ 95% lean ground turkey<br>__ 95% lean ham<br>__ Beans and peas<br>__ Chicken—white meat, skinless<br>__ Fat-free ice milk<br>__ Low-fat cottage cheese<br>__ Nonfried fish or seafood<br>__ Skim milk<br>__ Trimmed beef or pork roast<br>__ Turkey—white meat, skinless<br>__ White meat tuna in water<br>__ Whole grains<br>__ Yogurt from skim milk (no sugar) | __ 2% milk<br>__ 85% lean ground beef<br>__ 85% lean ground turkey<br>__ 85% lean ham<br>__ 85% lean encased meats<br>__ Low-fat cheese<br>__ Low-fat yogurt<br>__ Regular cottage cheese<br>__ Regular yogurt<br>__ Trimmed lamb<br>__ Trimmed beef brisket<br>__ Turkey bacon or sausage | __ Baked chicken strips or nuggets<br>__ Chicken—dark meat, skinless<br>__ Dark meat tuna in water<br>__ Frozen ice milk<br>__ Low-fat pudding<br>__ Nuts or seeds<br>__ Peanut butter<br>__ Ricotta cheese<br>__ Skim mozzarella cheese<br>__ Trimmed choice steaks<br>__ Trimmed pork chops<br>__ Turkey—dark meat, skinless | __ 75% lean ground beef<br>__ 75% lean ground turkey<br>__ Bacon<br>__ Beef or pork ribs<br>__ Chicken—with skin<br>__ Fried chicken<br>__ Fried fish or seafood<br>__ Ham on bone<br>__ Ice cream<br>__ Regular cheese<br>__ Regular encased meats<br>__ Whole eggs<br>__ Whole milk | **Things to remember!**<br>• Concentrate on best choice items as your source of protein.<br>• Remember every time the butcher processes the meat (i.e., skinless or boneless), the cost goes up. |

## Step 2: Alter Your Carbohydrate Intake Relative to Your Activity Level

Two types of nutrients found in food—carbohydrates and fats—supply most of the body's energy needs. (Protein also can supply a small amount of energy under certain circumstances.) In order for these nutrients to be used by the muscles, carbohydrates must be broken down into simple sugars called glucose, while fats are converted into fatty acids. Glucose and fatty acids are the final by-products of digestion that can then be converted by our cellular machinery (like mitochondria) into ATP. As you may recall from chapter 2, ATP is the only fuel product utilized for muscle contraction.

Glucose and fatty acids can be stored as glycogen and triglycerides, respectively. Glycogen is stored in the liver and muscle fibers and is readily available for quick energy needs. Triglycerides are stored in fat cells called adipose tissue. While fat can be stored in almost unlimited amounts, carbohydrate storage is limited to about a day's supply. Therefore, carbohydrate intake through the food you eat must be replenished daily to ensure the capability of maximum performance. When the energy demands of the body increase, the stored glycogen and triglycerides are called upon to meet energy needs (figure 8.1).

Carbohydrate and fat metabolism occur together simultaneously; however, the ratio of carbohydrate to fat utilization during activity depends on the intensity and volume of the overload. As the intensity of activity increases, the demand for carbohydrate utilization increases and fat demand decreases. Fuel for high-intensity, short-duration exercise is supplied predominantly from the breakdown of carbohydrates. During very low-intensity, long-duration activity levels, fat contributes up to 70 percent of the total energy needs. During sleep the energy demands for carbohydrates are the lowest and fat is utilized at an even higher ratio. So, while sitting in a chair reading this book you are burning primarily fat.

In chapter 1, we described the three energy systems as an interaction among three storage tanks. One tank represents the ATP-PC energy system. During a football play, the muscle fibers almost strictly utilize ATP stored in the muscle. The ATP-PC energy system is replenished by the oxygen system tank, seconds after a play is over, by supplying ATP by the breakdown of carbohydrates (blood glucose, muscle, and liver glycogen), fat, and to a small degree protein. Fat is converted into ATP from the oxygen tank during the 50 to 60 seconds between plays at nearly the same rate as at rest (50 to 70 percent). The other 30 to 50 percent is replaced by converting carbohydrate into ATP, also from the oxygen system. During a football game only the ATP-PC system during the play

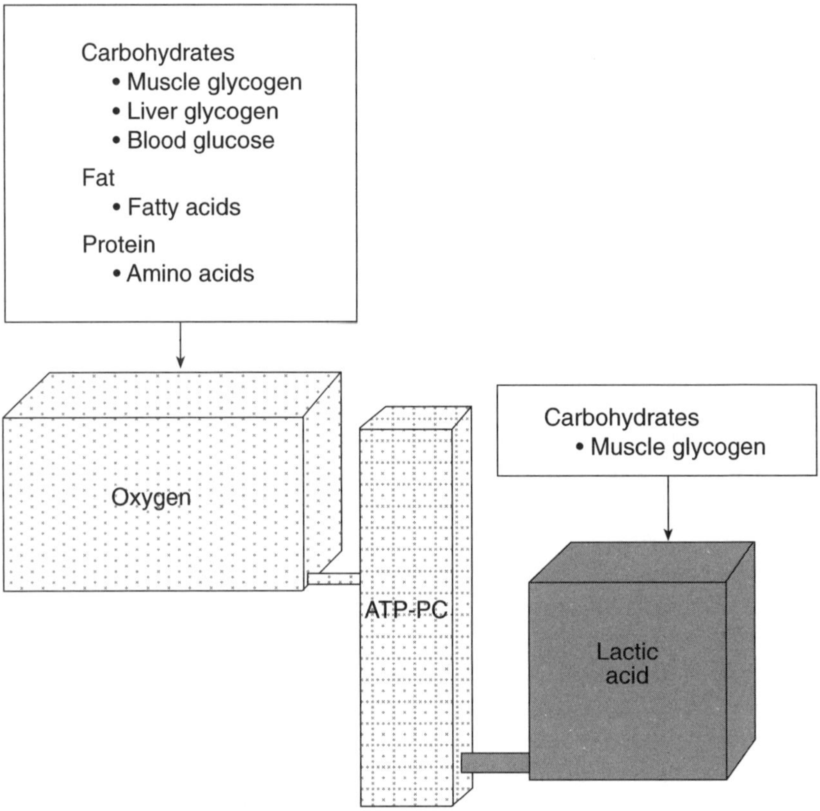


**Figure 8.1** Stored glycogen and triglycerides help meet the body's energy needs.

and the oxygen system during recovery between plays are called upon to a great degree; the lactic acid system is scarcely called into play.

There are times during strength and interval training that the demand on the lactic acid system to supply ATP by breaking down carbohydrates is higher. But the demands from a single workout are not enough to deplete the body's carbohydrate stores; only if you trained several days in a row without eating any carbohydrates would carbohydrate depletion be a problem. Following this three-step performance diet will supply enough carbohydrates to meet the energy demands of the high strength training programs outlined in this book.

It is important to regulate your carbohydrate intake according to your activity level, though. When activity levels are high eat more carbohydrates, and when low consume less. For instance, the high-energy demands during two-a-days are balanced by eating more carbohydrate foods. After two-a-days the energy demand is lower and is balanced by eating fewer carbohydrates. Because the body is not burning as many carbohydrates when practice is conducted once a day the muscles' storage tanks aren't emptied to as great a degree, and it doesn't take as much carbohydrate to refill the tanks. Eating a high-carbohydrate meal when your energy demands are low may throw your energy balance out of whack, as a certain percentage of the excess carbohydrate will be stored as fat. When inactive, reduce your total carbohydrate intake even more to balance the energy demand. To safely lose excess fat, reduce carbohydrate intake to slightly below your current energy demand. A reduced carbohydrate intake allows a higher ratio of fat to be burned during inactive periods.

Various carbohydrates release glucose into the bloodstream at different rates. The relative ability of individual foods to quickly raise blood glucose to a high level is known as the glycemic index. Foods such as potato chips, candy bars, cookies, and soda pop digest quickly, stimulating a fast addition of blood glucose. This gives the body a quick jolt of energy and the body responds by releasing massive quantities of insulin. Insulin is a hormone that quickly lowers the glucose level; in fact, sometimes it lowers glucose levels so quickly and so much that energy levels dip. The body then responds by creating an appetite for more carbohydrates to raise glucose levels and the cycle continues—more carbohydrates, more blood glucose, more insulin, more glucose stored as fat. Insulin not only converts excess glucose into fat in the body, it shuts down fat metabolism; thus, a cycle of high and low blood glucose levels leads to the storage of more and more fat. Carbohydrate foods with a high fiber and protein content, such as kidney beans, digest slowly, inducing a slow increase of blood glucose, a slow and steady insulin response, and therefore less carbohydrate stored as fat.

Table 8.1 gives three types of carbohydrate choices based on glycemic index:

Best Choice Carbohydrate—Low glycemic response

Second Choice Carbohydrate—Moderate glycemic response

Third Choice Carbohydrate—High glycemic response

The classification of carbohydrate sources by insulin response in the blood breaks from the traditional definitions of "simple" and "complex" carbohydrates. The majority of the fruits and vegetables listed as good sources of vitamin A and C are also listed as best choice carbohydrates. Vegetables that are also good carbohydrate choices are cucumbers, eggplant, mushrooms, onions, garlic, and summer squash. Some fruits such as cherries, pears, plums, nectarines, and blueberries are good carbohydrate choices. It is OK to eat second and third choice carbohydrates, especially during high activity periods. But it is important to consume them with a lean protein source to slow down the glucose release. Third choice carbohydrates that also have a fat content such as candy bars, cookies, and potato chips are especially fattening. These types of foods should be cut out altogether. There are some guys who seem to eat anything and as much as they want and still put on muscle. They are the exceptional, lucky few. Just keep track of your waist measurement to see what kinds of carbohydrates to add to or remove from your diet.

## Step 3: Select a Lean Protein Source

Protein is the building material for the development of muscle tissue. It also provides the structural framework for hormones that control metabolic processes. To adapt to high loads associated with football training, a player may have double the protein requirements of a sedentary person. However, most football players already eat more than double their protein requirement.

During digestion, proteins are broken down into amino acids and released into the bloodstream. There are 20 amino acids that form different protein combinations for growth and body functions. All 20 are necessary to support the metabolism necessary for life. There are two types of amino acids—essential and nonessential. The body manufactures the nonessential amino acids, but the eight essential amino acids must be supplied through the food we eat. Animal proteins are complete proteins, containing all eight of the essential amino acids. Most plant proteins, with the exception of isolated soy proteins, lack one or more of the eight amino acids and are not complete sources of protein. Plant proteins can supply the essential amino acids only if eaten in the proper combinations. We recommend including protein from an animal source with each meal to ensure an adequate intake of all eight amino acids.

The amount of protein you should eat is based on your body weight. Table 8.2 shows the approximate amount of protein to take for every 50 pounds of body weight. Basically it takes about four ounces of animal protein (approximately 35 grams protein), eight fluid ounces of milk (approximately eight grams protein), and one-half cup of beans (approximately eight grams protein) for every 50 pounds of body weight per day to meet the protein requirements of an athlete in training.

Some essential fatty acids, which your body cannot synthesize, can be obtained by selecting foods with high vitamin E content (see table 8.1). When foods with high vitamin E content are combined with protein consumed from animal sources, you may run the risk of eating too much

**Table 8.2 Protein Requirements Based on Body Weight**

| Body weight (lb.) | Fish, poultry, beef, or egg* (oz.) |
|---|---|
| 100 | 8 |
| 150 | 12 |
| 200 | 16 |
| 250 | 20 |
| 300 | 24 |

*1 egg = 1 oz.

fat. To help you identify calories from fat, table 8.1 classifies the sources of protein into three categories. If you select foods from the best choice list, you will satisfy both your protein and fat needs.

Best Choice Protein—Less than 10 grams of fat per serving

Second Choice Protein—11 to 20 grams of fat per serving

Third Choice Protein—Over 20 grams of fat per serving

The third choice proteins are also higher in saturated fat. It is especially important to limit third choice proteins when you aren't active. Nine calories are stuffed into one gram of fat, whereas one gram of carbohydrate and one gram of protein each have only four calories. A little too much fat can quickly translate into excess calorie intake and storage of fat. Especially eliminate second and third choice proteins from pretraining or precompetition meals. For example, eating BBQ ribs during a precompetition meal diverts a lot of blood to the digestive tract. In order for the muscles to perform at maximum capacity they must not compete for blood, which supplies oxygen and energy. A lower-fat protein source like fish or skinless chicken breast is digested quicker.

Eating large, high-protein meals requires lots of energy to digest and slows down the anabolic recovery processes. By spacing your protein intake with smaller, more frequent meals you'll promote less competition between the energy necessary for digestion and that needed for the recovery of muscle tissue after training. Protein uptake and glycogen storage are both maximized when proteins and carbohydrates, combined in an easy-to-digest form, are consumed together after training.

Even though the intake of fat must be moderated, don't be afraid of fat. When trying to completely eliminate fat from the diet you run the risk of not consuming enough essential amino acids necessary for maximum performance. While too many total calories increases the percentage of body fat and decreases performance capabilities, fat is a major contributor of muscle ATP during low-intensity activities. Fat spares liver and muscle glycogen, extending the endurance of the body. Fat also adds flavor to the foods we eat.

## DRINKING FLUIDS

Water makes up about 60 percent of a person's total body weight and is the nutrient most important to the body's functioning. Water is the main component of blood plasma. Without it oxygen, glucose, fatty acids, and amino acids can't be transported to your active muscles and catabolic waste products can't be eliminated from the body. Water loss is accelerated during exercise, and as little as a 4 percent reduction can have a devastating impact on performance. Be sure to drink plenty of water. Drinking a pint per pound body weight lost during exercise is recommended by the American College of Sports Medicine. Make sure that you are properly hydrated before conditioning workouts and football practices, and to ensure proper hydration, drink even more water than what your thirst indicates during heavy activity. Make it a lifestyle habit to drink fluids.

There has been a lot of advertising lately for several different carbohydrate drinks. A lot of these ads are geared toward football players. The consumption of these drinks is not going to give you more energy—unless, of course, you have not been eating properly. While the drinks may not give you an energy boost, they do help replace fluids. If water lost by sweating is not replaced, then you are going to have energy problems. It does not matter whether you drink water or a flavored drink as long as you replace the fluids. But if you prefer flavored drinks and they encourage you to drink more fluids, then by all means drink them. But remember, water is just as good and a lot cheaper.

Many athletes think that they can replace fluids by drinking a nice cold beer after a workout or practice. Alcohol is actually considered a nutrient, supplying seven calories of energy per gram. This is almost the same number of calories as a gram of fat, and the result of the consumption of too many total calories can be a "beer gut." Alcohol is also considered a drug because of its depressive effects on the nervous system. The biggest problem for an athlete is that it interferes with the metabolism of the other six important nutrients. When the liver is forced to metabolize alcohol it shuts down the metabolism of other nutrients critical to the recovery processes. Alcohol also suppresses the release of the antidiuretic hormone, which results in the excretion of more urine and potential dehydration.

## GETTING PLENTY OF SLEEP

While you sleep, the process of anabolism has a chance to recharge your body with new energy and tissue. Thus, it is important to get at least eight hours of sleep in order for your body to get recharged. Even a small loss of sleep will result in overtraining, general irritability, and possible illness. A primary factor of getting proper rest is going to bed the same time every night. By developing a daily routine to get to bed at the same time every night you can affect the structure of the rest of your day.

Part of getting proper rest is the ability to recognize and control your emotions. Emotions can cause muscle tension that drains the body of energy, or emotions can relax the muscles and enhance your energy supply. For example, competition usually stimulates an automatic reaction called the "fight or flight response"—an instinctive reaction to stress by either fighting or running for our lives. Adrenaline, cortisol, and growth hormone are released in the bloodstream in response to stress caused by the excitement of a football game. The adrenaline shifts blood from the digestive organs to the muscles. This is felt as stomach butterflies. Without this nervous feeling you know you're not physically or mentally ready. This nervous energy is best utilized by keeping mentally and physically relaxed and not allowing the nervousness to cause muscle tension. Muscle tension causes needless expenditure of energy and makes coordinated movements less efficient. In extreme cases it can cause nausea and vomiting. Fatigue sets in quicker and compromises powerful muscular contractions. When mistakes are made, tense muscles cause you to become angry and frustrated. In a relaxed state the muscles "sit back" and conserve energy for the exact moment when explosive action is required. In a relaxed state the mind is confident and focused on the present task, ready to excite the muscles into action in fractions of a second.

Negative emotions such as anger, depression, worry, and guilt can also cause the same "fight or flight response." The metabolic hormones adrenaline and cortisol remain in the blood at high levels for long periods of time. When cortisol is present in the blood it catabolizes muscle tissue while shutting down protein synthesis. While this is happening, adrenaline increases the heart rate and blood pressure. If these emotions catabolize muscle tissue over an extended period of time and never allow it to rebuild, energy stores are never replenished and the body is thrown out of balance into a permanent catabolic state. The body loses muscle tissue and the immune system is weakened, making us more susceptible to injury, illness, and disease.

Just as muscles grow stronger by adapting to an exercise overload, character strengthens by adapting to an emotional overload. Without problems in your life you could not develop your character to a great degree. Stress is not what happens to you, but how you react to what happens. Your character determines how you handle emotional stress in your everyday life. A good belief system is that by using your intellect you have control over a problem situation. With resolve, you know your destination and are committed. Discipline, courage, and perseverance help you cope with emotion. Unity, knowing that you are part of something larger than yourself, is especially important. You know that you are not alone and can rely on your teammates, coaches, parents, and clergy to help you through your problems.

Becoming aware of your negative emotions challenges you to face up to your problems and deal with them effectively. Once you have effectively dealt with a problem you feel relieved and have a relaxed calmness, or peace of mind. Your character is strengthened and you feel energized. This in return enhances your ability to perform. On the other hand, escaping from your problems through procrastination, sex, excessive television viewing, alcohol, drugs, and tobacco can lead to not following through on commitments, lying, cheating, stealing, unwanted pregnancies, abortions, and HIV. All of this drains you of both physical and emotional energy. This results in another downward cycle of depression, anxiety, and guilt. Character strength, conditioning levels, and performance all go in a downward spiral.

## BEHAVIOR MODIFICATION

Ultimately, your behaviors determine the outcome of your strength and conditioning program. Behavior is simply a response to a stimulus (figure 8.2). Behaviors repeated over and over develop into habits. One bad habit such as not eating properly, smoking, drinking alcohol, or taking drugs can destroy all the work that you have done in the weight room and out on the field. On the other hand, a good habit such as going to bed the same time every day and getting eight hours of sleep can accelerate the conditioning process. Most athletes are aware of these

### Alcohol, Drugs, and Tobacco Will Hurt Your Football Game

Consuming alcohol, taking drugs, and smoking are bad habits that will work against you and your football game. As drinking, using drugs, and smoking accelerate the process of catabolism, your body must work overtime to recover. It cannot keep pace trying to recover from both intense workouts *and* bad habits.

Steroids are well-known for their ability to help the body recover. That is why they are often referred to as anabolic steroids. However, the undesirable side effects of liver disease, impairment of the heart, sexual dysfunction, and stunted bone growth are simply not worth the risk of using them. Your body only has so much potential. You can reach your goals without steroids. You only have one body, so take the best care of it that you possibly can. Stay away from steroids. You don't need them.

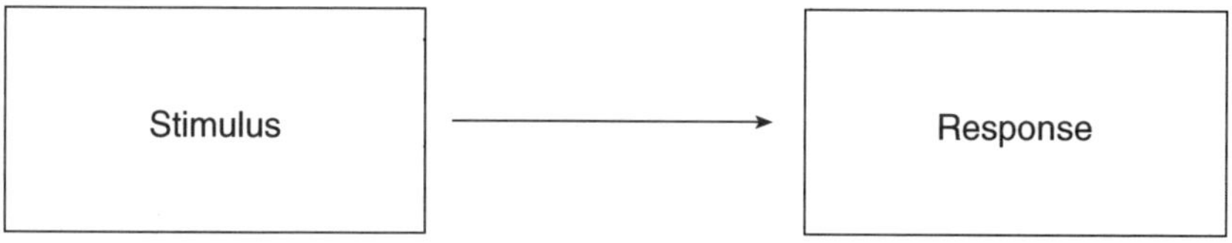


**Figure 8.2** One viewpoint of human behavior is that it is simply a conditioned response to a stimulus.

pitfalls but lack the control over themselves to modify their behavior. It's a shame when an athlete does not attain his absolute skill level because of bad habits. If you take charge of your behaviors, however, you can reach your goals.

## Conscious Versus Subconscious Behaviors

Behavior can be either conscious or subconscious. Conscious awareness allows you to respond to external and internal stimulus through your thoughts, actions, or speech. Subconscious control handles bodily functions such as your heart rate, digestion, and temperature regulation. Ninety percent of your daily functions are subconscious and, for the most part, this is desirable (especially when you are asleep!).

## Conditioned Responses

Many of your behaviors are conditioned responses. In other words, you can be programmed to respond in a specific way to a specific stimulus. Conditioned responses are similar to the way computers work. Computers have memory banks that store information. You can program the computer so that when a specific command is given it responds by bringing up specific information to the screen from its memory bank. With humans, memories are stored as sensory and emotional experiences. Memories can be used to program your muscles to respond to a stimulus automatically. For example, there are certain techniques used to make a proper block. You have to position your body in relation to the opponent by using exact foot and hand movements along proper ankle, knee, and hip angles. You must be prepared for a variety of situations so by the time you get in the game you have experienced everything possible. The only way to perfect the technique of blocking is through consistently conditioning your body to block, day after day, week after week, month after month.

The more often you receive a specific stimulus, the more established the nerve pathway becomes and the more muscle memory is established. That is why exercises and drills incorporated into the strength and interval training programs must stimulate nerve pathways similar to football movements. Once a bad technique has become established in the nervous system it is difficult to change. Once these muscle memories have been programmed they automatically react to a specific stimulus subconsciously. If you need to consciously think about a situation in a game, you lose valuable time. By the time you are done figuring out what to do, it's too late.

Though conditioned responses are necessary to develop football skills, your habits are also conditioned responses. Habits determine most of your daily behaviors and affect your character. Through intelligence you can program your body; that is, between the stimulus and the response, you have the freedom to choose your response. Thus, the key to modifying your behavior is to respond by consciously making a choice to reprogram your habits (figure 8.3 ).

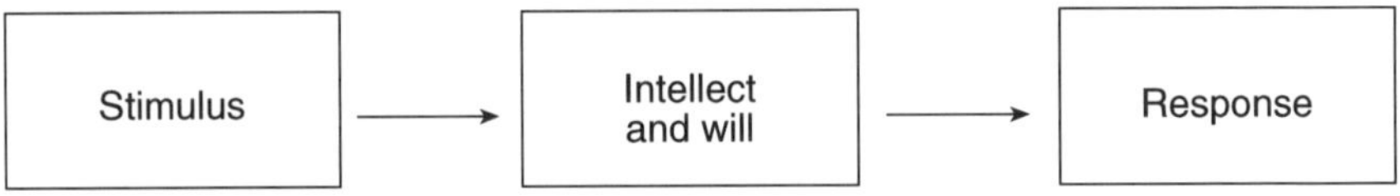


**Figure 8.3** You can consciously change your behavior by thinking about your actions before responding.

If your behavior is based on pleasure you are heading down the wrong road. Even though, for example, pizza tastes so good and your conditioned response is to eat several more pieces, overeating is harmful because it can lead to gaining excess fat. Discipline is the function of a strong conscience to subordinate impulses and behaviors not conducive to achieving your resolve. Without discipline you have a deadened conscience. You are "doped" by your lesser peers or emotional feelings into doing activities that keep you from being the most you can be.

How many times have you heard the saying "pain is gain"? Most strength workouts are painful, but this pain induces muscle growth. It is a lot easier and more pleasurable to skip a workout. It is emotionally painful to miss a good party and go to bed early so that you are fresh for an early morning training session. It is often physically painful to get up in the morning to make your workout. But these pains are the price you must pay for the gains you want.

To break a bad habit, use your intellect. First become consciously aware of the bad habit. Then use your discipline to substitute a good habit for it. Without doing this it is almost impossible to break a bad habit. Even by using discipline to force yourself into a good habit, your body will fight back. For example, one bad habit that affects many of you young football players is not getting enough sleep. Perhaps you are staying up late several nights a week watching television. You get up the next morning feeling tired and don't even remember what you watched the night before. You can substitute lying in bed and reading a relaxing book or studying your playbook for watching television. Before you know it, you will feel your eyelids getting heavy. The urge may be to watch television, but use your discipline to go to bed and read. It won't be long before you'll be in the habit of going to bed and getting your rest.

You may slip sometimes, but don't give in, keep fighting, use your discipline. Go back and read chapter 1 on character when a bad habit is giving you a hard time. Ask yourself before you do anything, "Is this helping me attain my goal?" Your beliefs determine your goals, your behaviors, and ultimately your character. If you do something that does not help you attain your goals, then you have a weakness in your belief system that you need to reevaluate.

CHAPTER 9

# CONDITIONING WORKOUTS AND PROGRAMS

This chapter describes the running and lifting programs that make up a complete conditioning program. The running program includes interval training guidelines and example workouts using the speed and agility drills detailed in chapters 6 and 7. The lifting program describes strength training guidelines using explosive, strength, and specialty exercises detailed in chapter 5.

## YOUR RUNNING PROGRAM

As we discussed in chapter 2, it is important to develop your running program in accordance with the demands of a football game. The average football play is 5 seconds of 100 percent intensity; the average rest between plays during a normal drive is about 50 seconds. The program to meet football's specific demands must therefore meet the following conditions:

1. Speed and agility drills requiring maximum intensity for 3 to 8 seconds.
2. Take approximately 10-second rest periods for every second of work. Thus, if a drill lasts 5 seconds, the rest period should last approximately 50 seconds.

## Interval Training Guidelines

The best way to set up a running program is to follow interval training principles. Interval training consists of a series of work bouts (called "intervals"), consisting of speed and agility drills alternated with a prescribed rest interval. One repetition consists of one work interval and one rest interval. To increase the intensity of a drill, it is helpful to perform the drill with someone else, turning it into a competition by racing each other. Another method of increasing intensity is to time each drill and compare your time with other athletes. If you are working with a group of players, only two players need to perform at the same time. The players resting give encouragement. As two players finish, the next two should be ready to go.

Each drill has a recommended rest interval dependent on the length of the speed or agility drill (10 seconds rest per 1 second of work, 10:1). To ensure that you are using the ATP-PC energy system, allow a two-minute rest period between each category of drills. This allows complete recovery and a chance to get a drink of water to ensure proper hydration. A common training error that athletes and coaches make in their running programs is making the rest intervals too short. To meet the demands of the next maximum-intensity effort, follow the recommended guidelines for the rest interval of each drill.

The total volume of repetitions for each running workout varies from phase to phase and from position to position. Do not include any running workouts during the base phase. Concentrate most of your effort on the weight room at this time; the first two weeks of the strength program will cause muscle soreness. Running backs, receivers, and defensive backs can add two days of agility drills during the first week of the development phase and two days of speed drills during the third week of the development phase. This allows for a gradual increase of repetitions, running only two days a week to start with and then increasing to four days. Linemen, however, should only do agility drills

... ... a week during the development phase. Linemen can then add two days of speed drills during the peak phase, allowing four running workouts a week. This allows linemen a little longer time to gradually adjust to the running workouts and to have more time to focus on strength and power in the weight room.

Do no more than 35 reps of agility drills and no more than 15 reps of speed drills (running backs, receivers, and defensive backs) during the development phase. During the peak phase the number of agility drills should not exceed 35 reps, and speed drills should not exceed 25. Gradually increase the number of repetitions by 2 or 3 each week. Keep the running program no longer than 30 minutes during the development phase and no longer than 45 minutes during the peak phase. Perform no more than 12 repetitions within any category of drills and no more than 5 repetitions for any individual drill. For example, 10 repetitions of bag drills can be divided into two straight runs, two lateral step drills, two weave drills, two wheel drills, and two zigzag drills. Always do one category of drills before proceeding to the next category. The categories of speed and agility drills and tables listing this program information for each position are shown later on in this chapter.

## Agility Drills

We recommend doing the agility drills on Tuesdays and Fridays in the following sequence:

1. Warm-up
2. Stretching
3. Rope and bag drills
4. Backpedal drills
5. Cone drills
6. Jump rope drills
7. Line drills
8. Mobility drills

Agility drills vary with each position. For example, only the defensive backs and linebackers do the backpedal drills. The line drills are more intense than the rest of the drills and should be done at the end of the workout; if you do them first you may not have enough energy to finish the rest of the drills explosively. Again, always conclude your workout with mobility drills to move the body through full ranges of motion and aid recovery. Table 9.1*a* displays a menu of agility drills and notes which drills are appropriate for which positions.

**Table 9.1a Agility Drills by Drill Type and Player Position**

| Drill name | Drill type | Position | Page |
|---|---|---|---|
| Backpedal weave | Backpedal | DB | 215 |
| Centerfield | Backpedal | DB | 211 |
| Comeback | Backpedal | LB, DB | 208 |
| Confidence | Backpedal | DB | 216 |
| 45-degree | Backpedal | LB, DB | 210 |
| Hip flip on line | Backpedal | LB, DB | 212 |
| Mirror | Backpedal | DB | 215 |
| 90-degree | Backpedal | LB, DB | 209 |
| Post/corner | Backpedal | DB | 210 |
| W backpedal-break | Backpedal | DB | 213 |
| Wet field | Backpedal | DB | 214 |
| Bunny hop rotation | Bag | OB, R | 204 |
| Change of direction | Bag | OL, DL, LB, OB, R | 200 |
| Combo lateral step/high knee | Bag | LB, OB, R | 207 |
| Combo lateral/forward-back | Bag | DL, LB | 202 |
| Forward with double chop | Bag | DL, LB, OB, R | 198 |
| Forward-back | Bag | OL, DL, LB, OB, R | 201 |
| Lateral speed | Bag | OB, R | 206 |
| Lateral step | Bag | DL, LB, OB, R | 199 |
| Lateral step with double chop | Bag | DL, LB, OB, R | 199 |
| Rotation | Bag | DL, LB, OB, R | 204 |
| Straight run | Bag | OL, DL, LB, OB, R | 198 |
| Tap | Bag | DL, LB | 200 |
| Wave | Bag | DL, LB | 203 |
| Wheel | Bag | DL, LB, OB | 205 |
| Zigzag or shuffle | Bag | OL, DL, LB, OB, R | 202 |
| Backward zigzag | Cone | OL, DB | 224 |
| Combo zigzag | Cone | OL, LB, DB | 225 |
| Dodging run | Cone | OL, OB | 223 |
| Four-corner carioca | Cone | OL, DL, LB, DB | 217 |
| Four-corner comeback | Cone | DL, LB, DB | 219 |
| Four-corner drop | Cone | LB, R, DB | 220 |
| Four-corner shuffle | Cone | OL, DL, DB | 218 |
| Four-corner square-in | Cone | OB, R, DB | 220 |
| Nebraska agility | Cone | OL, DL, LB, OB, R, DB | 225 |
| Rag | Cone | DL, LB, OB, R | 221 |
| Three-corner | Cone | LB, DB | 222 |
| Zigzag | Cone | OL | 223 |
| Ali shuffle | Jump rope | OL, OB, R | 235 |
| Double bunny hop | Jump rope | OL, OB, R | 233 |
| Scissors step | Jump rope | OL, OB, R | 235 |
| Shuffle step | Jump rope | OL, OB, R | 234 |

*(continued)*

Table 9.1a *(continued)*

| Drill name | Drill type | Position | Page |
|---|---|---|---|
| Single bunny hop | Jump rope | OL, OB, R | 233 |
| Three to nine | Jump rope | OL, OB, R | 236 |
| Ladder—5/10/5 backpedal-forward | Line | OL, DL, LB, OB, R, DB | 230 |
| Ladder—5/10/5 shuffle | Line | OL, DL, LB, OB, R, DB | 229 |
| Ladder—5/10/5 sprint | Line | OL, DL, LB, OB, R, DB | 229 |
| Ladder—backpedal-sprint | Line | OL, DL, LB, OB, R, DB | 231 |
| Pro agility | Line | OL, DL, LB, OB, R, DB | 227 |
| Squirm | Line | OL, DL, LB, OB, R, DB | 228 |
| Bunny hop | Rope | DL, LB, OB, R | 196 |
| Crossover step | Rope | DL, LB, OB, R | 196 |
| Double chop | Rope | OL, DL, LB, OB, R | 194 |
| Every hole | Rope | OL, DL, LB, OB, R | 194 |
| Every other hole | Rope | OL, DL, LB, OB, R | 193 |
| Lateral step | Rope | OL, DL, LB, OB, R | 195 |
| Lateral step with double chop | Rope | OL, DL, LB, OB, R | 195 |
| Rope weave | Rope | DL, LB, OB, R | 197 |

## Speed Drill Workouts

Do speed drill workouts on Mondays and Thursdays of each training phase using the interval training guidelines. The speed workout consists of the following categories of speed drills and should be done in this sequence:

1. Warm-up
2. Stretching
3. Starts
4. Sprints
5. Plyometrics
6. Resisted drills
7. Mobility drills

It is important to always warm up your muscles, ligaments, and tendons by doing the warm-up and partner stretch routines described in chapter 4 *before* starting your running workout. The warm-up routine not only warms up the body for the workout, but also helps with active flexibility of the hips and legs. These warm-up drills, if done properly, also develop speed mechanics.

Run the starts before the longer sprints; they serve as another phase of the warm-up. Begin easy on the first few runs, gradually increasing the intensity of succeeding runs. Stretch between the sprint drills and keep warm; hamstring injuries usually occur when the legs fatigue during sprint drills.

Don't perform any heavy legwork prior to running speed drills or you'll compromise the explosiveness required for starts. Moreover, we recommend heavy linemen only do light plyometric drills. Do resisted drills, such as the harness drills, stadium steps, or hill runs, at the end of your workout. Conclude your speed workouts with mobility drills (chapter 4) to take the body through full ranges of motion and aid recovery. Table 9.1*b* displays speed and acceleration drills.

## Position-Specific Workouts

Chapters 1 and 2 discussed the importance of doing exercises and drills specific to football movements. Certain movements are not only specific to football, but are specific to different positions. The following section discusses specific movement patterns used for specific positions. Included with each position are workouts telling what drills to do on which days, the numbers of repetitions to do, and the rest intervals. See chapter 6 for descriptions of the speed drills and chapter 7 for descriptions of the agility drills.

### Offensive Linemen

An offensive lineman is required to move quickly in a limited amount of space, with several changes of direction during a play. It is rare that a lineman gets to top speed running in a straight line. Therefore, agility drills constitute most of an offensive lineman's running program. However, the agility drills need to be modified, since to maintain their balance during a football play offensive linemen are taught to not lift their feet high off the ground. For the rope drills use ropes that are low to the ground, preferably no more than three inches high. Concentrate on quick feet, lifting them only high enough to clear the ropes. (Don't include any drills that require stepping over bags.) Emphasize keeping hands in front, eyes focused, hips low, back straight, and weight on the balls of the feet.

Keep the offensive linemen's speed drills short, exactly as they are described in this chapter, and keep the plyometric drills light to minimize the stress on tendons and ligaments. Tight ends should do most of

**Table 9.1b Speed Drills by Drill Type and Player Position**

| Drill name | Drill type | Position | Page |
|---|---|---|---|
| Bag jumps | Plyometrics | LB, OB, R, DB | 183 |
| Bounding | Plyometrics | OB, R, DB | 178 |
| Lateral bag jumps | Plyometrics | OB, DB | 182 |
| Power skips for distance | Plyometrics | LB, OB, R, DB | 180 |
| Power skips for height | Plyometrics | LB, OB, R, DB | 179 |
| Right, left, jump | Plyometrics | LB, OB, R, DB | 186 |
| Single leg hops | Plyometrics | OB, R, DB | 184 |
| Speed skips | Plyometrics | OB, R, DB | 181 |
| 10/10 hopping | Plyometrics | LB, OB, R, DB | 184 |
| Harness (10 yards) | Resisted speed | OL, DL | 188 |
| Harness (10-25 yards) | Resisted speed | LB | 188 |
| Harness (10-40 yards) | Resisted speed | OB, R, DB | 188 |
| Harness drill | Resisted speed | OL, DL, LB, OB, R, DB | 188 |
| Harness starts | Resisted speed | OL, DL | 187 |
| Hill sprints | Resisted speed | OL, DL, LB, OB, R, DB | 189 |
| Hill sprints (10-20 yards) | Resisted speed | OL, DL | 189 |
| Hill sprints (10-40 yards) | Resisted speed | LB, OB, R, DB | 189 |
| Stadium steps | Resisted speed | OL, DL, LB, OB, R, DB | 190 |
| Buildups | Acceleration | OL, DL, LB, OB, R, DB | 174 |
| Buildups (30 yards) | Acceleration | OL, DL | 174 |
| Buildups (40 yards) | Acceleration | LB | 174 |
| Buildups (40-60 yards) | Acceleration | OB, R, DB | 174 |
| Flying 10s | Acceleration | OL, DL, LB, OB, R, DB | 174 |
| Flying 20s | Acceleration | DL, LB, OB, R, DB | 175 |
| Flying 30s | Acceleration | OB, DB | 176 |
| 40-yard sprints | Acceleration | OB, R, DB | 177 |
| Hollow sprints | Acceleration | OL, DL, LB, OB, R, DB | 177 |
| Form starts | Speed | OL, DL, LB, OB, R, DB | 172 |
| Position starts | Speed | OL, DL, LB, OB, R, DB | 173 |

the running program with the offensive line and some workouts with the receivers. Table 9.2 (also refer to table 9.1, *a* and *b*) shows an example of daily workouts for offensive linemen during each phase.

## Defensive Linemen

Rush ends or defensive ends who start in a down position and whose major responsibility is rushing the quarterback should work with defensive linemen. Defensive linemen are required to step over other players frequently during a play. Therefore, do the rope drills with the ropes a foot or more off the ground. Defensive linemen also move laterally,

**Table 9.2 Offensive Lineman Daily Workout**

| Speed drills | Monday and Thursday | | |
|---|---|---|---|
| | Sets | Development | Peak |
| Warm-up | | | Warm-up routine |
| Stretching | | | Stretching routine |
| Starts | 6-10 | None | Form starts × 5 reps<br>Position starts × 5 reps |
| Sprints | 6-10 | None | Buildups × 3-5 reps<br>Flying 10s × 3-5 reps |
| Resisted drills | 6-10 | None | Harness starts × 3-5 reps<br>Stadium steps × 3-5 reps |
| Mobility drills | | | Mobility routine |
| **Agility drills** | **Tuesday and Friday** | | |
| Warm-up | | Warm-up routine | Warm-up routine |
| Stretching | | Stretching routine | Stretching routine |
| Rope drills | 6-10 | Every other hole × 2 reps<br>Every hole × 2 reps<br>Lateral step × 2 reps<br>Lateral step with double chop × 2 reps | Every other hole × 2 reps<br>Every hole × 2 reps<br>Double chop × 2 reps<br>Lateral step × 2 reps<br>Lateral step with double chop × 2 reps |
| Bag drills | 4-8 | Forward-back × 2 reps<br>Shuffle × 2 reps | Forward-back × 2 reps<br>Zigzag × 2 reps |
| Cone drills | 4-8 | Zigzag × 2 reps<br>Backward zigzag × 2 reps<br>Nebraska agility × 2 reps | Zigzag × 2 reps<br>Backward zigzag × 2 reps<br>Nebraska agility × 2 reps<br>Four-corner shuffle × 2 reps |
| Jump rope drills | | Jump rope routine | Jump rope routine |
| Line drills | 4-8 | Ladder—5/10/5 sprint × 2 reps<br>Ladder—5/10/5 shuffle × 2 reps | Ladder—5/10/5 sprint × 2 reps<br>Ladder—5/10/5 shuffle × 2 reps<br>Ladder—5/10/5 backpedal-forward × 2 reps |
| Mobility drills | | Mobility routine | Mobility routine |

shuffle stepping as they pursue a play. Do a variety of bag drills that require both going over and shuffling around the bags.

Defensive linemen must visually react to the ball as it is snapped and to the movement of the play. Therefore, include some drills requiring reactions to a coach's or friend's visual signal. Emphasize quick feet on all drills, and keep the speed drills short. We recommend limiting plyometric drills for defensive linemen because of the great stress on the tendons and ligaments of the knees at their body weight. Because they are required to jump high to knock passes down, do some of the plyometric drills in the vertical plane. If pass protection is required, they can do some workouts with the linebackers. Table 9.3 (also refer to table 9.1, *a* and *b*) gives some suggestions and examples of workouts for defensive linemen during the development and peak phases.

## Linebackers

The linebacker is basically a combination of a defensive lineman and a defensive back, and his movement patterns are more varied than those of any other position. (See also the descriptions of these two positions in this chapter.) The ability to plug a hole, blitz a quarterback, move laterally from sideline to sideline, and backpedal to cover a receiver are all requirements of a linebacker. Therefore, a wide range of drills including movement in all directions is required to prepare a linebacker. On all drills recommended in table 9.4 (also refer to table 9.1, *a* and *b*), emphasize keeping the hips low, back straight, shoulders square, head up, and weight on the balls of the feet.

## Offensive (Running) Backs

The requirements of a back demand a combination of acceleration, power, agility, and balance. The ability to stop quickly, change directions, and accelerate is paramount. Often offensive backs are required to step or jump over players during a play. A variety of rope, bag, and cone drills requiring movements both over and around them make up the bulk of the running back program. Many times a running back is knocked off balance and must regain it again by putting a hand to the ground. The rag and squirm drills (chapter 7) were devised especially for the running back. Note our recommended workouts for running backs and example program in table 9.5 (also refer to table 9.1, *a* and *b*).

## Receivers

Receivers spend most of their time during a football play running routes. The ability to stop quickly, change directions, and accelerate quickly to top speed are the most important requirements of a receiver. This requires a good breakdown position (bending at the knees, lowering the hips, keeping the back straight and head up, and chopping the feet) to enable quick stops and starts. Include rope, bag, and cone drills, and emphasize a good breakdown position when changing directions. A receiver must also be a good blocker, which requires the ability to shuffle step as he blocks a linebacker or defensive back, so include drills that require shuffle steps. Keep the ropes on the rope drills low to the ground to emphasize quick feet in a balanced position. Include bag drills requiring movements going around them and not over them. Do the jump rope routine year-round to develop quick foot movements. See table 9.6 for workout recommendations and examples (also refer to table 9.1, *a* and *b*).

### Defensive Backs

Defensive backs start most plays by backpedaling. Develop good backpedaling technique by keeping the hips low, head up, back straight, and feet quick and low to the ground. Off the backpedal, defensive backs must be able to react to the receiver's movement in any direction. The backpedal drills require a coach or friend to signal the direction of movement off the backpedal. Therefore, concentrate most of your effort doing backpedal drills that require you to react to these visual movements. See table 9.7 (also refer to table 9.1, *a* and *b*) for drill selections, repetition guidelines, and example workouts for defensive backs.

## YOUR LIFTING PROGRAM

A lifting program can accomplish many different goals whether you are weight training for fitness, bodybuilding to build large muscles, or Olympic weightlifting and power lifting for competition. When a lifting program is done to improve sports performance it is called strength training. The improvements in strength training have made the single most positive contribution to football in the last two decades. Players now find it absolutely necessary to lift weights to better prepare themselves for the sport. The number one purpose of the following strength training workouts is to improve the athletic abilities of each player according to his position.

### Workout Selection

The strength workouts are based on your level of physical development and skill. There are two workout levels: beginner and advanced. The beginner workouts are for athletes who have no or very little lifting

**Table 9.3 Defensive Lineman Daily Workout**

| Speed drills | Monday and Thursday | | |
|---|---|---|---|
| | **Sets** | **Development** | **Peak** |
| Warm-up | | | Warm-up routine |
| Stretching | | | Stretching routine |
| Starts | 6-10 | None | Form starts × 5 reps<br>Position starts × 5 reps |
| Sprints | 6-10 | None | Buildups × 3-5 reps<br>Flying 10s × 3-5 reps |
| Resisted drills | 6-10 | None | Harness starts × 3-5 reps<br>Stadium steps × 3-5 reps |
| Mobility drills | | | Mobility routine |
| **Agility drills** | **Tuesday and Friday** | | |
| Warm-up | | Warm-up routine | Warm-up routine |
| Stretching | | Stretching routine | Stretching routine |
| Rope drills | 6-10 | Every other hole × 2 reps<br>Every hole × 2 reps<br>Lateral step × 2 reps<br>Lateral step with double chop × 2 reps | Every other hole × 2 reps<br>Every hole × 2 reps<br>Double chop × 2 reps<br>Lateral step × 2 reps<br>Lateral step with double chop × 2 reps |
| Bag drills | 4-8 | Straight run × 2 reps<br>Lateral step × 2 reps<br>Wave × 2 reps<br>Tap × 2 reps | Straight run × 2 reps<br>Lateral step × 2 reps<br>Forward-back × 2 reps<br>Wave × 2 reps<br>Shuffle × 2 reps |
| Cone drills | 4-8 | Zigzag × 2 reps<br>Backward zigzag × 2 reps<br>Nebraska agility × 2 reps | Zigzag × 2 reps<br>Backward zigzag × 2 reps<br>Nebraska agility × 2 reps<br>Four-corner shuffle × 2 reps |
| Line drills | 4-8 | Ladder—5/10/5 sprint × 2 reps<br>Ladder—5/10/5 shuffle × 2 reps | Ladder—5/10/5 sprint × 2 reps<br>Ladder—5/10/5 shuffle × 2 reps<br>Ladder—5/10/5 backpedal-forward × 2 reps |
| Mobility drills | | Mobility routine | Mobility routine |

**Table 9.4 Linebacker Daily Workout**

| Speed drills | | Monday and Thursday | |
|---|---|---|---|
| | Sets | Development | Peak |
| Warm-up | | | Warm-up routine |
| Stretching | | | Stretching routine |
| Starts | 6-10 | None | Form starts × 5 reps<br>Position starts × 5 reps |
| Sprints | 6-10 | None | Buildups × 3-5 reps<br>Flying 10s × 3-5 reps |
| Resisted drills | 6-10 | None | Harness drill × 3-5 reps<br>Stadium steps × 3-5 reps |
| Mobility drills | | | Mobility routine |
| **Agility drills** | | **Tuesday and Friday** | |
| Warm-up | | Warm-up routine | Warm-up routine |
| Stretching | | Stretching routine | Stretching routine |
| Rope drills | 6-10 | Every other hole × 2 reps<br>Every hole × 2 reps<br>Lateral step × 2 reps<br>Lateral step with double chop × 2 reps | Every other hole × 2 reps<br>Every hole × 2 reps<br>Double chop × 2 reps<br>Lateral step × 2 reps |
| Bag drills | 4-8 | Lateral step × 2 reps<br>Shuffle × 2 reps<br>Tap × 2 reps | Lateral step × 2 reps<br>Forward-back × 2 reps<br>Tap × 2 reps<br>Shuffle × 2 reps |
| Backpedal drills | 4-8 | Hip flips on line × 2 reps<br>45-degree × 2 reps<br>Backpedal weave × 2 reps | Hip flips on line × 2 reps<br>45-degree × 2 reps<br>Backpedal weave × 2 reps<br>90-degreee × 2 reps |
| Cone drills | 4-6 | Zigzag × 2 reps<br>Backward zigzag × 2 reps | Zigzag × 2 reps<br>Backward zigzag × 2 reps<br>Nebraska agility × 2 reps |
| Line drills | 4-6 | Pro agility × 2 reps<br>Ladder—5/10/5 shuffle × 2 reps | Pro agility × 2 reps<br>Ladder—5/10/5 shuffle × 2 reps<br>Ladder—5/10/5 backpedal-forward × 2 reps |
| Mobility drills | | Mobility routine | Mobility routine |

**Table 9.5 Offensive Back Daily Workout**

| Speed drills | | Monday and Thursday | |
|---|---|---|---|
| | **Sets** | **Development** | **Peak** |
| Warm-up | | | Warm-up routine |
| Stretching | | | Stretching routinc |
| Starts | 6-10 | Form starts × 5 reps<br>Position starts × 5 reps | Form starts × 5 reps<br>Position starts × 5 reps |
| Sprints | 6-10 | Buildups × 4 reps<br>Hollow sprints × 2 reps | Buildups × 2 reps<br>Hollow sprints × 2 reps<br>Flying 10s × 2 reps<br>Flying 20s × 2 reps<br>Flying 30s × 2 reps |
| Plyometrics | 6-10 | Power skips for distance × 2 reps<br>Bounding × 2 reps | Power skips for distance × 2 reps<br>Bounding × 2 reps<br>Right, left, jump × 2 reps<br>Bag jumps × 2 reps |
| Resisted drills | 6-10 | None | Harness drill × 3-5 reps<br>Stadium steps × 3-5 reps |
| Mobility drills | | Mobility routine | Mobility routine |
| **Agility drills** | | **Tuesday and Friday** | |
| Warm-up | | Warm-up routine | Warm-up routine |
| Stretching | | Stretching routine | Stretching routine |
| Rope drills | 6-10 | Every other hole × 2 reps<br>Every hole × 2 reps<br>Lateral step × 2 reps<br>Rope weave × 2 reps | Every other hole × 2 reps<br>Every hole × 2 reps<br>Lateral step × 2 reps<br>Bunny hop × 2 reps<br>Rope weave × 2 reps |
| Bag drills | 4-8 | Straight run × 2 reps<br>Lateral step × 2 reps<br>Change of direction × 2 reps | Straight run × 2 reps<br>Lateral step × 2 reps<br>Change of direction × 2 reps<br>Wheel × 2 reps |
| Cone drills | 4-8 | Rag × 2 reps<br>Dodging run × 2 reps<br>Nebraska agility × 2 reps | Zigzag × 2 reps<br>Rag × 2 reps<br>Nebraska agility × 2 reps<br>Four-corner carioca × 2 reps |
| Jump rope drills | | Jump rope routine | Jump rope routine |

**Table 9.6 Receiver Daily Workout**

| Speed drills | | Monday and Thursday | |
|---|---|---|---|
| | **Sets** | **Development** | **Peak** |
| Warm-up | | | Warm-up routine |
| Stretching | | | Stretching routine |
| Starts | 6-10 | Form starts × 5 reps<br>Position starts × 5 reps | Form starts × 5 reps<br>Position starts × 5 reps |
| Sprints | 6-10 | Buildups × 4 reps<br>Hollow sprints × 4 reps | Buildups × 2 reps<br>Hollow sprints × 2 reps<br>Flying 10s × 2 reps<br>Flying 20s × 2 reps<br>Flying 30s × 2 reps |
| Plyometrics | 6-10 | Power skips for height × 2 reps<br>Bounding × 2 reps | Power skips for height × 2 reps<br>Bounding × 2 reps<br>Right, left, jump × 2 reps<br>Bag jumps × 2 reps |
| Resisted drills | 6-10 | None | Harness drill × 3-5 reps<br>Stadium steps × 3-5 reps |
| Mobility drills | | Mobility routine | Mobility routine |
| **Agility drills** | | **Tuesday and Friday** | |
| Warm-up | | Warm-up routine | Warm-up routine |
| Stretching | | Stretching routine | Stretching routine |
| Rope drills | 6-10 | Every other hole × 2 reps<br>Double chop × 2 reps<br>Lateral step × 2 reps<br>Lateral step with double chop × 2 reps | Every other hole × 2 reps<br>Double chop × 2 reps<br>Lateral step × 2 reps<br>Lateral step with double chop × 2 reps<br>Bunny hop × 2 reps |
| Bag drills | 4-8 | Forward-back × 2 reps<br>Shuffle × 2 reps<br>Change of direction × 2 reps | Forward-back × 2 reps<br>Shuffle × 2 reps<br>Change of direction × 2 reps |
| Cone drills | 4-8 | Zigzag × 2 reps<br>Dodging run × 2 reps | Zigzag × 2 reps<br>Dodging run × 2 reps<br>Combo zigzag × 2 reps |
| Jump rope drills | | Jump rope routine | Jump rope routine |

**Table 9.7 Defensive Back Daily Workout**

| Speed drills | | Monday and Thursday | |
|---|---|---|---|
| | Sets | Development | Peak |
| Warm-up | | | Warm-up routine |
| Stretching | | | Stretching routine |
| Starts | 6-10 | Form starts × 5 reps<br>Position starts × 5 reps | Form starts × 5 reps<br>Position starts × 5 reps |
| Sprints | 6-10 | Buildups × 4 reps<br>Hollow sprints × 4 reps | Buildups × 2 reps<br>Hollow sprints × 2 reps<br>Flying 10s × 2 reps<br>Flying 20s × 2 reps<br>Flying 30s × 2 reps |
| Plyometrics | 6-10 | Power skips × 2 reps<br>Bounding × 2 reps | Power skips × 2 reps<br>Bounding × 2 reps<br>Right, left, jump × 2 reps<br>Bag jumps × 2 reps |
| Resisted drills | 6-10 | None | Harness drill × 3-5 reps<br>Stadium steps × 3-5 reps |
| Mobility drills | | Mobility routine | Mobility routine |
| **Agility drills** | | **Tuesday and Friday** | |
| Warm-up | | Warm-up routine | Warm-up routine |
| Stretching | | Stretching routine | Stretching routine |
| Backpedal drills | 6-10 | Hip flips on line × 2 reps<br>45-degree × 2 reps<br>Backpedal weave × 2 reps<br>W backpedal-break × 2 reps<br>Mirror backpedal × 2 reps | Hip flips on line × 2 reps<br>45-degree × 2 reps<br>Backpedal weave × 2 reps<br>90-degree × 2 reps<br>Wet field × 2 reps |
| Cone drills | 4-8 | Four-corner drop × 2 reps<br>Four-corner comeback × 2 reps<br>Nebraska agility × 2 reps | Four-corner drop × 2 reps<br>Four-corner comeback × 2 reps<br>Nebraska agility × 2 reps<br>Three-corner × 2 reps |
| Line drills | 4-8 | Pro agility × 2 reps<br>Ladder—5/10/5 sprint × 2 reps | Pro agility × 2 reps<br>Ladder—5/10/5 sprint × 2 reps<br>Ladder—5/10/5 shuffle × 2 reps |
| Mobility drills | | Mobility routine | Mobility routine |

experience. The advanced workouts are for lifters with at least one year of training at the beginner level. The main difference between the workout levels is the skill involved in executing the exercises. Therefore, it is important to start off at the beginning level to develop the muscles, tendons, and ligaments to handle the stress of more intense exercises. Many athletes use heavier weights before learning proper technique. If proper technique is not practiced, there will not be any transfer of training to performance of football skills. Proper technique is the number one objective before moving to advanced workouts.

During the off-season do the phases in the order listed: base phase, development phase, and peak phase. Do each phase for four weeks before proceeding to the next phase.

The off-season workouts outlined below use a split routine with the explosive lifts on Monday and Thursday and the base strength lifts on Tuesday and Friday. Wednesday is a rest day and no workouts are scheduled. It is best to have the heavy lifting days on Monday and Friday and the easy days on Tuesday and Thursday, so Monday is a heavy explosive day and Thursday an easy explosive day. Tuesday is an easy base strength day, allowing you to lift more explosively on Thursday. Friday is the hard base strength day, allowing two days of rest (Saturday and Sunday) before doing the heavy explosive day on Monday of the following week.

## Beginner Off-Season—Base Phase

This workout is for football players with little or no lifting experience (table 9.8*a*). No explosive lifts are included during the base phase. This program prepares you for explosive lifting in the following development phase. You should experience some weight gain of lean body tissue during this phase.

## Beginner Off-Season—Development Phase

This workout follows the base phase for beginner lifters (table 9.8*b*). Some of the explosive lifts are introduced during this phase (rack cleans and jammer extensions or power presses). With this program you have choices between doing the free weight exercises or exercises using a Jammer machine. The choices are power presses or Jammer extensions, and trunk twists or Jammer rotations. Most weight rooms may not have a Jammer machine, developed by Hammer Strength. If you do have a Jammer, you can do it on both Monday and Thursday or alternate it with the power press on different days. You also have a choice between two free weight exercises, good mornings or Romanian dead lifts, on Tuesday and Friday. There is not a beginner's peak phase program. After doing the beginner base and development phases, proceed to the intermediate base phase program.

**Table 9.8a Beginner Off-Season—Base Phase**

| | Week 1 | Week 2 | Week 3 | Week 4 |
|---|---|---|---|---|
| **Monday and Thursday** | | | | |
| Clean shrug | 10/10 | 10/10/10 | 10/10/10 | 10/10/10 |
| Clean dead lift | 10/10 | 10/10/10 | 10/10/10 | 10/10/10 |
| Standing shoulder press | 10/10 | 10/10/10 | 10/10/10 | 10/10/10 |
| Back extension | 10/10 | 10/10/10 | 10/10/10 | 10/10/10 |
| Jammer rotation or trunk twist | 10/10 | 10/10 | 10/10 | 10/10 |
| Crunches | | | | |
| **Tuesday and Friday** | | | | |
| Squat | 10/10 | 10/10/10 | 10/10/10 | 10/10/10 |
| Bench press | 10/10 | 10/10/10 | 10/10/10 | 10/10/10 |
| Triceps extension | 10/10 | 10/10/10 | 10/10/10 | 10/10/10 |
| Barbell curl | 10/10 | 10/10/10 | 10/10/10 | 10/10/10 |
| Neck machine | 10/10 | 10/10 | 10/10 | 10/10 |

**Table 9.8b Beginner Off-Season—Development Phase**

| | Week 1 | Week 2 | Week 3 | Week 4 |
|---|---|---|---|---|
| **Monday and Thursday** | | | | |
| Rack clean | 5/5/5 | 5/5/5 | 5/5/5 | 5/5/5 |
| Power press or Jammer extension | 5/5/5 | 5/5/5 | 5/5/5 | 5/5/5 |
| Trunk twist or Jammer rotation | 5/5/5 | 5/5/5 | 5/5/5 | 5/5/5 |
| Crunches | | | | |
| **Tuesday and Friday** | | | | |
| Squat | 5/5/5 | 5/5/5 | 5/5/5 | 5/5/5 |
| Good morning or RDL | 10/10 | 10/10 | 10/10 | 10/10 |
| Bench press | 5/5/5 | 5/5/5 | 5/5/5 | 5/5/5 |
| Triceps extension | 10/10 | 10/10 | 10/10 | 10/10 |
| Barbell curl | 10/10 | 10/10 | 10/10 | 10/10 |
| Neck machine | 10/10 | 10/10 | 10/10 | 10/10 |

## Beginner In-Season

This workout is for younger players who have done both the beginner off-season base and development phases in preparation for the in-season program (table 9.8*c*). This is a two-day-per-week schedule used to maintain strength during the season. Monday's workout is a heavy

**Table 9.8c Beginner In-Season**

| | Week 1 | Week 2 | Week 3 | Week 4 |
|---|---|---|---|---|
| **Monday and Wednesday** | | | | |
| Bench press | 5/5/5 | 5/5/5 | 5/5/5 | 5/5 |
| Squat | 5/5/5 | 5/5/5 | 5/5/5 | 5/5 |
| Rack clean (or upright row) | 5/5/5 | 5/5/5 | 5/5/5 | 5/5 |
| Lat pulldown | 10/10 | 10/10 | 10/10 | 10/10 |
| Neck machine | 10/10 | 10/10 | 10/10 | 10/10 |
| Crunches | | | | |

workout and Wednesday's is lighter. The important objective is to train twice a week, once heavy and once light. Allow at least one day of rest before the game. The minimum number of exercises to work all the major muscle groups have been included. You have a choice between doing rack cleans or upright rows. If your technique is good, do the rack clean. If hand, wrist, elbow, or shoulder problems prevent you from doing rack cleans, the upright row would be a better exercise. A strength coach can show the proper technique for upright rows.

## Intermediate Off-Season—Base Phase

The program in table 9.9*a* is for lifters who have completed both the beginner base (four weeks) and beginner development (four weeks) phases. If you have some experience doing the explosive lifts you can skip the beginner programs and start this intermediate program.

## Intermediate Off-Season—Development Phase

The exercises done during the development phase (table 9.9*b*) are not much different than those done during the base phase. What changes is the number of repetitions on squats and bench presses on Tuesday and Friday, switching from sets of 10 to 5, so the weight will get heavier. Do rack cleans on both Mondays and Thursdays. It is easier to learn the clean exercises before doing the snatch exercises. If your technique with the rack cleans improves and you want to add some variety, replace the rack cleans on Thursday with box snatches.

## Intermediate Off-Season—Peak Phase

Many of the exercises done during the peak phase are similar to those done during the base and development phases, except hang cleans are

**Table 9.9a Intermediate Off-Season—Base Phase**

| | Week 1 | Week 2 | Week 3 | Week 4 |
|---|---|---|---|---|
| **Monday and Thursday** | | | | |
| Snatch squat | 5/5 | 5/5 | 5/5 | 5/5 |
| Rack clean | 5/5/5 | 5/5/5 | 5/5/5 | 5/5/5 |
| Power press or Jammer extension | 5/5/5 | 5/5/5 | 5/5/5 | 5/5/5 |
| Trunk twist or Jammer rotation | 10/10 | 10/10 | 10/10 | 10/10 |
| Crunch | | | | |
| **Tuesday and Friday** | | | | |
| Squats | 10/10/10 | 10/10/10 | 10/10/10 | 10/10/10 |
| Good morning or RDL | 10/10 | 10/10 | 10/10 | 10/10 |
| Bench press | 10/10/10 | 10/10/10 | 10/10/10 | 10/10/10 |
| Jammer press | 10/10/10 | 10/10/10 | 10/10/10 | 10/10/10 |
| Lat pulldown | 10/10/10 | 10/10/10 | 10/10/10 | 10/10/10 |
| Triceps extension | 10/10/10 | 10/10/10 | 10/10/10 | 10/10/10 |
| Barbell curl | 10/10/10 | 10/10/10 | 10/10/10 | 10/10/10 |
| Neck machine | 10/10/10 | 10/10/10 | 10/10/10 | 10/10/10 |

done in place of rack cleans (table 9.9*c*). The intensity of the bench press is increased by using heavy sets of four, three, and two repetitions.

## Intermediate In-Season

This workout is for players who have prior experience doing explosive exercises in preparation for the season (table 9.9*d*). This two-days-per-week schedule is used to maintain strength during the season by having one heavy and one light workout. Monday's workout should be heavier than Wednesday's. Allow at least one day of rest before the game. The minimum number of exercises to work all the major muscles groups are included. Do one explosive lift, based on your prior lifting experience, at the start of the workout followed by squats.

## Advanced Off-Season—Base Phase

The advanced workouts are only for experienced lifters. The advanced program includes snatch movements. The base phase is especially difficult because of the metabolic circuit done on Tuesday and Friday (table 9.10*a*).

The metabolic circuit is a strong stimulator of the endocrine system (testosterone and growth hormone) to get the greatest increase in muscle

**Table 9.9b Intermediate Off-Season—Development Phase**

| | Week 1 | Week 2 | Week 3 | Week 4 |
|---|---|---|---|---|
| **Monday and Thursday** | | | | |
| Snatch squat | 5/5 | 5/5 | 5/5 | 5/5 |
| Rack clean | 5/5/5 | 5/5/5 | 5/5/5 | 5/5/5 |
| Power press or Jammer extension | 5/5/5 | 5/5/5 | 5/5/5 | 5/5/5 |
| Trunk twist or Jammer rotation | 10/10 | 10/10 | 10/10 | 10/10 |
| Crunch | | | | |
| **Tuesday** | | | | |
| Squat | 5/5/5 | 5/5/5 | 5/5/5 | 5/5/5 |
| Good morning or RDL | 10/10 | 10/10 | 10/10 | 10/10 |
| Bench press | 5/5/5 | 5/5/5 | 5/5/5 | 5/5/5 |
| Jammer press | 10/10/10 | 10/10/10 | 10/10/10 | 10/10/10 |
| Low lat pull | 10/10/10 | 10/10/10 | 10/10/10 | 10/10/10 |
| Triceps extension | 10/10/10 | 10/10/10 | 10/10/10 | 10/10/10 |
| Barbell curl | 10/10/10 | 10/10/10 | 10/10/10 | 10/10/10 |
| Neck machine | 10/10/10 | 10/10/10 | 10/10/10 | 10/10/10 |
| **Friday** | | | | |
| Squat | 5/5/5 | 5/5/5 | 5/5/5 | 5/5/5 |
| Good morning or RDL | 10/10 | 10/10 | 10/10 | 10/10 |
| Incline press | 5/5/5 | 5/5/5 | 5/5/5 | 5/5/5 |
| Jammer press | 10/10/10 | 10/10/10 | 10/10/10 | 10/10/10 |
| Low lat pull | 10/10/10 | 10/10/10 | 10/10/10 | 10/10/10 |
| Triceps extension | 10/10/10 | 10/10/10 | 10/10/10 | 10/10/10 |
| Barbell curl | 10/10/10 | 10/10/10 | 10/10/10 | 10/10/10 |
| Neck machine | 10/10/10 | 10/10/10 | 10/10/10 | 10/10/10 |

size. Do these exercises in the order that they're listed: leg exercises, then chest and back exercises. The multiple joint exercises precede the single joint exercises. This program differs from other programs in that there is only a 1-minute rest between exercises and sets. (The greatest amount of growth hormone release has been observed when the rest period is 1 minute as opposed to 3 or more minutes.) The 1-minute rest period makes the metabolic circuit very demanding, and enables you to complete the entire workout within 40 minutes. Use poundage that allows three sets of 10 repetitions. More growth hormone is released when you do 10 repetitions as opposed to doing 5 or fewer repetitions. Each set of 10 repetitions should take only 20 seconds to complete, though squats may take 30 to 40 seconds. Use this type of training only during the base phase when you are trying to develop lean muscle.

**Table 9.9c Intermediate Off-Season—Peak Phase**

| | Week 1 | Week 2 | Week 3 | Week 4 |
|---|---|---|---|---|
| **Monday** | | | | |
| Snatch squat | 5/5 | 5/5 | 5/5 | 5/5 |
| Hang clean | 5/5/5 | 5/5/5 | 5/5/5 | 5/5/5 |
| Power press or Jammer extension | 5/5/5 | 5/5/5 | 5/5/5 | 5/5/5 |
| Trunk twist or Jammer rotation | 10/10 | 10/10 | 10/10 | 10/10 |
| Crunch | | | | |
| **Tuesday** | | | | |
| Squat | 5/5/5 | 5/5/5 | 5/5/5 | 5/5/5 |
| Good morning or RDL | 10/10 | 10/10 | 10/10 | 10/10 |
| Bench press | 4/3/2 | 4/3/2 | 4/3/2 | 4/3/2 |
| Jammer press | 10/10/10 | 10/10/10 | 10/10/10 | 10/10/10 |
| Low lat pull | 10/10/10 | 10/10/10 | 10/10/10 | 10/10/10 |
| Triceps extension | 10/10/10 | 10/10/10 | 10/10/10 | 10/10/10 |
| Barbell curl | 10/10/10 | 10/10/10 | 10/10/10 | 10/10/10 |
| Neck machine | 10/10/10 | 10/10/10 | 10/10/10 | 10/10/10 |
| **Thursday** | | | | |
| Snatch squat | 5/5 | 5/5 | 5/5 | 5/5 |
| Rack clean | 5/5/5 | 5/5/5 | 5/5/5 | 5/5/5 |
| Power press or Jammer extension | 5/5/5 | 5/5/5 | 5/5/5 | 5/5/5 |
| Trunk twist or Jammer rotation | 10/10 | 10/10 | 10/10 | 10/10 |
| Crunch | | | | |
| **Friday** | | | | |
| Squat | 5/5/5 | 5/5/5 | 5/5/5 | 5/5/5 |
| Good morning or RDL | 10/10 | 10/10 | 10/10 | 10/10 |
| Incline press | 4/3/2 | 4/3/2 | 4/3/2 | 4/3/2 |
| Jammer press | 10/10/10 | 10/10/10 | 10/10/10 | 10/10/10 |
| Low lat pull | 10/10/10 | 10/10/10 | 10/10/10 | 10/10/10 |
| Triceps extension | 10/10/10 | 10/10/10 | 10/10/10 | 10/10/10 |
| Barbell curl | 10/10/10 | 10/10/10 | 10/10/10 | 10/10/10 |
| Neck machine | 10/10/10 | 10/10/10 | 10/10/10 | 10/10/10 |

## Advanced Off-Season—Development Phase

The metabolic circuit is dropped during this phase; the rest periods are as long as it takes to recover between sets. Front squats and inclines are added on Friday to give some variety to the workout (table 9.10*b*). This should allow you to continue to get stronger.

**Table 9.9d Intermediate In-Season**

| | Week 1 | Week 2 | Week 3 | Week 4 |
|---|---|---|---|---|
| **Monday** | | | | |
| Hang clean or Jammer extension | 5/5 | 5/5 | 5/5 | 5/5 |
| Bench press or Jammer press | 5/5/5 | 5/5/5 | 5/5/5 | 5/5 |
| Squat | 5/5/5 | 5/5/5 | 5/5/5 | 5/5 |
| Neck machine | 10/10 | 10/10 | 10/10 | 10/10 |
| Crunch | | | | |
| **Wednesday** | | | | |
| Hang clean or Jammer extension | 5/5 | 5/5 | 5/5 | 5/5 |
| Bench press or Jammer press | 5/5 | 5/5 | 5/5 | 5/5 |
| Squat | 5/5 | 5/5 | 5/5 | 5/5 |
| Neck machine | 10/10 | 10/10 | 10/10 | 10/10 |
| Crunch | | | | |

## Advanced Off-Season—Peak Phase

Only do this peak phase four weeks before two-a-days start. It is a high-intensity, low-volume workout, with the volume lowered to allow more running and to ensure proper recovery between workouts (table 9.10*c*).

## Advanced In-Season

This workout is for players who have lots of experience doing explosive exercises in preparation for the season. This four-days-per-week schedule is for teams that play their games on Saturdays. The workouts on Monday and Tuesday should be heavier than on Wednesday and Thursday (table 9.10*d*). Allow at least one day of rest from the weights before the game. This program uses a split routine with explosive lifts on Mondays and Tuesdays and the base strength lifts on Tuesdays and Thursdays. These workouts should take no longer than 15 minutes to complete.

# Determining Workout Load

Determine your strength level for each exercise of the program that you have selected by following these simple procedures while referring to table 9.11.

After finding your 1RM for each lift, find the weight to lift for each set. The first three columns under the "10" headings show the weight you

*3rd year*

**Table 9.10a Advanced Off-Season—Base Phase**

| | Week 1 | Week 2 | Week 3 | Week 4 |
|---|---|---|---|---|
| **Monday** | | | | |
| Snatch squat | 5/5 | 5/5 | 5/5 | 5/5 |
| Rack clean | 5/5/5 | 5/5/5 | 5/5/5 | 5/5/5 |
| Power press or Jammer extension | 5/5/5 | 5/5/5 | 5/5/5 | 5/5/5 |
| Trunk twist or Jammer rotation | 5/5/5 | 5/5/5 | 5/5/5 | 5/5/5 |
| Neck machine | 10/10 | 10/10 | 10/10 | 10/10 |
| Crunch | | | | |
| **Tuesday—Metabolic circuit** | | | | |
| Squat | 10/10 | 10/10/10 | 10/10/10 | 10/10/10 |
| Leg curl | 10/10 | 10/10/10 | 10/10/10 | 10/10/10 |
| Leg extension | 10/10 | 10/10/10 | 10/10/10 | 10/10/10 |
| Bench press | 10/10 | 10/10/10 | 10/10/10 | 10/10/10 |
| Seated shoulder press | 10/10 | 10/10/10 | 10/10/10 | 10/10/10 |
| Triceps extension | 10/10 | 10/10/10 | 10/10/10 | 10/10/10 |
| Low lat pull | 10/10 | 10/10/10 | 10/10/10 | 10/10/10 |
| Lat pulldown | 10/10 | 10/10/10 | 10/10/10 | 10/10/10 |
| Barbell curl | 10/10 | 10/10/10 | 10/10/10 | 10/10/10 |
| **Thursday** | | | | |
| Snatch squat | 5/5 | 5/5 | 5/5 | 5/5 |
| Box snatch | 5/5/5 | 5/5/5 | 5/5/5 | 5/5/5 |
| Power press or Jammer extension | 5/5/5 | 5/5/5 | 5/5/5 | 5/5/5 |
| Trunk twist or Jammer rotation | 10/10 | 10/10 | 10/10 | 10/10 |
| Neck machine | 10/10 | 10/10 | 10/10 | 10/10 |
| Crunch | | | | |
| **Friday—Metabolic circuit** | | | | |
| Squat | 10/10 | 10/10/10 | 10/10/10 | 10/10/10 |
| Leg curl | 10/10 | 10/10/10 | 10/10/10 | 10/10/10 |
| Leg extension | 10/10 | 10/10/10 | 10/10/10 | 10/10/10 |
| Incline press | 10/10 | 10/10/10 | 10/10/10 | 10/10/10 |
| Seated shoulder press | 10/10 | 10/10/10 | 10/10/10 | 10/10/10 |
| Triceps extension | 10/10 | 10/10/10 | 10/10/10 | 10/10/10 |
| Low lat pull | 10/10 | 10/10/10 | 10/10/10 | 10/10/10 |
| Lat pulldown | 10/10 | 10/10/10 | 10/10/10 | 10/10/10 |
| Barbell curl | 10/10 | 10/10/10 | 10/10/10 | 10/10/10 |

should lift for each of three sets of 10 repetitions (reps). The next three columns under the "5" headings (columns three through five) show the amount of weight to lift for each of three sets of five reps. The columns under the "4," "3," and "2" headings show the amount to lift for each of three sets of three reps.

**Table 9.10b Advanced Off-Season—Development Phase**

| | Week 1 | Week 2 | Week 3 | Week 4 |
|---|---|---|---|---|
| **Monday** | | | | |
| Snatch squat | 5/5 | 5/5 | 5/5 | 5/5 |
| Hang clean | 5/5/5 | 5/5/5 | 5/5/5 | 5/5/5 |
| Power press or Jammer extension | 5/5/5 | 5/5/5 | 5/5/5 | 5/5/5 |
| Trunk twist or Jammer rotation | 5/5/5 | 5/5/5 | 5/5/5 | 5/5/5 |
| Neck machine | 10/10 | 10/10 | 10/10 | 10/10 |
| Crunch | | | | |
| **Tuesday** | | | | |
| Squat | 5/5/5 | 5/5/5 | 5/5/5 | 5/5/5 |
| Good morning or RDL | 10/10 | 10/10 | 10/10 | 10/10 |
| Bench press | 5/5/5 | 5/5/5 | 5/5/5 | 5/5/5 |
| Jammer press | 10/10/10 | 10/10/10 | 10/10/10 | 10/10/10 |
| Lat pulldown | 10/10/10 | 10/10/10 | 10/10/10 | 10/10/10 |
| Triceps extension | 10/10/10 | 10/10/10 | 10/10/10 | 10/10/10 |
| Barbell curl | 10/10/10 | 10/10/10 | 10/10/10 | 10/10/10 |
| **Thursday** | | | | |
| Snatch squat | 5/5 | 5/5 | 5/5 | 5/5 |
| Hang snatch | 5/5/5 | 5/5/5 | 5/5/5 | 5/5/5 |
| Power press or Jammer extension | 5/5/5 | 5/5/5 | 5/5/5 | 5/5/5 |
| Trunk twist or Jammer rotation | 10/10 | 10/10 | 10/10 | 10/10 |
| Neck machine | 10/10 | 10/10 | 10/10 | 10/10 |
| Crunch | | | | |
| **Friday** | | | | |
| Front squat | 5/5/5 | 5/5/5 | 5/5/5 | 5/5/5 |
| Good morning or RDL | 10/10 | 10/10 | 10/10 | 10/10 |
| Incline press | 5/5/5 | 5/5/5 | 5/5/5 | 5/5/5 |
| Jammer press | 10/10/10 | 10/10/10 | 10/10/10 | 10/10/10 |
| Lat pulldown | 10/10/10 | 10/10/10 | 10/10/10 | 10/10/10 |
| Triceps extension | 10/10/10 | 10/10/10 | 10/10/10 | 10/10/10 |
| Barbell curl | 10/10/10 | 10/10/10 | 10/10/10 | 10/10/10 |

*Note*. The poundage at the 100 1RM shows the intensity of each set. For example, three sets of 10 repetitions are done at 65, 70, and 75 percent maximum, and three sets of five repetitions are done at 75, 80, and 85 percent maximum.

**Table 9.10c Advanced Off-Season—Peak Phase**

| | Week 1 | Week 2 | Week 3 | Week 4 |
|---|---|---|---|---|
| **Monday** | | | | |
| Snatch squat | 5/5 | 5/5 | 5/5 | 5/5 |
| Power clean | 4/3/2 | 4/3/2 | 4/3/2 | 4/3/2 |
| Power press or Jammer extension | 4/3/2 | 4/3/2 | 4/3/2 | 4/3/2 |
| Trunk twist or Jammer rotation | 5/5/5 | 5/5/5 | 5/5/5 | 5/5/5 |
| Neck machine | 10/10 | 10/10 | 10/10 | 10/10 |
| Crunch | | | | |
| **Tuesday** | | | | |
| Squat | 4/3/2 | 4/3/2 | 4/3/2 | 4/3/2 |
| Good morning or RDL | 10/10 | 10/10 | 10/10 | 10/10 |
| Bench press | 4/3/2 | 4/3/2 | 4/3/2 | 4/3/2 |
| Jammer press | 5/5/5 | 5/5/5 | 5/5/5 | 5/5/5 |
| Lat pulldown | 10/10 | 10/10 | 10/10 | 10/10 |
| Triceps extension | 10/10 | 10/10 | 10/10 | 10/10 |
| Barbell curl | 10/10 | 10/10 | 10/10 | 10/10 |
| **Thursday** | | | | |
| Snatch squat | 5/5 | 5/5 | 5/5 | 5/5 |
| Power snatch | 4/3/2 | 4/3/2 | 4/3/2 | 4/3/2 |
| Power press or Jammer extension | 5/5/5 | 5/5/5 | 5/5/5 | 5/5/5 |
| Trunk twist or Jammer rotation | 10/10 | 10/10 | 10/10 | 10/10 |
| Neck machine | 10/10 | 10/10 | 10/10 | 10/10 |
| Crunch | | | | |
| **Friday** | | | | |
| Squat | 4/3/2 | 4/3/2 | 4/3/2 | 4/3/2 |
| Good morning or RDL | 5/5/5 | 5/5/5 | 5/5/5 | 5/5/5 |
| Incline press | 4/3/2 | 4/3/2 | 4/3/2 | 4/3/2 |
| Jammer press | 10/10 | 10/10 | 10/10 | 10/10 |
| Lat pulldown | 10/10 | 10/10 | 10/10 | 10/10 |
| Triceps extension | 10/10 | 10/10 | 10/10 | 10/10 |
| Barbell curl | 10/10 | 10/10 | 10/10 | 10/10 |

## Increasing Workout Weight

On Monday and Tuesday (heavy days) do as many repetitions as possible on the last set. If the workout calls for five reps on the last set and you achieve six reps with good form, this shows that you are getting

**Table 9.10d Advanced In-Season** * 3rd Season

| | Week 1 | Week 2 | Week 3 | Week 4 |
|---|---|---|---|---|
| **Monday** | | | | |
| Bench press | 5/5 | 5/5 | 5/5 | 5/5 |
| Squat | 5/5 | 5/5 | 5/5 | 5/5 |
| **Tuesday** | | | | |
| Hang clean | 5/5 | 5/5 | 5/5 | 5/5 |
| Jammer extension | 5/5 | 5/5 | 5/5 | 5/5 |
| Jammer rotation | 5/5 | 5/5 | 5/5 | 5/5 |
| **Wednesday** | | | | |
| Incline press | 5/5 | 5/5 | 5/5 | 5/5 |
| Squat | 5/5 | 5/5 | 5/5 | 5/5 |
| **Thursday** | | | | |
| Hang clean | 5/5 | 5/5 | 5/5 | 5/5 |
| Jammer extension | 5/5 | 5/5 | 5/5 | 5/5 |
| Jammer rotation | 5/5 | 5/5 | 5/5 | 5/5 |

stronger. When you achieve six reps you can move up to the next 1RM to find your workout poundage. For example, if at the 230-pound workout you get 195 pounds for six reps, move up to the 235-pound workout. If you only get four repetitions, the poundage is too heavy and you probably should do the 225-pound workout next time or stay at the 230-pound workout. If you get five reps on the last set, stay at the current 1RM until you can achieve six reps. Remember—technique first, don't try to increase poundage too fast.

## TRAINING FOR MULTISPORT ATHLETES

Twenty-two different sports strength train during the in-season at the University of Nebraska, and all coaches realize the benefits of conditioning for performance and injury prevention. Regardless of what sport you participate in, strength training is going to benefit your performance, especially in the power sports (basketball, wrestling, baseball, soccer, and track and field events). Even endurance athletes can benefit from strength training.

Our strength program is the same for all sports; the common thread of every skill in each sport is the triple extension of the ankle, knees, and

**Table 9.11 Poundage Chart**

| 1RM | 10 | 10 | 10 5 | 5 4 | 5 3 | 2 | 1RM | 10 | 10 | 10 5 | 5 4 | 5 3 | 2 | 1RM | 10 | 10 | 10 5 | 5 4 | 5 3 | 2 |
|---|---|---|---|---|---|---|---|---|---|---|---|---|---|---|---|---|---|---|---|---|
| 45 | 30 | 30 | 35 | 35 | 40 | 40 | 220 | 145 | 155 | 165 | 175 | 185 | 200 | 395 | 255 | 275 | 295 | 315 | 335 | 355 |
| 50 | 30 | 35 | 35 | 40 | 40 | 45 | 225 | 145 | 155 | 170 | 180 | 190 | 200 | 400 | 260 | 280 | 300 | 320 | 340 | 360 |
| 55 | 35 | 40 | 40 | 45 | 45 | 50 | 230 | 150 | 160 | 170 | 185 | 195 | 205 | 405 | 265 | 285 | 305 | 325 | 345 | 365 |
| 60 | 40 | 40 | 45 | 50 | 50 | 55 | 235 | 150 | 165 | 175 | 190 | 200 | 210 | 410 | 265 | 285 | 305 | 330 | 350 | 370 |
| 65 | 40 | 45 | 50 | 50 | 55 | 60 | 240 | 155 | 170 | 180 | 190 | 205 | 215 | 415 | 270 | 290 | 310 | 330 | 350 | 375 |
| 70 | 45 | 50 | 50 | 55 | 60 | 65 | 245 | 160 | 170 | 185 | 195 | 210 | 220 | 420 | 275 | 295 | 315 | 335 | 355 | 380 |
| 75 | 50 | 50 | 55 | 60 | 65 | 65 | 250 | 160 | 175 | 185 | 200 | 210 | 225 | 425 | 275 | 295 | 320 | 340 | 360 | 380 |
| 80 | 50 | 55 | 60 | 65 | 70 | 70 | 255 | 165 | 180 | 190 | 205 | 215 | 230 | 430 | 280 | 300 | 320 | 345 | 365 | 385 |
| 85 | 55 | 60 | 65 | 70 | 70 | 75 | 260 | 170 | 180 | 195 | 210 | 220 | 235 | 435 | 280 | 305 | 325 | 350 | 370 | 390 |
| 90 | 60 | 65 | 65 | 70 | 75 | 80 | 265 | 170 | 185 | 200 | 210 | 225 | 240 | 440 | 285 | 310 | 330 | 350 | 375 | 395 |
| 95 | 60 | 65 | 70 | 75 | 80 | 85 | 270 | 175 | 190 | 200 | 215 | 230 | 245 | 445 | 290 | 310 | 335 | 355 | 380 | 400 |
| 100 | 65 | 70 | 75 | 80 | 85 | 90 | 275 | 180 | 190 | 205 | 220 | 235 | 245 | 450 | 290 | 315 | 335 | 360 | 380 | 405 |
| 105 | 70 | 75 | 80 | 85 | 90 | 95 | 280 | 180 | 195 | 210 | 225 | 240 | 250 | 455 | 295 | 320 | 340 | 365 | 385 | 410 |
| 110 | 70 | 75 | 80 | 90 | 95 | 100 | 285 | 185 | 200 | 215 | 230 | 240 | 255 | 460 | 300 | 320 | 345 | 370 | 390 | 415 |
| 115 | 75 | 80 | 85 | 90 | 95 | 105 | 290 | 190 | 205 | 215 | 230 | 245 | 260 | 465 | 300 | 325 | 350 | 370 | 395 | 420 |
| 120 | 80 | 85 | 90 | 95 | 100 | 110 | 295 | 190 | 205 | 220 | 235 | 250 | 265 | 470 | 305 | 330 | 350 | 375 | 400 | 425 |
| 125 | 80 | 85 | 95 | 100 | 105 | 110 | 300 | 195 | 210 | 225 | 240 | 255 | 270 | 475 | 310 | 330 | 355 | 380 | 405 | 425 |
| 130 | 85 | 90 | 95 | 105 | 110 | 115 | 305 | 200 | 215 | 230 | 245 | 260 | 275 | 480 | 310 | 335 | 360 | 385 | 410 | 430 |
| 135 | 85 | 95 | 100 | 110 | 115 | 120 | 310 | 200 | 215 | 230 | 250 | 265 | 280 | 485 | 315 | 340 | 365 | 390 | 410 | 435 |
| 140 | 90 | 100 | 105 | 110 | 120 | 125 | 315 | 205 | 220 | 235 | 250 | 265 | 285 | 490 | 320 | 345 | 365 | 390 | 415 | 440 |
| 145 | 95 | 100 | 110 | 115 | 125 | 130 | 320 | 210 | 225 | 240 | 255 | 270 | 290 | 495 | 320 | 345 | 370 | 395 | 420 | 445 |
| 150 | 95 | 105 | 110 | 120 | 125 | 135 | 325 | 210 | 225 | 245 | 260 | 275 | 290 | 500 | 325 | 350 | 375 | 400 | 425 | 450 |

| | | | | | | | | | | | | | | | | | | | | |
|---|---|---|---|---|---|---|---|---|---|---|---|---|---|---|---|---|---|---|---|---|
| 155 | 100 | 110 | 115 | 125 | 130 | 140 | 330 | 215 | 230 | 245 | 265 | 280 | 295 | 505 | 330 | 355 | 380 | 405 | 430 | 455 |
| 160 | 105 | 110 | 120 | 130 | 135 | 145 | 335 | 215 | 235 | 250 | 270 | 285 | 300 | 510 | 330 | 355 | 380 | 410 | 435 | 460 |
| 165 | 105 | 115 | 125 | 130 | 140 | 150 | 340 | 220 | 240 | 255 | 270 | 290 | 305 | 515 | 335 | 360 | 385 | 410 | 435 | 465 |
| 170 | 110 | 120 | 125 | 135 | 145 | 155 | 345 | 225 | 240 | 260 | 275 | 295 | 310 | 520 | 340 | 365 | 390 | 415 | 440 | 470 |
| 175 | 115 | 120 | 130 | 140 | 150 | 155 | 350 | 225 | 245 | 260 | 280 | 295 | 315 | 525 | 340 | 365 | 395 | 420 | 445 | 470 |
| 180 | 115 | 125 | 135 | 145 | 155 | 160 | 355 | 230 | 250 | 265 | 285 | 300 | 320 | 530 | 345 | 370 | 395 | 425 | 450 | 475 |
| 185 | 120 | 130 | 140 | 150 | 155 | 165 | 360 | 235 | 250 | 270 | 290 | 305 | 325 | 535 | 345 | 375 | 400 | 430 | 455 | 480 |
| 190 | 125 | 135 | 140 | 150 | 160 | 170 | 365 | 235 | 255 | 275 | 290 | 310 | 330 | 540 | 350 | 380 | 405 | 430 | 460 | 485 |
| 195 | 125 | 135 | 145 | 155 | 651 | 175 | 370 | 240 | 260 | 275 | 295 | 315 | 335 | 545 | 355 | 380 | 410 | 435 | 465 | 490 |
| 200 | 130 | 140 | 150 | 160 | 170 | 180 | 375 | 245 | 260 | 280 | 300 | 320 | 335 | 550 | 355 | 385 | 410 | 440 | 465 | 495 |
| 205 | 135 | 145 | 155 | 165 | 175 | 185 | 380 | 245 | 265 | 285 | 305 | 325 | 340 | 555 | 360 | 390 | 415 | 445 | 470 | 500 |
| 210 | 135 | 145 | 155 | 170 | 180 | 190 | 385 | 250 | 270 | 290 | 310 | 325 | 345 | 560 | 365 | 390 | 420 | 450 | 475 | 505 |
| 215 | 140 | 150 | 160 | 170 | 180 | 195 | 390 | 255 | 275 | 290 | 310 | 330 | 350 | 565 | 365 | 395 | 425 | 450 | 480 | 510 |

65% 70% 75%

hips explosively applying force against the ground. Thus, the same exercises that apply to football relate to all power sports. Only one program is necessary to develop explosive power, so if you participate in another sport during the football off-season there is no need to develop specialty programs for your other sports.

Likewise, the improvement of the four performance indicators of speed, power, agility, and endurance is the goal of every sport. For example, reacting to the movements of the opponent is common to football, basketball, and wrestling. Basketball, wrestling, baseball, sprints, and field events have a high anaerobic component. Change of direction and acceleration are basic requirements of every sport. Therefore, even though the running programs presented in this book may not specifically meet the biomechanical and energy system needs of each sport, the characteristics of one sport will have transfer value to others. Using the football running program for other sports is unquestionably better than doing absolutely nothing at all.

If you are a three-sport athlete, your sports probably overlap and you do not have time to incorporate an off-season football-training program during the school year. But it is important that you strength train the entire school year regardless of what sport you are participating in. Making sure this happens may require that all the sport coaches involved communicate with each other and agree on the strength training program for the entire year. Since you are in-season the entire year, you need an in-season program to maintain strength while not detracting from your performance in other sports. This objective can be accomplished by strength training at least twice a week, once heavy and once easy with the easy workout prior to the competition. Allow at least one day of no lifting before any competition and have at least one day of rest between workouts.

Table 9.12*a* outlines an in-season strength training program for multisport athletes. Of course, doing the same program the entire year may get a little tedious, so you may want to change it, such as by doing heavy strength exercises the first workout of the week and doing explosive lifts the second workout of the week (see table 9.12*b*). Regardless of what program you do, squat heavy at least once a week and do at least one explosive exercise movement once a week. The explosive exercises can vary from workout to workout. You do not need to have a maintenance running program. Participating in the sport itself will be adequate enough in place of the running program.

As a two-sport athlete you have at least one season in which you are not competing and you may want to take a few weeks off after one sport is over before starting an off-season program. The biggest mistake you

**Table 9.12a In-Season Strength Training for Multisport Athletes**

| | Program #1 | | | |
|---|---|---|---|---|
| | Week 1 | Week 2 | Week 3 | Week 4 |
| **Workout 1—Hard** | | | | |
| Hang clean | 5/5 | 5/5 | 5/5 | 5/5 |
| Bench press | 5/5/5 | 5/5/5 | 5/5/5 | 5/5 |
| Squat | 5/5/5 | 5/5/5 | 5/5/5 | 5/5 |
| Sit-up | | | | |
| **Workout 2—Easy** | | | | |
| Hang clean | 5/5 | 5/5 | 5/5 | 5/5 |
| Bench press | 5/5 | 5/5 | 5/5 | 5/5 |
| Squat | 5/5 | 5/5 | 5/5 | 5/5 |
| Sit-up | | | | |

**Table 9.12b In-Season Strength Training for Multisport Athletes**

| | Program #2 | | | |
|---|---|---|---|---|
| | Week 1 | Week 2 | Week 3 | Week 4 |
| **Workout 1—Strength** | | | | |
| Squat | 5/5/5 | 5/5/5 | 5/5/5 | 5/5 |
| Bench press | 5/5/5 | 5/5/5 | 5/5/5 | 5/5 |
| Sit-up | | | | |
| **Workout 2—Explosive** | | | | |
| Hang clean | 5/5 | 5/5 | 5/5 | 5/5 |
| Jammer rotation | 5/5 | 5/5 | 5/5 | 5/5 |
| Sit-up | | | | |

can make is to take the entire time off with no strength training or running at all. This is the only time you have to make improvement, so don't let it slip by. When not participating in a sport, do any of the off-season programs outlined previously based on your experience and position.

# ABOUT THE AUTHORS

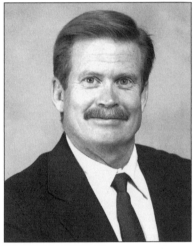

**Mike J. Arthur**, CSCS, is regarded as one of the most knowledgeable strength coaches in the nation. He joined the University of Nebraska staff as an assistant strength and conditioning coach in 1976. In 1994 he was named assistant director of athletic performance at Nebraska. During his tenure at Nebraska, the university has produced many advances in the strength programs used by athletes throughout the nation. His research helps Nebraska stay on the cutting edge of football conditioning. In 1995 Arthur was named National Collegiate Strength and Conditioning Coach of the Year by the Professional Football Strength and Conditioning Society.

An AAU wrestling champion at 123 pounds for Nebraska in 1970, Arthur was a collegiate and junior national powerlifting champion in the 132-pound weight class in 1977. A ten-time Nebraska powerlifting champion, he set a world record with a 540.25-pound dead lift in the 132-pound class.

He and his wife Reena have two daughters, Tara and Rachel, and a son, John.

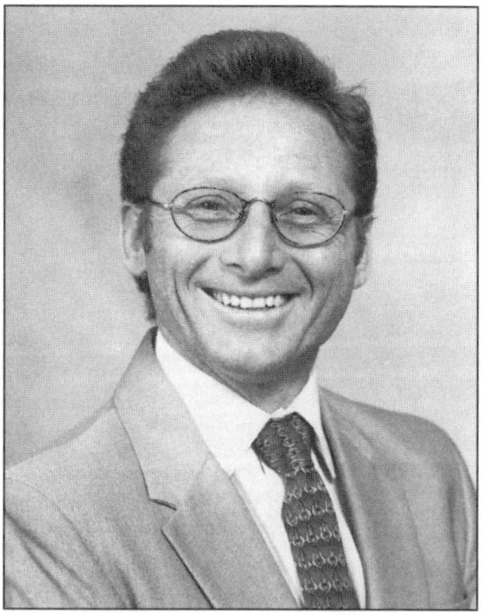

**Bryan L. Bailey**, CSCS, specializes in reconditioning athletes. He has served as an assistant strength and conditioning coach on the University of Nebraska staff since 1987. Nationally recognized for his innovative training methods for reconditioning, Bryan works with doctors and trainers to modify injured athletes' strength and conditioning programs.

Bryan received a BS degree in exercise physiology from the University of Nebraska and an MS degree in exercise science from the United States Sports Academy.

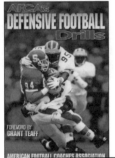